Molecules at Play in Neurological Diseases

Molecules at Play in Neurological Diseases

Guest Editor

Dumitru A. Iacobas

MDPI

Basel • Beijing • Wuhan • Barcelona • Belgrade • Novi Sad • Cluj • Manchester

Guest Editor
Dumitru A. Iacobas
Undergraduate Medical Academy
Prairie View A&M University
Prairie View, TX
USA

Editorial Office
MDPI AG
Grosspeteranlage 5
4052 Basel, Switzerland

This is a reprint of the Special Issue, published open access by the journal *Current Issues in Molecular Biology* (ISSN 1467-3045), freely accessible at: https://www.mdpi.com/journal/cimb/special_issues/ZA13E5993K.

For citation purposes, cite each article independently as indicated on the article page online and as indicated below:

Lastname, A.A.; Lastname, B.B. Article Title. *Journal Name* **Year**, *Volume Number*, Page Range.

ISBN 978-3-7258-5021-1 (Hbk)
ISBN 978-3-7258-5022-8 (PDF)
https://doi.org/10.3390/books978-3-7258-5022-8

Contents

About the Editor

Dumitru A. Iacobas

Dumitru A. Iacobas is currently a Research Professor of Personalized Genomics at the Texas Undergraduate Medial Academy of Prairie View A&M University. An expert in both experimental and computational genomics, he has been involved in numerous studies on human and animal (mouse, rat, rabbit, dog, chicken) tissues and cells, elucidating the molecular mechanisms of several types of cancers, cardiomyopathies, and neurological disorders. Beyond the biomedical significance of his works, Iacobas' contributions to the field include the optimization of several wet protocols, introduction of the Genomic Fabric Paradigm and Principle of Transcriptomic Stoichiometry, and development of advanced mathematical algorithms and computer software. The Genomic Fabric Paradigm offers the most (theoretically possible) comprehensive characterization of the transcriptome, while the Principle of Transcriptomic Stoichiometry identifies the most statistically significant transcriptomic network of a functional pathway.

Preface

This Reprint, “Molecules at Play in Neurological Diseases”, is a collection of the articles included in the Special Issue of the same name aiming to discuss the roles of specific molecules in the etiology and progression of some major disturbances of the nervous system. Beyond professionals in the field, this body of work is addressed to members of the wider public with interest in understanding how the nervous system works, what occurs during neurodegeneration, and what the medical solutions might be. The invitation to collaborate was honored by prominent researchers from Bulgaria, Croatia, Italy, Israel, Japan, Poland, Romania, and the U.S.A., who delved into the intricate interplay of the biochemical, genetic, and epigenetic elements of neuropathology, illuminating potential therapeutic targets. Their contributions present interesting results on epilepsy, infantile spasms, spine and brain degeneration, hypomyelination leukodystrophy, unipolar and bipolar depression, and Alzheimer’s and Parkinson disease. Genetic population studies are complemented by careful molecular and genomic investigations performed on human blood, surgically removed tissues, and standard cell lines, as well as on engineered (mouse and rat) animal models. In summary, "Molecules at Play in Neurological Diseases" offers a comprehensive portrayal of the molecular landscape of brain and spine afflictions, providing invaluable insights that may pave the way for the future development of more efficacious treatments of such debilitating diseases.

Dumitru A. Iacobas
Guest Editor

current issues in molecular biology

MDPI

Editorial

Special Issue "Molecules at Play in Neurological Diseases"

Dumitru Andrei Iacobas [1,2]

1 Personalized Genomics Laboratory, Undergraduate Medical Academy, School of Public and Allied Health, Prairie View A&M University, Prairie View, TX 77446, USA; daiacobas@pvamu.edu

2 DP Purpura Department of Neuroscience, Albert Einstein College of Medicine, Bronx, New York, NY 10461, USA

Pending the approval of the Institutional Review Boards (IRBs), researchers can access clinicians' tools to explore the molecular phenomena affected by neurological disorders in living humans. Among others, they can use various imaging techniques (e.g., [1]) and also could analyze blood (e.g., [2,3]), bodily waste (urine and feces, e.g., [4]) or surgically removed tissues (e.g., [5]). However, testing novel therapeutic avenues on living humans faces drastic legal, moral and religious constrains beyond the ethics rules established by the Declaration of Helsinki [6] and needs a long chain of approvals before being accepted for clinical trials. Therefore, frequent choices are use of cell cultures isolated from surgically removed tissues of diseased persons (e.g., [7]) or replication of the disorder's major symptoms on animal models (e.g., [8–10]). An intermediate choice is use of genetically engineered animal precursor cell line (e.g., [11]).

Both cell cultures and animal models were instrumental for our incremental understanding of nervous system pathology and it is hard to imagine what level of knowledge and medicine we would have today without them. Particularly, primary cell cultures have been essential tools for investigating the roles of various cell phenotypes in brain normal and disease states. For example, many key functions of central glial cells in metabolism and intercellular calcium signaling were uncovered through tissue culture methods, and most of these findings were later validated in vivo (e.g., [12]). Animal models were also indispensable systems for exploring novel therapeutic avenues for infantile spasms (e.g., [13]), and many other severe pathologies. However, neither cell cultures, nor animal models can perfectly reproduce the complexity of the human nervous system and one needs to take into account and finds ways to overcome their limitations. This Editorial summarizes part of the challenges experienced when investigating neurological disorders in cell lines purchased from authorized vendors or in (genetically, chemically, or mechanically) engineered animal models.

The four major aspects one has to consider when using standard cell lines to study the neurological disorders are:

(1) The cell lines were formed by culturing cells collected either from cancer tumors of the nervous system (like neuroblastoma, astrocytoma, lymphoma, brain metastases of prostate adenocarcinoma etc.) or immortalized for better preservation after collection from an affected (but not cancerous) tissues. In all cases, the cell cycle was considerably modified, so that translating the results into what might happen inside the real tissue of the living person is questionable owing to a totally different dynamics and outputs of the biological processes (e.g., [14]).

(2) In a monoculture, the cells are missing the normal hetero-cellular environment from the tissue that strongly affects all the inner molecular processes. In previous studies,

we reported that the transcriptomes of astrocytes and oligodendrocytes were substantially different when profiled in separate cultures than when profiled co-cultured in insert systems [15,16], sharing the same medium even without physically touching each-other. The differences were not only in the expression levels of the genes but also in the strength of the homeostatic control of the transcripts' abundances and in the gene networking, indicating profound remodeling of the functional pathways. This limitation of the monocultures got a partial solution through the development of the very promising technology of constructing human brain organoids (e.g., [17,18]).

(3) In addition to race, sex and age, the concrete manifestation of a disease depends on the never repeatable combination of the personal characteristics of the patients that includes but is not limited to the medical history, diet, exposure to stress and toxins, climate etc. Therefore, the donor of the selected cell line should match as many as possible characteristics of the studied person or of the homogeneous population.

(4) Any genetic manipulation of the sequence, 3d spatial configuration or expression level of a gene has ripple effects on hundreds other genes, presumably because of their integration in functional pathways. Owing to the uniqueness of the local conditions, the combination and the amplitudes of all other affected genes is never repeatable. Moreover, about 1/1000 of the nucleotides are randomly mutated just because of the stochastic nature of the chemical reactions involved in the DNA replication, making difficult to blame solely the targeted gene for the observed phenotype. Sometimes, the manipulated gene is just one out of several other potential triggers of cascades of similar molecular mechanisms.

Despite being limited by the welfare rules included in the Declaration of Helsinki and subjected to protocol approval by the Institutional Animal Care and Use Committee, an animal model still allows otherwise never acceptable investigations on humans.

However, animal modelling have many challenges too. Like humans, animal features depend on species, strain, sex, age/developmental stage and hormonal status, exposure to oxygen deprivation and toxins, diet, external stimuli, medical history, and treatment (e.g., [19,20]). Importantly, the subcellular localization of certain proteins not only differs between sexes but also changes during the estrogen cycle [21], making the female animal models much more difficult to manage and interpret than their male counterparts. Therefore, choosing the right animal model is far from an easy task. Furthermore, sanitary precautions and housing conditions (e.g.,: distribution of cages and vicinity of other caged males, diet chow and water abundance and quality, environmental temperature, humidity, day and night lighting cycles) are also major modulators of the experimental results.

Nevertheless, the molecular characteristics of the model are not uniform across different regions of the organ and are affected by tissue hetero-cellular organization. We have profiled the transcriptomes of various regions of the brain, spinal cord and retina. The tissues were collected from wildtype and in-house engineered mice, rats and rabbits that modeled neuroblastoma, glioma, autism, epilepsy, glaucoma, intraventricular hemorrhage, infantile spasms, multiple sclerosis, neuroblastoma, neuropsychiatric lupus erythematosus, Charcot–Marie–Tooth disease, and oculodentodigital dysplasia. In rat experiments, we found substantial transcriptomic differences among the hippocampal dentate gyrus, CA1, CA2 and CA3 regions, as well as between the hypothalamic arcuate and periventricular nuclei. Therefore it is very important to select the right region to study and also to have a very skilled neuroanatomist in the team.

It is a widespread belief that many diseases are caused by altered sequence or/and expression level of certain critical gene(s), termed (gene) biomarker(s) (e.g., [22]). Most genomists assumed that, by engineering the same alteration in the genome of an animal, one can reproduce the key features of human disease. On this line, we induced some diseases by manipulating genes like *Gja1*, *Gjb1*, *Gjd2* that encode the connexins forming the gap junction channels in astrocytes, oligodendrocytes and neurons, and the *Fas* gene, whose loss of function mutation leads to a systemic lupus-like phenotype. In all these engineered mice, we found hundreds other genes as significantly regulated and many major functional pathways remodeled, whose alterations, dependent on the type of manipulation, were different between strains, sexes, hormonal status, and age groups. Even informative for that particular animal model, translating the results to humans should remain in hypothetical qualitative terms.

Other animal models might be acquired through chemical or mechanical treatment. For instance, glaucoma was derived in rats by crushing the optic nerve. Infantile Spasms were induced in prenatally betamethasone primed rats with NMDA, status epilepticus was induced in rats with intraperitoneal injection of kainic acid, while multiple sclerosis symptoms were satisfactorily replicated in mouse adoptive transfer experimental autoimmune encephalomyelitis obtained by injecting myelin basic protein (Mbp). Intraventricular hemorrhage was triggered in rabbit premature pups by intraperitoneal injection with 50% glycerol. However, although these animal models mimicked satisfactorily the symptoms of the corresponding human disorders, their occurrence and dynamics were different, requiring careful interpretation of the results.

In summary, albeit very useful to get an idea about the molecular phenomena that might be responsible for the development of neurological disorders, one should consider the limitations of standard cell lines and animal models to reproduce the phenomena in the human nervous system.

Conflicts of Interest: The author declares no conflicts of interest.

References

1. Capotosti, F. a-synuclein PET Imaging: From Clinical Utility in Multiple System Atrophy to the Possible Diagnosis of Parkinson's Disease. *Cells* **2025**, *14*, 834. [CrossRef]
2. Bagarić, T.; Mihaljević-Peleš, A.; Skočić Hanžek, M.; Živković, M.; Kozmar, A.; Rogić, D. Serum Levels of Zinc, Albumin, Interleukin-6 and CRP in Patients with Unipolar and Bipolar Depression: Cross Sectional Study. *Curr. Issues Mol. Biol.* **2024**, *46*, 4533–4550. [CrossRef]
3. Klein, B.Y.; Gofrit, O.N.; Greenblatt, C.L. Testing Protein Stress Signals in Peripheral Immunocytes Under the Same Treatment Capable of Decreasing the Incidence of Alzheimer's Disease in Bladder Cancer Patients. *Curr. Issues Mol. Biol.* **2025**, *47*, 392. [CrossRef]
4. Algahtani, H.; Shirah, B.; Algahtani, O.; Alassiri, A.H. Unraveling the enigma of spinal cord schistosomosis: Clinical spectrum, diagnosis, and therapeutic insights. *Ann. Parasitol.* **2025**, *71*, 1–9. [CrossRef]
5. Staszkiewicz, R.; Gładysz, D.; Sobański, D.; Bolechała, F.; Golec, E.; Sobańska, M.; Strojny, D.; Turek, A.; Grabarek, B.O. Assessment of the Concentration of Transforming Growth Factor Beta 1–3 in Degenerated Intervertebral Discs of the Lumbosacral Region of the Spine. *Curr. Issues Mol. Biol.* **2024**, *46*, 12813–12829. [CrossRef] [PubMed]
6. World Medical Association. World Medical Association Declaration of Helsinki: Ethical principles for medical research involving human subjects. *Jama* **2013**, *310*, 2191–2194. [CrossRef] [PubMed]
7. Pecoraro, M.; Serra, A.; Pascale, M.; Franceschelli, S. The ER Stress Induced in Human Neuroblastoma Cells Can Be Reverted by Lumacaftor, a CFTR Corrector. *Curr. Issues Mol. Biol.* **2024**, *46*, 9342–9358. [CrossRef]
8. Shishmanova-Doseva, M.; Barbutska, D. BDNF/Cyclin D1 Signaling System and Cognitive Performance After Perampanel and Lacosamide Treatment Singly or in Combination in an Experimental Model of Temporal Lobe Epilepsy. *Curr. Issues Mol. Biol.* **2024**, *46*, 14010–14032. [CrossRef]
9. Meca, A.D.; Boboc, I.K.S.; Mititelu-Tartau, L.; Bogdan, M. Unlocking the Potential: Semaglutide's Impact on Alzheimer's and Parkinson's Disease in Animal Models. *Curr. Issues Mol. Biol.* **2024**, *46*, 5929–5949. [CrossRef]

10. Iacobas, D.A.; Veliskova, J.; Chachua, T.; Chern, C.R.; Vieira, K.; Iacobas, S.; Velíšek, L. Neurotransmission Sex Dichotomy in the Rat Hypothalamic Paraventricular Nucleus in Healthy and Infantile Spasm Model. *Curr. Issues Mol. Biol.* **2025**, *47*, 380. [CrossRef] [PubMed]
11. Sawaguchi, S.; Ishida, M.; Miyamoto, Y.; Yamauchi, J. Hypomyelination Leukodystrophy 16 (HLD16)-Associated Mutation p.Asp252Asn of TMEM106B Blunts Cell Morphological Differentiation. *Curr. Issues Mol. Biol.* **2024**, *46*, 8088–8103. [CrossRef]
12. Li, X.; Ding, L.; Nie, H.; Deng, D.Y.B. Calcium Signaling in Astrocytes and Its Role in the Central Nervous System Injury. *Mol. Neurobiol.* **2025**, *Epub ahead of print*. [CrossRef]
13. CUREInfantile Spasms Consortium; CURE Staff; Lubbers, L.; Iyengar, S.S.; Vezzani, A.; Berg, A.T.; Lowenstein, D.H.; Klitgaard, H.; Goodkin, H.P.; Rho, J.M.; et al. A team science approach to discover novel targets for infantile spasms (IS). *Epilepsia Open* **2020**, *6*, 49–61. [CrossRef]
14. Fallot, L.B.; Pinc, J.R.; Buselmeier, J.E.; Palchak, J.C.; Shroff, S.S.; Zang, K.; Rinauro, D.J.; Bacon, K.M.; Nguyen, M.; Schleck, M.C.; et al. An aminosterol breaks the autocatalytic cycle of Aβ42 aggregation and protects cell membranes from its soluble aggregates. *Proc. Natl. Acad. Sci. USA* **2025**, *122*, e2417944122. [CrossRef]
15. Iacobas, S.; Iacobas, D.A. Astrocyte proximity modulates the myelination gene fabric of oligodendrocytes. *Neuron Glia Biol.* **2010**, *6*, 157–169. [CrossRef]
16. Iacobas, D.A.; Iacobas, S.; Stout, R.F.; Spray, D.C. Cellular Environment Remodels the Genomic Fabrics of Functional Pathways in Astrocytes. *Genes* **2020**, *11*, 520. [CrossRef]
17. Kshirsagar, A.; Mnatsakanyan, H.; Kulkarni, S.; Guo, J.; Cheng, K.; Ofria, L.D.; Bohra, O.; Sagar, R.; Mahairaki, V.; Badr, C.E.; et al. Multi-Region Brain Organoids Integrating Cerebral, Mid-Hindbrain, and Endothelial Systems. *Adv. Sci.* **2025**, e03768. *Online ahead of print*. [CrossRef]
18. Zhou, M.; Cao, Y.; Yue, K.; Wu, W.; Xie, Y.; Hu, D.; Zhao, J.; Xu, F.; Guo, J.; Li, Z.; et al. Brain organoids and genome editing: A new era in understanding human brain development and disorders. *Neural Regen. Res.* **2025**, *Epub ahead of print*. [CrossRef] [PubMed]
19. DeFranco, J.P.; Telling, G.C. The Evolution of Experimental Rodent Models for Prion Diseases. *J. Neurochem.* **2025**, *169*, e70039. [CrossRef] [PubMed]
20. Diederich, K.; Steinfath, M.; Bannach-Brown, A.; Bert, B.; Butzke, D.; Wildner, P.L.; Wurm, M.; Schadock, I.; Heinl, C. Protocol for the systematic review of age and sex in preclinical models of age-correlated diseases. *F1000Research* **2024**, *13*, 858. [CrossRef] [PubMed]
21. Thomas, N.M.; Jasmin, J.F.; Lisanti, M.P.; Iacobas, D.A. Sex Differences in Expression and subcellular Localization of Heart Rhythm Determinant Proteins. *Biochem. Biophys. Res. Commun.* **2011**, *406*, 117–122. [CrossRef] [PubMed]
22. Sapana, T.; Zhuo, Z. Biomarkers for diagnosis and prognosis of myelin oligodendrocyte glycoprotein antibody-associated disease-review article. *Front. Immunol.* **2025**, *16*, 1594960. [CrossRef] [PubMed]

current issues in molecular biology

MDPI

Article

Serum Levels of Zinc, Albumin, Interleukin-6 and CRP in Patients with Unipolar and Bipolar Depression: Cross Sectional Study

Tihana Bagarić [1,*], Alma Mihaljević-Peleš [1,2], Milena Skočić Hanžek [1,2], Maja Živković [1,2], Ana Kozmar [1,3] and Dunja Rogić [1,3]

1 Department for Psychiatry and Psychological Medicine, University Hospital Centre Zagreb, 10000 Zagreb, Croatia; apeles@mef.hr (A.M.-P.); mskocic@kbc-zagreb.hr (M.S.H.); maja.zivkovic@kbc-zagreb.hr (M.Ž.); akozmar@kbc-zagreb.hr (A.K.); dunjarogic@hotmail.com (D.R.)
2 School of Medicine, University of Zagreb, 10000 Zagreb, Croatia
3 Faculty of Pharmacy and Biochemistry, University of Zagreb, 10000 Zagreb, Croatia
* Correspondence: tihana.bagaric@kbc-zagreb.hr; Tel.: +385-9-8955-2867

Abstract: Unipolar (UD) and bipolar depression (BDD) show a high degree of similarity in clinical presentations, which complicates the differential diagnosis of these disorders. The aim of this study was to investigate the serum levels of interleukin 6 (IL-6), C-reactive protein (CRP), albumin (Alb), and zinc (Zn) in patients with UD, BDD, and healthy controls (HC). A total of 211 samples were collected: 131 patient samples (65 UD and 68 BDD) and 80 HC. The Montgomery–Asberg Depression Rating Scale (MADRS), along with the Hamilton Depression Rating Scale (HAMD-17), were administered to patient groups to evaluate symptoms. A cross-sectional study was performed to analyse the serum levels of IL-6, CRP, albumin, and zinc. The concentration of CRP was determined using the immunoturbidimetry method, zinc using the colorimetric method, and albumin using the colorimetric method with bromocresol green on the Alinity c device. IL-6 cytokine concentration in serum samples was ascertained using a commercial enzyme immunoassay, ELISA. We found no significant differences in serum concentrations of zinc, albumin, CRP, and IL-6 between the groups of patients with unipolar and bipolar depression. There was a significant statistical difference ($p < 0.001$) between serum levels of all investigated parameters in both groups of depressed patients in comparison with HC. Furthermore, correlations with specific items on HAMD-17; (namely, hypochondrias, work and activities, somatic symptoms-general, and weight loss) and on MADRS (concentration difficulties, lassitude) were observed in both patient groups. These findings confirm the presence of low-grade inflammation in depression, thus adding better insight into the inflammation hypothesis directed to explain the aetiology of depressive disorders. Our results do not indicate potential biomarkers for distinguishing between unipolar and bipolar depression.

Keywords: bipolar depression; unipolar depression; zinc; albumin; CRP; IL-6; inflammation

1. Introduction

At least 20% of the general population, at some point in their lives, experience an episode of mood swings, or even develop a mood disorder. Within mood disorders, bipolar disorder (BD) and depressive disorder (DD) are the most common and most disabling disorders [1,2]. Among patients who clinically present with depression, there is a significant number of those who later turn out to have bipolar disorder, that is, who belong on the bipolar spectrum [3–5]. Namely, a depressive episode in unipolar depression and a depressive episode in BD are clinically presented almost identically. Without insight into the longitudinal course of the disorder, it is difficult to distinguish which disorder it is at first. Even then, it should be taken into account that the onset of BD is characterized by alternations of depressive episodes (before the development of a hypomanic or manic episode) that can last for several years [6]. Furthermore, BD is clinically demanding to diagnose due to subsyndromal states that often occur between major episodes of the disorder [7].

Timely diagnostic differentiation of these disorders is important because pharmacotherapeutic treatment is fundamentally different. While unipolar depression is primarily treated with antidepressants, they are not a good therapeutic choice for bipolar disorder. Treatment with antidepressants in undiagnosed bipolar patients causes mixed states, faster exchanges of polarity, but also increases the risk of suicide, especially in younger age groups of patients [8,9].

Apart from anamnestic and hetero-anamnestic data and a clinical examination, for now, there is no objective measurable indicator that would help in the differential diagnosis of these two disorders.

The prevailing paradigm is that unipolar and bipolar depression are qualitatively and etiologically different [10]. This duality is also represented in the DSM 5 diagnostic manual, which categorizes them as separate disorders [11].

In recent years, numerous studies have suggested the involvement of the immune system and inflammatory processes in mood disorders [12–14].

Research indicates that both unipolar depression (UD) and bipolar disorder (BD) are associated with an inflammatory state characterized by imbalances in proinflammatory and anti-inflammatory cytokines [15,16]. While some studies report no significant differences in inflammatory markers like IL-6 and TNFR between UD and BD, other research highlights distinct immunological profiles for each disorder [13,17]. Specifically, patients with UD have shown elevated levels of cytokines such as IL-1β, TNF-α, and IL-12, whereas those with BD exhibit higher levels of IL-6, IL-18, IL-33, and sST2. These findings suggest differential immune-inflammatory involvement in the pathogenesis of UD and BD, although the data remain somewhat inconsistent across studies.

Biomarkers such as IL-6 [18–21], CRP [22,23], albumin [24,25], and zinc [26–29] have been subject of numerous studies aimed to shed light into complex interplay between inflammatory process and depressive symptoms. However, the differences in these biomarkers have not previously been evaluated in patients with UD and BD, and the relationship between these biomarkers and symptoms in BD and UD had not yet been studied.

Our study was designed to include a wider range of biological parameters in groups of hospitalized patients with BDD and hospitalized patients with UD and HC.

Four biological parameters were selected that in earlier research were found to be associated with inflammatory events in mood disorders: IL-6, CRP, Zn, and albumin levels [30,31].

The hypothesis was that, respecting the paradigm of the etiological diversity of these two disorders [32], there would be a significant difference in the concentration of the mentioned parameters between all examined groups.

We additionally considered, if one of the researched parameters would prove to be a good and clinically relevant biological marker for the distinction of these two disorders, it would be of great importance in daily clinical work and a great help when establishing a diagnosis.

2. Materials and Methods

2.1. Participants and Procedures

A total of 211 participants of both genders aged 18 to 60 were included in this cross-sectional study conducted in the period between 2016 and 2023: 65 patients with unipolar depression (UD), 68 patients with bipolar depression (BDD) treated in the Psychiatric Hospital "Dr. Ivan Barbot" in Popovača and in the Clinic for Psychiatry and Psychological Medicine, UHC Zagreb, and 80 healthy controls (HC). The diagnosis of UD and BDD was confirmed using a structured clinical interview based on the DSM 5 criteria [11]. All patients were experiencing an acute depressive episode at the time of admission to the hospital. We chose a consecutive sample of patients by the order of their arrival at the hospital treatment. The purpose of the research was explained to all participants who were suitable for participation in the study, and their informed consent was obtained. To assess the severity of depressive symptoms among patients, we used the Montgomery–Asberg Depression Rating Scale (MADRS) [33] and the Hamilton Rating Scale for Depression (HAMD-17) [34]. The study included patients whose depressive episode was evaluated at least as moderately severe using the clinical scales used (MADRS > 20, HAMD-17 > 18). The exclusion criteria were: refusal to give informed consent or withdrawal of informed consent to participate in research, clear manifestation of infection, physical diagnoses such as autoimmune diseases or malignant diseases, other psychiatric disorders or intellectual disability, and pregnancy and lactation. Also, we excluded participants on an extreme diet, those with an eating disorder, and those who abused psychoactive substances. The use of regular pharmacotherapy (according to the protocol for UD and BD) that patients used before the onset of the depressive episode was not in the exclusion criteria. As a control group, 80 healthy individuals matched by age and gender were recruited. The control group participants had no history of psychiatric disorders, and participation was voluntary in all cases. The same exclusion criteria were used for both the experimental and control groups. The study protocol was approved by the Ethics Committees of Psychiatric Hospital "Dr. Ivan Barbot" Popovača, University Hospital Centre Zagreb and Medical School of the University of Zagreb. The study complied with World Medical Association Declaration of Helsinki 2013 (World Medical Association 2013).

2.2. Collection of Blood Samples

From the patients diagnosed with UD and BDD blood samples were taken for the analysis of serum levels of interleukin 6 (IL-6), C-reactive protein (CRP), albumin (Alb), and zinc (Zn). Blood samples were taken from the cubital vein at around 8 am in tubes with a gel separator of 8 mL (Greiner Bio-One International GmbH, Kremsmünster, Austria).

The samples were then centrifuged for 10 min at 3000 rpm (Hettich Rotofix 32, Andreas Hetich Gmb & Co. KG, Tuttlingen, Germany). The obtained serum was divided into plastic tubes (1.5 mL; Kartell, Noviglio, Italy) which were stored at −20 °C for determination of interleukin 6 (IL-6). The serum sample for C-reactive protein (CRP), zinc, and albumin tests were analysed using centrifugation.

2.3. Statistical Analysis

Categorical data are represented by absolute and relative frequencies. Differences in categorical variables were tested with the Chi-square test and, if necessary, with Fisher's exact test. The normality of the distribution of numerical variables was tested with the Shapiro–Wilk test. Numerical data are described by the median and the limits of the interquartile range. Differences of numerical variables between two independent groups was performed using the Mann–Whitney U test (with the Hodges–Lehmann median difference and 95% confidence interval of the difference shown). The internal reliability of the scales (HAM-D and MADRS) was expressed through the Cronbach Alpha coefficient. The association of continuous variables was assessed using Spearman's correlation coefficient ρ (rho). For all multiple testing, the Bonferroni correction was used. The influence of independent factors on the severity of a depressive episode and changes in depressive illness were tested using bivariate and multivariate logistic regression (without correction and with correction for taking antidepressants). All p values are two-sided. The significance level was set at alpha (α) = 0.05. The statistical program MedCalc® Statistical Software version 22.006 (MedCalc® Statistical Software version 22.018 (MedCalc Software Ltd., Ostend, Belgium); https://www.medcalc.org (accessed on 6 May 2024)) and SPSS (ver.23.0, SPSS Inc., Chicago, IL, USA) were used for statistical analysis.

2.4. Determination of CRP, Zinc, and Albumin

The concentration of CRP was determined using the immunoturbidimetry method, zinc using the colorimetric method, and albumin using the bromcresol green colorimetric method on the Alinity c device (Abbott Laboratories, Chicago, IL, USA). All methods for CRP and albumin were implemented and validated according to [35].

2.5. Determination of IL-6

IL-6 cytokine concentration in serum samples was determined using a commercial enzyme immunoassay, ELISA (Enzyme-linked immunosorbent assay). Assays were performed according to the manufacturer's instructions (Invitrogen, Thermo Fisher Scientific Inc., Waltham, MA, USA).

2.6. Performing an ELISA Test

The wells of the microtiter plate coated with monoclonal antibody to human IL-6 were washed twice with 300 μL of washing solution each. After washing, add 100 μL of the standard (concentration range 5.0–0.05 pg/mL) to the wells and 50 μL of the serum diluent and 50 μL of the sample to the serum wells. Then, 50 μL biotin-labelled monoclonal anti-human IL-6 antibody was added to all wells and incubated at room temperature for two hours on a Mini-Shaker PSU-2T mixer (BioSan, Riga, Latvia). After incubation, the plate was washed six times, and 100 μL of freshly prepared streptavidin-HRP conjugate was added to the wells and incubated at room temperature for one hour on a mixer. After washing again, add 100 μL of amplification solution I to all wells and incubate for 15 min at room temperature on a mixer. Washing the plate again precedes adding 100 μL of amplification solution II to all wells and incubation for 30 min on a mixer. After the final washing, 100 μL of tetramethyl benzidine (TBM) substrate was added to the wells and incubated for 20 min protected from light. The reaction was stopped by adding 100 μL of 1 M phosphoric acid. The absorbance of the resulting developed colour is immediately read at 450 nm with a reference wavelength of 620 nm on a Sunrise microtiter plate reader (Tecan Trading AG, Männedorf, Switzerland). The measurement results were calculated according to the standard curve (software support Magellan 7.3 STD Tecan Trading AG, Männedorf, Switzerland) and multiplied using the appropriate dilution factor and expressed in pg/mL. The standard curve was obtained from standards of known concentrations.

3. Results

3.1. Sociodemographic and General Medical Characteristics of Study Participants

This research was conducted on 211 participants, of whom 131 (62.1%) were patients with depression. In total, 66 subjects (50.4%) had bipolar and 65 subjects (49.6%) had unipolar depression. The healthy control group consisted of 80 participants. We found no significant difference in relation to the gender and mean age between the control group and the patient group (Table 1).

Table 1. General characteristics of the study population.

	Healthy Control (HC)	Patient Groups	Total	p *
Gender [n (%)]				
Female	60 (75)	84 (64.1)	144 (68.2)	0.10
Male	20 (25)	47 (35.9)	67 (31.8)	
Age (years) [Median (IQR)]	53 (44–57)	55 (47–58)	54 (42–57)	0.06 †

* χ^2 test; † Mann–Whitney U test.

In total, 84 (64%) participants are women and 47 (36%) are men, with no significant difference in relation to the spectrum.

The most common diagnosis is bipolar depression—moderately severe depressive episode in 60 (46%) subjects, and depressive disorder—moderately severe depressive episode in 44 (34%) subjects.

Median age of the participants is 55 (interquartile range from 47 to 58 years) in the range from 52 to 60 years, without a significant difference in relation to the spectrum. In total, 103 (79%) respondents have children, with no significant difference in the number of children compared to the examined groups. In total, 75 (56%) participants have a high school education, and 17 (13%) have a university degree, of which there are significantly more, 16 (24%) of them from the group of participants with bipolar depression (χ^2 test, $p = 0.004$). In total, 59 (45%) participants are employed, and 40 (31%) are retired. In total, 78 (60%) participants are married, 24 (18%) are single, 22 (17%) participants are divorced, and 7 (5%) are widowed. Again, no statistically significant difference between examined groups was found in all of the above listed parameters.

Psychiatric heredity was noted in 42 (32%) participants.

Interestingly, in the group of subjects with bipolar depression who smoked tobacco cigarettes, we found a significantly higher number of packs of cigarettes per day (Mann–Whitney U test, $p = 0.023$) and "pack years" (Mann–Whitney U test, $p = 0.018$) compared to group of study participants who have unipolar depression (Table 2).

Table 2. General characteristics of the study population distribution according to general characteristics and psychiatric heredity.

	Percentage of Participants (%)			p *
	Unipolar Depression	**Bipolar Depression**	**Total**	
Educational Level				
No formal education	1 (2)	1 (2)	2 (2)	0.004
Elementary school	10 (15)	9 (14)	19 (15)	
High school	44 (67)	31 (47)	75 (56)	
College (short program)	9 (14)	9 (13)	18 (14)	
University degree	1 (2)	16 (24)	17 (13)	
Employment Status				
Employed	27 (42)	32 (48)	59 (45)	0.633
Unemployed	18 (28)	14 (21)	32 (24)	
Retired	20 (30)	20 (31)	40 (31)	
Marital Status				
Married	41 (64)	37 (55)	78 (60)	0.418 †
Divorced	9 (15)	13 (20)	22 (17)	
Single	10 (15)	14 (22)	24 (18)	
Widowed	5 (7.6)	2 (3)	7 (5)	
Psychiatric Heredity	18 (28)	24 (36)	42 (32)	0.288
Family History of Psychiatric Illness (n = 40)				
Mother—depressive disorder	6 (33.3)	12 (54.5)	18 (45)	0.498 †
Father—depression	1 (5.6)	1 (4.5)	2 (5)	
Father—alcoholism, suicide	1 (5.6)	0	1 (3)	
Father—alcoholism	4 (22)	5 (22.7)	9 (23)	
Mother—bipolar disorder	0	2 (9.1)	2 (5)	
Sister—depression	1 (5.6)	1 (4.5)	2 (5)	
Sister—schizophrenia	1 (5.6)	0	1 (3)	
Father—suicide	1 (5.6)	0	1 (3)	
Sister and mother suicide, father alcoholic	1 (5.6)	0	1 (3)	
Brother PTSD, brother alcoholism, mother BAP	0	1 (4.5)	1 (3)	
Father and brother depression and suicide	1 (5.6)	0	1 (3)	
Aunt depressive disorder	1 (5.6)	0	1 (3)	

* χ^2 test; † Fisher's exact test.

3.2. Serum Levels of Il-6, CRP, Alb and Zn in Patients and Healthy Control Subjects

The values of IL-6 (Mann–Whitney U test, $p = 0.006$), CRP (Mann–Whitney U test, $p = 0.002$), and zinc (Mann–Whitney U test, $p = 0.013$) were significantly higher in the patient group compared to the control group, while albumin values were significantly lower in the patient group compared to the control (Mann–Whitney U test, $p = 0.002$) (Table 3).

Table 3. Comparison of serum levels of IL-6, CRP-u, albumin, and zinc between the healthy control group and patient group.

	Median (Interquartile Range)		Difference	95% CI (Confidence Interval)	p *
	Healthy Controls	Patients			
IL-6	0.95 (0.296–2.518)	1.54 (0.871–2.35)	0.41	0.14–0.76	0.006
CRP	1.40 (0.90–2.15)	2.90 (1.10–6.0)	0.80	0.10–2.20	0.002
Albumin	46.0 (44.0–48.0)	44.05 (42.0–47.0)	−2	−3–(−1)	0.002
Zinc	12.20 (10.67–14.02)	13.20 (11.43–15.38)	1.22	0.23–2.11	0.013

* Mann–Whitney U test.

3.3. Comparison of Serum Levels of Il-6, CRP, Alb, and Zn in Patients with Depressive Episode of Bipolar Disorder (DBD), Unipolar Depression (UD), and Healthy Control Group (HC)

There are significantly lower values in the control group compared to patients with unipolar or bipolar spectrum in levels of IL-6 (Kruskal–Wallis test, $p = 0.020$) and CRP (Kruskal–Wallis test, $p = 0.008$), while albumin values are significantly higher (Kruskal–Wallis test, $p = 0.007$). Zinc values are significantly lower in the control group compared to the group of patients with unipolar spectrum (Kruskal–Wallis test, $p = 0.013$), while they do not significantly differ from the values of patients with bipolar spectrum (Table 4).

Table 4. Differences between IL-6, CRP, albumin, and zinc between healthy the control group and patient group, considering the spectrum of the disorder (unipolar; bipolar).

	Median (Interquartile Range)			p *
	Control Group	Unipolar Depression	Bipolar Depression	
IL-6	0.95 (0.296–2.518)	1.54 (0.82–2.76)	1.53 (0.96–2.26)	0.020 †
CRP	1.40 (0.90–2.15)	3.40 (1.0–5.70)	2.45 (1.10–6.80)	0.008 †
Albumin	46.0 (44.0–48.0)	44.80 (42.10–47.0)	44.0 (42.0–47.0)	0.007 †
Zinc	12.20 (10.67–14.02)	13.40 (11.9–15.5)	13.15 (10.40–15.0)	0.013 ‡

* Kruskal Wallis test (post hoc Conover); † $p < 0.05$ significantly lower values in controls vs. unipolar and bipolar spectrum; ‡ $p < 0.05$ significantly lower values in controls vs. unipolar spectrum.

3.4. Comparison of Serum Levels of Il-6, CRP, Albumin, and Zinc in BD and UD Subjects

There are no significant differences in the values of zinc, albumin, CRP, and IL-6 with respect to the examined groups of patients (Table 5).

Table 5. Comparison of serum levels of zinc, albumin, CRP, and IL-6 between groups of participants with unipolar and bipolar depression.

	Median (Interquartile Range)		Difference	95% CI (Confidence Interval)	p *
	Unipolar Depression	Bipolar Depression			
Zinc	13.4 (11.9–15.5)	13.2 (10.4–15)	−0.8	−1.7–0.3	0.134
Albumin	44.8 (42.1–47.0)	44.0 (42–47)	0	−1.6–1.0	0.825
CRP	3.4 (1.0–5.7)	2.5 (1.1–6.8)	0.1	−0.7–0.8	0.718
IL-6	1.54 (0.82–2.76)	1.53 (0.96–2.26)	−0.006	−0.44–0.36	0.962

* Mann–Whitney U test.

3.5. Association between Serum Levels of IL-6, Zn, Alb, CRP, and Severity of Depressive Episode According to HAMD-17 and MADRS

The researched parameters were compared in each examined group considering the severity of the depressive episode on the Hamilton and Montgomery–Asberg Rating Scales.

Comparing depressive episodes of equal clinical severity (moderate or severe according to HAMD-17) in the studied patient groups (UD and BDD), there were no significant differences in serum levels of IL-6, Zn, CRP, and albumin.

In the groups of participants classified according to the diagnosis of affective disorder (UD or BD), with regard to the severity of the depressive episode assessed on the Hamilton Rating Scale for Depression, there were no significant differences in serum levels of IL-6, Zn, CRP, or Alb.

Interestingly, in patients with bipolar depression, severe depressive episode (evaluated according to Hamilton Scale), albumin values were significantly lower compared to the moderately severe depressive episode of the same participants group (Mann–Whitney U test, $p = 0.042$).

On this basis, there were no differences in the group with unipolar depression. Similarly, no significant differences were found when comparing moderate or severe depressive episodes assessed using the MADRAS between patients with bipolar and unipolar depression.

3.6. Correlations of Zn, Alb, CRP, and IL-6, with Items on the HAMD-17 and MADRS

Spearman's correlation coefficient was used to evaluate the association of serum values of zinc, albumin, CRP, and IL-6 with individual items and the total score of HAMD-17 and MADRS.

We must underline the statistically significant positive and somewhat statistically weaker relationship between albumin and somatic anxiety (Rho = 0.264), and a negative and significant relationship with "hypochondriasis" (Rho = −0.303) in the group of subjects with unipolar depression (items on HAMD-17 scale). In addition, there is a significant and positive relation of CRP values to items "work and activities" (Rho = 0.253), "somatic symptoms, general" (Rho = 0.281), and item "weight loss" (Rho = 0.364). Interleukin-6 is significantly positively related to "work and activity" (Rho = 0.319), with "somatic symptoms, general" (Rho = 0.424) and with "weight loss" (Rho = 0.277), but negatively and significantly related to the scale item "guilt feelings" (Rho = −0.293). The total scale of HAM-D-17 in subjects with unipolar depression is not significantly related to the observed values (Table 6).

Table 6. Association between items on HAMD-17 in groups of patients with unipolar depression (Spearman's correlation coefficient).

Unipolar Depression Items on HAMD-17 Scale	Spearman's Correlation Coefficient Rho (*p* Value)			
	Zinc	Albumin	CRP	IL-6
Depressed mood	0.085 (0.50)	−0.087 (0.49)	0.019 (0.88)	−0.035 (0.79)
Guilt feelings	0.019 (0.88)	−0.103 (0.42)	0.006 (0.96)	−0.293 (0.02)
Suicide thoughts	0.040 (0.75)	−0.160 (0.21)	0.037 (0.77)	0.074 (0.56)
Insomnia-early	0.093 (0.46)	0.060 (0.64)	0.020 (0.88)	0.093 (0.47)
Insomnia-middle	−0.031 (0.80)	0.049 (0.70)	−0.024 (0.85)	0.002 (0.99)
Insomnia-late	0.130 (0.30)	0.160 (0.21)	0.014 (0.91)	−0.112 (0.38)
Work and activities	−0.226 (0.07)	−0.238 (0.06)	0.253 (0.04)	0.319 (0.01)
Retardation psychomotor	0.008 (0.95)	−0.193 (0.13)	0.166 (0.19)	0.221 (0.08)
Agitation	0.238 (0.06)	0.077 (0.55)	−0.115 (0.36)	−0.063 (0.62)
Anxiety-psychic	−0.035 (0.78)	0.079 (0.54)	0.249 (0.05)	0.114 (0.37)
Anxiety-somatic	0.217 (0.08)	0.264 (0.04)	0.011 (0.93)	−0.054 (0.67)
Gastrointestinal symptoms	−0.247 (0.05)	−0.104 (0.41)	0.064 (0.61)	0.091 (0.48)
Somatic symptoms. general	−0.227 (0.07)	−0.159 (0.21)	0.281 (0.02)	0.424 (<0.001)
Sexual disturbances	−0.082 (0.52)	−0.016 (0.90)	0.083 (0.51)	0.107 (0.41)
Hypochondriasis (somatization)	−0.109 (0.39)	−0.303 (0.01)	0.095 (0.45)	0.122 (0.34)
Weight loss	−0.231 (0.06)	−0.249 (0.05)	0.364 (<0.001)	0.277 (0.03)
Insight	−0.074 (0.56)	−0.164 (0.19)	0.046 (0.72)	0.166 (0.19)
HAMD−17 total	−0.027 (0.83)	−0.091 (0.47)	0.227 (0.07)	0.177 (0.16)

In groups of subjects with bipolar depression on the HAMD-17 scale, there was found a significant, positive, and slightly weaker relationship of zinc serum levels with scale items "gastrointestinal symptoms" (Rho = −0.366), "somatic symptoms, general" (Rho = −0.253), "weight loss" (Rho = −0.327), and also a positive and significant relationship with "anxiety-psychic" (Rho = 0.396). Albumin serum values were found to have a statistically significant and negative relation with "guilt feelings" (Rho = −0.341), and "work and activity" (Rho = −0.342). In addition, IL-6 serum values were found to be significantly statistically positively related to the items "gastrointestinal symptoms" (Rho = 0.254), "somatic symptoms, general" (Rho = 0.458), and with "work and activity" (Rho = 0.250), while a significant negative relationship with "anxiety-psychic" (Rho = −0.307) was calculated. The total HAMD-17 scale in subjects with bipolar depression is not significantly related to the observed values (Table 7).

Table 7. Association of serum levels of Zn, Albumin, CRP, and IL-6 to HAMD-17 items in a group of patients with bipolar depression.

Bipolar Depression	Spearman's Correlation Coefficient Rho (*p* Value)			
	Zinc	Albumin	CRP	IL-6
Depressed mood	−0.072 (0.57)	−0.239 (0.05)	0.052 (0.68)	0.133 (0.29)
Guilt feelings	−0.110 (0.38)	−0.341 (0.01)	0.145 (0.25)	0.050 (0.69)
Suicidal thoughts	−0.001 (0.99)	−0.174 (0.16)	−0.071 (0.57)	0.037 (0.77)
Insomnia: initial	0.050 (0.69)	−0.069 (0.58)	0.154 (0.22)	−0.053 (0.68)
Insomnia: middle	0.082 (0.51)	0.124 (0.32)	0.194 (0.12)	−0.104 (0.41)

Table 7. *Cont.*

Bipolar Depression	Spearman's Correlation Coefficient Rho (*p* Value)			
	Zinc	Albumin	CRP	IL-6
Insomnia: late	0.164 (0.19)	0.205 (0.1)	0.187 (0.13)	−0.084 (0.51)
Work and activities	−0.182 (0.14)	−0.342 (<0.001)	0.093 (0.46)	0.250 (0.04)
Psychomotor retardation	0.125 (0.32)	0.043 (0.73)	−0.008 (0.95)	0.039 (0.76)
Psychomotor agitation	0.176 (0.16)	−0.062 (0.62)	0.019 (0.88)	−0.225 (0.07)
Anxiety. psychic	0.396 (<0.001)	0.059 (0.64)	0.040 (0.75)	−0.307 (0.01)
Anxiety. somatic	0.088 (0.48)	0.082 (0.51)	0.202 (0.10)	−0.150 (0.23)
Gastrointestinal symptoms	−0.366 (<0.001)	−0.231 (0.06)	0.225 (0.07)	0.254 (0.04)
Somatic symptoms. general	−0.253 (0.04)	−0.270 (0.03)	0.206 (0.10)	0.458 (<0.001)
Sexual disturbances	0.035 (0.78)	0.075 (0.55)	0.046 (0.71)	−0.009 (0.94)
Hypochondriasis (somatization)	−0.111 (0.38)	−0.011 (0.93)	0.206 (0.10)	0.032 (0.80)
Weight loss	−0.327 (0.01)	−0.129 (0.30)	0.122 (0.33)	0.152 (0.23)
Insight	−0.018 (0.89)	−0.095 (0.45)	0.028 (0.82)	−0.105 (0.40)
HAMD-17 total	−0.082 (0.51)	−0.211 (0.09)	0.239 (0.05)	0.024 (0.85)

Subjects with unipolar depression have a significant and positive relationship of CRP serum levels with the "concentration difficulties" item (Rho = 0.262), and IL-6 also with the items "concentration difficulties" (Rho = 0.278) and "lassitude" (Rho = 0.345) on the MADRS Depression Rating Scale (Table 8).

Table 8. Association of items on MADRS to serum levels of Zn, albumin, CRP, and IL-6 in groups of patients with unipolar depression.

Unipolar Depression	Spearman's Correlation Coefficient Rho (*p* Value)			
	Zinc	Albumin	CRP	IL-6
Apparent sadness	0.079 (0.53)	0.068 (0.59)	0.238 (0.06)	0.113 (0.38)
Reported sadness	0.171 (0.17)	0.003 (0.98)	0.087 (0.49)	−0.059 (0.65)
Inner tension	−0.019 (0.88)	−0.200 (0.11)	0.138 (0.27)	0.160 (0.21)
Reduced sleep	0.135 (0.28)	−0.045 (0.73)	0.165 (0.19)	0.056 (0.67)
Reduced appetite	0.006 (0.96)	−0.167 (0.19)	−0.065 (0.61)	0.081 (0.53)
Concentration difficulties	−0.170 (0.18)	−0.181 (0.15)	0.262 (0.04)	0.278 (0.03)
Lassitude	−0.191 (0.13)	−0.051 (0.69)	0.228 (0.07)	0.345 (0.01)
Inability to feel	−0.115 (0.36)	−0.029 (0.82)	0.114 (0.37)	0.109 (0.39)
Pessimistic thoughts	−0.049 (0.70)	−0.163 (0.20)	0.200 (0.11)	0.070 (0.59)
Suicidal thoughts	−0.109 (0.39)	−0.053 (0.68)	0.221 (0.08)	0.238 (0.06)
MADRS total	−0.005 (0.97)	−0.124 (0.33)	0.219 (0.08)	0.184 (0.15)

In subjects with bipolar depression, zinc values are significantly and negatively related to reduced appetite (Rho = −0.338). Albumin has a negative and significant relationship with noticeable grief (Rho = −0.259), reduced appetite (Rho = −0.264), concentration difficulties (Rho = 0.272), and the total MADRS (Rho = −0.253), and CRP has a positive and significant relationship related to fatigue (Rho = 0.384) (Table 9).

Table 9. Association of items on MADRS to serum levels of Zn, albumin, CRP, and IL-6 in groups of patients with bipolar depression.

Bipolar Depression	Spearman's Correlation Coefficient Rho (*p* Value)			
	Zinc	**Albumin**	**CRP**	**IL-6**
Apparent sadness	0.029 (0.82)	−0.259 (0.04)	0.120 (0.34)	0.062 (0.62)
Reported sadness	−0.055 (0.66)	−0.201 (0.11)	0.167 (0.18)	0.070 (0.58)
Inner tension	0.002 (0.99)	−0.062 (0.62)	0.099 (0.43)	−0.153 (0.22)
Reduced sleep	0.096 (0.44)	−0.130 (0.30)	0.118 (0.34)	−0.012 (0.92)
Reduced appetite	−0.338 (0.01)	−0.264 (0.03)	0.159 (0.20)	0.151 (0.23)
Concentration difficulties	−0.051 (0.69)	−0.272 (0.03)	0.135 (0.28)	0.101 (0.42)
Lassitude	−0.174 (0.16)	−0.231 (0.06)	0.384 (<0.001)	0.245 (0.05)
Inability to feel	−0.165 (0.19)	−0.221 (0.08)	0.131 (0.29)	0.073 (0.57)
Pessimistic thoughts	−0.068 (0.59)	−0.183 (0.14)	0.136 (0.28)	−0.046 (0.72)
Suicidal thoughts	−0.156 (0.21)	−0.172 (0.17)	0.075 (0.55)	0.102 (0.42)
MADRS total	−0.066 (0.60)	−0.253 (0.04)	0.185 (0.14)	0.064 (0.61)

3.7. The Influence of Sociodemographic Data, General Medical Conditions and Substance Abuse Including Tobacco Smoking on the Severity of Depressive Episode According to HAMD and MADRS (Logistic Regression)

Bivariate and multivariate logistic regression analyses were conducted to predict the likelihood of a severe depressive episode using the Hamilton Depression Rating Scale (HAMD score of 25–52) and the Montgomery–Åsberg Depression Rating Scale (MADRS score of 35–60).

In the group of subjects with unipolar depression, a significant model in the bivariate regression for predicting a severe depressive episode was "pack years" (Odds Ratio [OR] = 1.15), while no significant model emerged in the multivariate regression. After correcting for the use of antidepressants, "pack years" remained a significant predictor in the unipolar depression group, indicating that patients with higher "pack years" had a 1.15 times greater chance of experiencing a severe depressive episode.

In the multivariate regression analysis, adjusted for antidepressant use, a significant model emerged that was entirely significant (χ^2 test = 9.5, df = 1, p = 0.002) and explained between 35% (according to Cox & Snell) and 51% (according to Negelkerke) of the variance in severe depressive episodes, accurately classifying 77% of cases. In this model, "pack years" was a significant predictor (OR = 1.15).

In the group of subjects with bipolar depression, no significant predictors were found in the bivariate regression without antidepressant correction for predicting a severe depressive episode, nor did any significant model emerge in the multivariate regression. However, in the bivariate regression adjusted for antidepressant use, albumin levels were a significant predictor in the bipolar depression group, reducing the likelihood of a severe depressive episode (OR = 0.86).

In predicting the probability of a severe depressive episode, both with and without correction for antidepressant use, in the group of subjects with unipolar depression, no significant predictors or models were identified that would support the prediction of a severe depressive episode according to MADRS (total score 35–60).

4. Discussion

4.1. Comparison of Serum Levels of Zinc, Albumin, IL-6, and CRP between the Group of Depressive Subjects (UD and BDD) and Healthy Controls (HC)

In the first step, the difference in biological parameters between the group of patients and the group of healthy subjects was examined. The patient group displayed elevated levels of inflammatory markers IL-6 and CRP compared to healthy controls. This finding aligns with studies suggesting a key role for systemic inflammation in mood disorders, pointing towards immune dysregulation as a significant aspect of their pathophysiology and progression [13,14,36–38].

An interesting finding is the reduced level of zinc in the group of healthy controls.

This finding deviates from established patterns observed in previous studies, where individuals with depression typically exhibited lower serum zinc levels compared to healthy controls [26,39,40].

This is supported by research that investigated the therapeutic potential of zinc and consistently supported the effectiveness of zinc supplementation as an adjunctive treatment, showing improved mood in both depressed and healthy individuals [41–44]. Notably, zinc supplementation has also demonstrated benefits in improving mood among individuals with treatment-resistant depression [42].

Conventionally, depression is associated with reduced serum zinc levels, attributed to factors such as poor nutrition, increased physiological stress, and inflammation [45].

Possible explanations of these findings may be dietary variations that were not included in the study design, and which resulted in a lower zinc intake in the control group, influencing their serum levels. Additionally, there could be inherent physiological differences between the groups, particularly in how their bodies absorb and metabolize zinc, unrelated to the presence of depression. Another interesting angle to consider is the body's response to stress in depression. It is conceivable that in depressed individuals, a unique stress response mechanism could paradoxically elevate zinc levels due to complex interaction between zinc, serotonin, and stress-related hormones in depression. These factors, individually or combined, might account for the unexpected findings and warrant further investigation to fully understand their implications [45].

Another finding was decreased albumin levels in the patient group (both UD and BD groups). This can be attributed to different influences including poor nutritional status, chronic inflammation, or acute phase response. Albumin, a key protein synthesized by the liver, is often reduced in chronic diseases and inflammatory states [46]. Its lower levels in the patient group could reflect the overall impact of mood disorders on physical health and metabolic function. The finding of significantly lower albumin levels in mood disorder [47] patients compared to healthy controls underscores the impact of these conditions on systemic health. Lower albumin levels in patients could indicate a state of chronic inflammation [46] or altered metabolism, a common occurrence in mood disorders [48].

4.2. Comparison of Serum Levels of Zinc, Albumin, IL-6, and CRP between the Groups of Unipolar Depressive Subjects (UD), Bipolar Depressive Subjects (BDD), and Healthy Controls (HC)

In the next step, the concentrations of zinc, albumin a, CRP, and IL-6 were compared between the groups of patients with unipolar depression (UD), bipolar depression (BDD), and the group of healthy subjects (HC).

This analysis found significantly lower serum levels of the inflammatory parameters IL-6 and CRP in the group of healthy subjects compared to both groups of patients (UD and BD), which is in accordance with our previous analysis, but also with existing the literature, suggesting the presence of an inflammatory component in mood disorders [49–55].

Elevated IL-6 and CRP levels have been associated with the pathophysiology of both unipolar and bipolar disorders, indicating systemic inflammation as a common characteristic in these conditions [14,56,57].

Perhaps the most striking finding is the lower zinc levels in the HC group compared to the UD group, diverging from the typical pattern where depressive states are often linked to reduced zinc due to poor nutrition or increased stress [26,45]. This suggests a complex interaction between zinc levels and mood disorders, potentially influenced by compensatory mechanisms in response to depression [58], dietary variations, or treatment effects [42,59].

Interestingly, zinc levels do not significantly differ between the BDD group and HC, suggesting unique aspects of zinc metabolism or homeostasis in BD [60]. This lack of difference could reflect specific physiological or compensatory responses in BD related to zinc regulation, distinct from those in UD [29]. Also, the impact of psychotropic medications on zinc levels might differ between unipolar and bipolar patients, partly due to the difference in medication regimens typically used in these conditions. Bipolar patients, who are often prescribed a combination of mood stabilizers, antipsychotics, and sometimes antidepressants, may experience more complex interactions affecting zinc levels compared to unipolar patients, who are more commonly treated with antidepressants alone. For instance, the fluctuating nature of bipolar disorder, with its manic and depressive episodes, may impact the immune system differently compared to the typically more persistent depressive state in unipolar depression [29].

4.3. Comparison of Serum Levels of Zinc, Albumin, IL-6, and CRP between the Groups of Unipolar Depressive Subjects (UD) and Bipolar Depressive Subjects (BDD)

A critical examination of inflammatory markers, nutritional elements, and protein levels has revealed a notable absence of significant differences between these two groups (UD and BDD) in parameters such as interleukin-6 (IL-6), C-reactive protein (CRP), zinc, and albumin.

This finding challenges the traditional dichotomy of unipolar and bipolar disorders, suggesting a more unified pathophysiological spectrum [61–64].

Both unipolar and bipolar disorders exhibit similar profiles in key inflammatory markers, IL-6 and CRP. This observation underscores a common inflammatory basis in mood disorders, as suggested by Bai et al. (2015) [14]. The elevated levels of these cytokines in both groups point toward a shared underlying inflammatory pathogenesis, potentially contributing to the symptomatology of both disorders. This convergence of inflammatory pathways in mood disorders echoes the growing recognition of immune dysregulation as a central aspect of psychiatric conditions [65–68].

Zinc levels, crucial for neurotransmitter function and neuroplasticity, have similarly shown no significant variance between unipolar and bipolar groups. The findings of Siwek et al. (2016) [29] lend credence to the hypothesis that alterations in zinc metabolism are a characteristic feature of depressive disorders, irrespective of their specific classification. This uniformity in zinc levels suggests that the role of zinc in mood regulation and brain function transcends the traditional diagnostic boundaries, hinting at a universal aspect of mood disorders.

Furthermore, the similarity in albumin levels across these groups might reflect a shared aspect of metabolic alteration in mood disorders. Albumin serum levels can be influenced by factors like nutrition, systemic inflammation, and overall health status [47,69]. The consistent levels across unipolar and bipolar disorders suggest parallel impacts on these physiological parameters.

The overarching implication of these findings is that unipolar and bipolar depression may share more common ground in their biological basis than previously acknowledged. This supports a more nuanced understanding of mood disorders as a continuum with shared biological mechanisms.

4.4. Comparison of the Results on Depression Rating Scales (HAMD-17 and MADRS) between the Examined Groups of Depressive Patients (UD and BD)

Both groups of patients were compared with respect to the scores on the Hamilton Scale and the MADRAS Scale for depression. The lack of significant differences in most HAMD-17 items between unipolar and bipolar depression groups suggests that the depressive episodes in these disorders manifest with similar symptom profiles. This finding aligns with previous research indicating overlapping features in the depressive phases of these mood disorders [9,32,70]. In clinical practice, UD and BDD can be difficult to diagnose.

The significant elevation of somatic anxiety in bipolar depression, compared to unipolar depression, as measured on the MADRS, could be attributed to the unique neurobiological and psychological aspects of bipolar disorder.

The heightened somatic anxiety in bipolar depression might be linked to the fluctuating nature of the disorder, where episodes of mania or hypomania precede or follow depressive phases, potentially leading to a heightened state of physiological arousal and anxiety [71,72]. Additionally, bipolar disorder may involve more pronounced dysregulation of stress response systems, which can manifest as somatic anxiety [73].

In conclusion, while unipolar and bipolar depression share many depressive symptoms, as shown in HAMD-17, the distinct increase in somatic anxiety in bipolar depression on the MADRAS highlights a key difference between these disorders. This underscores the importance of careful assessment in distinguishing between unipolar and bipolar depression, particularly considering the broader impact of bipolar disorder on somatic and psychological wellbeing.

4.5. Comparison of the Results of the Examined Groups of Depressive Patients (UD and BD) on the HAMD-17 and MADRS Rating Scales for Depression with Respect to the Severity of the Depressive Episode

The similarity in IL-6, Zn, CRP, and albumin levels between UD and BD during depressive episodes of similar severity suggests common underlying pathophysiological processes in mood disorders. This observation aligns with the growing evidence that mood disorders, irrespective of their specific type, may share fundamental inflammatory and metabolic disturbances [14].

The similar levels across UD and BD could indicate that these physiological aspects are consistently altered in depressive states. The shared biochemical profile in depressive episodes of UD and BD could be due to similar alterations in neuro-immune pathways, stress response mechanisms, or nutritional status associated with depressive states. It might also reflect the homogenizing effect of similar clinical severity on these biomarkers, regardless of the mood disorder subtype. This lack of distinction in key immuno-inflammatory markers between UD and BD depressive episodes challenges the long-held notion of these conditions as entirely separate entities. Instead, it proposes a continuum model of mood disorders where shared biological processes are involved [9,74]. Zinc, essential for neuroplasticity and immune function, further underscores the potential overlap in the neuro-immune pathways affected in both UD and BD [42,44]. However, the unique observation of lower albumin levels in severe episodes compared to moderate episodes within the BDD group may suggest that metabolic demands corelate with the severity of a depressive episode. Its reduction in severe BD episodes could reflect more pronounced systemic changes or stress responses, distinguishing severe BD from UD [58,75].

4.6. Correlations of the Examined Parameters (Zn, Albumin, IL-6, and CRP) in Both Groups of Depressive Subjects (UD and BD) with Items on the Depression Rating Scales (HAMD-17 and MADRS)

In the context of the research findings on unipolar and bipolar depression, a striking parallel emerges between the symptomatology of depression and so-called 'sickness behaviour'. This comparison is particularly evident in the significant correlations found in unipolar depression between symptoms like somatic anxiety, hypochondriacal symptoms, general somatic symptoms, work and activity limitations, weight loss, concentration difficulties, and lassitude with levels of albumin, C-reactive protein (CRP), and interleukin-6 (IL-6) [76–78]. These correlations illuminate the critical role of inflammation (as indicated by CRP and IL-6 levels) and metabolic factors (as indicated by albumin levels) in the manifestation of depressive symptoms. Symptoms such as fatigue, reduced activity, physical discomforts, cognitive challenges, and negative emotional states are hallmark characteristics of 'sickness behaviour', underscoring a biological underpinning for these manifestations in depression.

In bipolar depression, the intricate relationship of zinc, albumin, IL-6, and CRP with the symptoms assessed using the HAMD-17 and MADRS scales reveals a more complex interaction. Lower zinc levels correlating with physical symptoms like gastrointestinal issues and weight loss, along with heightened psychic anxiety, are particularly noteworthy [79]. Moreover, the negative correlations of albumin with feelings of guilt, sadness, reduced appetite, and concentration difficulties, and the positive correlation of CRP with lassitude, closely mirror 'sickness behaviour' symptoms [76,77]. These findings suggest a significant contribution of both inflammatory processes and metabolic status to the breadth of depressive symptoms, resonating with the physical and psychological aspects of 'sickness behaviour'.

The common thread running through both unipolar and bipolar depression is the overlap of symptoms such as lassitude, weight loss, gastrointestinal problems, reduced activity, and cognitive challenges with those typically associated with 'sickness behaviour'. This overlap indicates that similar biological processes, including inflammation and metabolic alterations, might underpin these symptoms in both forms of depressive states and in 'sickness behaviour'.

Understanding the nature of these correlations provides valuable insights into the mechanisms underlying depression and its resemblance to 'sickness behaviour'. This knowledge lays a foundation for the exploration of targeted treatments that focus on these underlying biological factors. Recognizing the shared aspects of these conditions can lead to more effective management and treatment strategies, acknowledging the significant influence of biological markers on the symptomatology of depression. This perspective promotes a more holistic approach, addressing not just the psychological dimensions of depression, but also its biological aspects. This study is not without its limitations. First, the cross-sectional design of the research inhibits our ability to establish cause and effect relationships between the investigated biological parameters and depressive symptoms. Such designs can only provide a snapshot of data at a single point in time, which limits our understanding of how these relationships may evolve or respond to changes over time. Additionally, our study did not account for the onset of the disorders, nor the number of previous depressive episodes experienced by patients. This study design may have implications to the generalizability of our findings, as the trajectory and recurrence of depressive episodes can significantly influence biological markers and symptom presentation. These limitations should be carefully considered when interpreting the results, and should guide future research directions that might overcome these constraints.

5. Conclusions

The findings of our study confirm the presence of low-grade inflammation in depression. The results provide a better insight into the inflammatory hypothesis about the aetiology of depressive disorders. According to our findings, we cannot recommend zinc, albumin, interleukin-6, and CRP as specific biomarkers for distinguishing unipolar and bipolar depressive episodes.

Author Contributions: Conceptualization, T.B. and A.M.-P.; methodology, T.B., A.M.-P. and A.K.; software, T.B., A.K. and D.R.; validation, A.K., D.R. and A.M.-P.; formal analysis, A.M.-P.; investigation, T.B.; resources, T.B., A.K., D.R., M.Ž. and M.S.H.; data curation, T.B.; writing—original draft preparation, T.B.; writing—review and editing, T.B., A.M.-P. and M.S.H.; visualization, A.M.-P.; supervision, A.M.-P.; project administration, M.Ž. and M.S.H. All authors have read and agreed to the published version of the manuscript.

Funding: This research retrieved no external fundings.

Institutional Review Board Statement: The study was conducted in accordance with the Declaration of Helsinki and approved by the Ethics Committee of the University Hospital Centre Zagreb (protocol code 8.1-16/141-2 number 02/21 AG and date of approval 3 October 2016) and by the Ethics Committee of the Psychiatric Hospital Popovača (protocol code ZH/MS 2176-128-16/3271-2/15 and date of approval 6 November 2015).

Informed Consent Statement: Informed consent was obtained from all subjects involved in the study. Written informed consent has been obtained from the patient(s) to publish this paper.

Data Availability Statement: Data is unavailable due to privacy or ethical restrictions.

Conflicts of Interest: The authors declare no conflict of interest.

References

1. Merikangas, K.R.; Akiskal, H.S.; Angst, J.; Greenberg, P.E.; Hirschfeld, R.M.A.; Petukhova, M.; Kessler, R.C. Lifetime and 12-month prevalence of bipolar spectrum disorder in the National Comorbidity Survey replication. *Arch. Gen. Psychiatry* **2007**, *64*, 543–552. [CrossRef] [PubMed]
2. Mihaljević-Peleš, A.; Šagud, M.; Janović, M.B. Do We Recognize and Diagnose Bipolar Affective Disorder? *Medicus* **2017**, *26*, 167–172.
3. Hirschfeld, R.M.A.; Lewis, L.; Vornik, L.A. Perceptions and Impact of Bipolar Disorder: How Far Have We Really Come? Results of the National Depressive and Manic-Depressive Association 2000 Survey of Individuals With Bipolar Disorder. *J. Clin. Psychiatry* **2003**, *64*, 161–174. [CrossRef] [PubMed]
4. Smith, D.J.; Craddock, N. Unipolar and bipolar depression: Different or the same? *Br. J. Psychiatry* **2011**, *199*, 272–274. [CrossRef]
5. Hashimoto, K. Metabolomics of Major Depressive Disorder and Bipolar Disorder: Overview and Future Perspective. *Adv. Clin. Chem.* **2018**, *84*, 81–99. [CrossRef]
6. Fire and Darkness: On the Assessment and Management of Bipolar Disorder. Available online: https://pubmed.ncbi.nlm.nih.gov/36402499/ (accessed on 28 March 2024).
7. Grande, I.; Berk, M.; Birmaher, B.; Vieta, E. Bipolar disorder. *Lancet* **2016**, *387*, 1561–1572. [CrossRef] [PubMed]
8. Stahl, S.M. *Stahl's Essential Psychopharmacology: Neuroscientific Basis and Practical Applications*, 5th ed.; Cambrige University Press: Cambrige, UK, 2021.
9. Rolin, D.; Whelan, J.; Montano, C.B. Is it depression or is it bipolar depression? *J. Am. Assoc. Nurse Pract.* **2020**, *32*, 703–713. [CrossRef]
10. Cassano, G.B.; Rucci, P.; Frank, E.; Fagiolini, A.; Dell'Osso, L.; Shear, M.K.; Kupfer, D.J. The mood spectrum in unipolar and bipolar disorder: Arguments for a unitary approach. *Am. J. Psychiatry* **2004**, *161*, 1264–1269. [CrossRef] [PubMed]
11. American Psychiatric Association. *Diagnostic and Statistical Manual of Mental Disorders*, 5th ed.; American Psychiatric Association: Arlington, VA, USA, 2013.
12. Shattuck, E.C.; Muehlenbein, M.P. Towards an integrative picture of human sickness behavior. *Brain Behav. Immun.* **2016**, *57*, 255–262. [CrossRef] [PubMed]
13. Brunoni, A.R.; Supasitthumrong, T.; Teixeira, A.L.; Vieira, E.L.; Gattaz, W.F.; Benseñor, I.M.; Lotufo, P.A.; Lafer, B.; Berk, M.; Carvalho, A.F.; et al. Differences in the immune-inflammatory profiles of unipolar and bipolar depression. *J. Affect. Disord.* **2020**, *262*, 8–15. [CrossRef]
14. Bai, Y.-M.; Su, T.-P.; Li, C.-T.; Tsai, S.-J.; Chen, M.-H.; Tu, P.-C.; Chiou, W.-F. Comparison of pro-inflammatory cytokines among patients with bipolar disorder and unipolar depression and normal controls. *Bipolar Disord.* **2015**, *17*, 269–277. [CrossRef] [PubMed]
15. Beurel, E.; Toups, M.; Nemeroff, C.B. The Bidirectional Relationship of Depression and Inflammation: Double Trouble. *Neuron* **2020**, *107*, 234–256. [CrossRef] [PubMed]
16. Kalin, N.H. New Insights into Major Depression and the Treatment of Bipolar Depression. *Am. J. Psychiatry* **2021**, *178*, 1071–1074. [CrossRef]
17. Mao, R.; Zhang, C.; Chen, J.; Zhao, G.; Zhou, R.; Wang, F.; Xu, J.; Yang, T.; Su, Y.; Huang, J.; et al. Different levels of pro- and anti-inflammatory cytokines in patients with unipolar and bipolar depression. *J. Affect. Disord.* **2018**, *237*, 65–72. [CrossRef]
18. Hunter, C.A.; Jones, S.A. IL-6 as a keystone cytokine in health and disease. *Nat. Immunol.* **2015**, *16*, 448–457. [CrossRef] [PubMed]
19. Kim, Y.-K.; Jung, H.-G.; Myint, A.-M.; Kim, H.; Park, S.-H. Imbalance between pro-inflammatory and anti-inflammatory cytokines in bipolar disorder. *J. Affect. Disord.* **2007**, *104*, 91–95. [CrossRef] [PubMed]
20. Maes, M.; Scharpé, S.; Meltzer, H.Y.; Bosmans, E.; Suy, E.; Calabrese, J.; Cosyns, P. Relationships between interleukin-6 activity, acute phase proteins, and function of the hypothalamic-pituitary-adrenal axis in severe depression. *Psychiatry Res.* **1993**, *49*, 11–27. [CrossRef] [PubMed]
21. Schiepers, O.J.G.; Wichers, M.C.; Maes, M. Cytokines and major depression. *Prog. Neuropsychopharmacol. Biol. Psychiatry* **2005**, *29*, 201–217. [CrossRef]
22. Dargél, A.A.; Godin, O.; Kapczinski, F.; Kupfer, D.J.; Leboyer, M. C-reactive protein alterations in bipolar disorder: A meta-analysis. *J. Clin. Psychiatry* **2015**, *76*, 142–150. [CrossRef] [PubMed]
23. Fernandes, B.S.; Steiner, J.; Molendijk, M.L.; Dodd, S.; Nardin, P.; Gonçalves, C.-A.; Jacka, F.; Köhler, C.A.; Karmakar, C.; Carvalho, A.F.; et al. C-reactive protein concentrations across the mood spectrum in bipolar disorder: A systematic review and meta-analysis. *Lancet Psychiatry* **2016**, *3*, 1147–1156. [CrossRef] [PubMed]
24. Kaysen, G.A.; Dubin, J.A.; Müller, H.G.; Rosales, L.M.; Levin, N.W. The acute-phase response varies with time and predicts serum albumin levels in hemodialysis patients. The HEMO Study Group. *Kidney Int.* **2000**, *58*, 346–352. [CrossRef]

25. Heinrich, P.C.; Castell, J.V.; Andus, T. Interleukin-6 and the acute phase response. *Biochem. J.* **1990**, *265*, 621–636. [CrossRef] [PubMed]
26. McLoughlin, I.J.; Hodge, J.S. Zinc in depressive disorder. *Acta Psychiatr. Scand.* **1990**, *82*, 451–453. [CrossRef]
27. Correlation between Dietary Zinc Intakes and Its Serum Levels with Depression Scales in Young Female Students. Available online: https://pubmed.ncbi.nlm.nih.gov/20013161/ (accessed on 19 February 2024).
28. Maes, M.; Vandoolaeghe, E.; Neels, H.; Demedts, P.; Wauters, A.; Meltzer, H.Y.; Altamura, C.; Desnyder, R. Lower serum zinc in major depression is a sensitive marker of treatment resistance and of the immune/inflammatory response in that illness. *Biol. Psychiatry* **1997**, *42*, 349–358. [CrossRef]
29. Siwek, M.; Sowa-Kućma, M.; Styczeń, K.; Szewczyk, B.; Reczyński, W.; Misztak, P.; Topór-Mądry, R.; Nowak, G.; Dudek, D.; Rybakowski, J.K. Decreased serum zinc concentration during depressive episode in patients with bipolar disorder. *J. Affect. Disord.* **2016**, *190*, 272–277. [CrossRef] [PubMed]
30. Biomarkers and Surrogate Endpoints: Preferred Definitions and Conceptual Framework. Available online: https://pubmed.ncbi.nlm.nih.gov/11240971/ (accessed on 19 February 2024).
31. Schmidt, H.D.; Shelton, R.C.; Duman, R.S. Functional biomarkers of depression: Diagnosis, treatment, and pathophysiology. *Neuropsychopharmacology* **2011**, *36*, 2375–2394. [CrossRef]
32. Cuellar, A.K.; Johnson, S.L.; Winters, R. Distinctions between bipolar and unipolar depression. *Clin. Psychol. Rev.* **2005**, *25*, 307–339. [CrossRef]
33. Montgomery, S.A.; Asberg, M. A new depression scale designed to be sensitive to change. *Br. J. Psychiatry* **1979**, *134*, 382–389. [CrossRef] [PubMed]
34. Hamilton, M. A rating scale for depression. *J. Neurol. Neurosurg. Psychiatry* **1960**, *23*, 56–62. [CrossRef]
35. *ISO 15189*; 2012 Medical Laboratories—Requirements for Quality and Competence. ISO (International Organization for Standardization): Geneva, Switzerland, 2012.
36. Miller, A.H.; Raison, C.L. Cytokines, p38 MAP Kinase and the Pathophysiology of Depression. *Neuropsychopharmacology* **2006**, *31*, 2089–2090. [CrossRef] [PubMed]
37. Dantzer, R.; Kelley, K.W. Twenty years of research on cytokine-induced sickness behavior. *Brain Behav. Immun.* **2007**, *21*, 153–160. [CrossRef] [PubMed]
38. Lu, Y.-R.; Rao, Y.-B.; Mou, Y.-J.; Chen, Y.; Lou, H.-F.; Zhang, Y.; Zhang, D.-X.; Xie, H.-Y.; Hu, L.-W.; Fang, P. High concentrations of serum interleukin-6 and interleukin-8 in patients with bipolar disorder. *Medicine* **2019**, *98*, e14419. [CrossRef]
39. Maes, M.; D'Haese, P.C.; Scharpé, S.; D'Hondt, P.; Cosyns, P.; De Broe, M.E. Hypozincemia in depression. *J. Affect. Disord.* **1994**, *31*, 135–140. [CrossRef]
40. Swardfager, W.; Herrmann, N.; Mazereeuw, G.; Goldberger, K.; Harimoto, T.; Lanctôt, K.L. Zinc in depression: A meta-analysis. *Biol. Psychiatry* **2013**, *74*, 872–878. [CrossRef] [PubMed]
41. Ranjbar, E.; Shams, J.; Sabetkasaei, M.; M-Shirazi, M.; Rashidkhani, B.; Mostafavi, A.; Bornak, E.; Nasrollahzadeh, J. Effects of zinc supplementation on efficacy of antidepressant therapy, inflammatory cytokines, and brain-derived neurotrophic factor in patients with major depression. *Nutr. Neurosci.* **2014**, *17*, 65–71. [CrossRef]
42. Siwek, M.; Dudek, D.; Paul, I.A.; Sowa-Kućma, M.; Zieba, A.; Popik, P.; Pilc, A.; Nowak, G. Zinc supplementation augments efficacy of imipramine in treatment resistant patients: A double blind, placebo-controlled study. *J. Affect. Disord.* **2009**, *118*, 187–195. [CrossRef] [PubMed]
43. Sawada, T.; Yokoi, K. Effect of zinc supplementation on mood states in young women: A pilot study. *Eur. J. Clin. Nutr.* **2010**, *64*, 331–333. [CrossRef]
44. Nowak, G.; Szewczyk, B.; Wieronska, J.M.; Branski, P.; Palucha, A.; Pilc, A.; Sadlik, K.; Piekoszewski, W. Antidepressant-like effects of acute and chronic treatment with zinc in forced swim test and olfactory bulbectomy model in rats. *Brain Res. Bull.* **2003**, *61*, 159–164. [CrossRef] [PubMed]
45. The Emerging Role for Zinc in Depression and Psychosis. Available online: https://www.ncbi.nlm.nih.gov/pmc/articles/PMC5492454/ (accessed on 26 March 2024).
46. Soeters, P.B.; Wolfe, R.R.; Shenkin, A. Hypoalbuminemia: Pathogenesis and Clinical Significance. *JPEN J. Parenter. Enter. Nutr.* **2019**, *43*, 181–193. [CrossRef]
47. Van Hunsel, F.; Wauters, A.; Vandoolaeghe, E.; Neels, H.; Demedts, P.; Maes, M. Lower total serum protein, albumin, and beta- and gamma-globulin in major and treatment-resistant depression: Effects of antidepressant treatments. *Psychiatry Res.* **1996**, *65*, 159–169. [CrossRef]
48. Wysokiński, A.; Margulska, A.; Strzelecki, D.; Kłoszewska, I. Levels of C-reactive protein (CRP) in patients with schizophrenia, unipolar depression and bipolar disorder. *Nord. J. Psychiatry* **2015**, *69*, 346–353. [CrossRef] [PubMed]
49. Lyu, N.; Zhao, Q.; Fu, B.; Li, J.; Wang, H.; Yang, F.; Liu, S.; Huang, J.; Zhang, X.; Zhang, L.; et al. Hormonal and inflammatory signatures of different mood episodes in bipolar disorder: A large-scale clinical study. *BMC Psychiatry* **2023**, *23*, 449. [CrossRef]
50. Pape, K.; Tamouza, R.; Leboyer, M.; Zipp, F. Immunoneuropsychiatry - novel perspectives on brain disorders. *Nat. Rev. Neurol.* **2019**, *15*, 317–328. [CrossRef] [PubMed]
51. Jones, G.H.; Vecera, C.M.; Pinjari, O.F.; Machado-Vieira, R. Inflammatory signaling mechanisms in bipolar disorder. *J. Biomed. Sci.* **2021**, *28*, 45. [CrossRef] [PubMed]

52. Howren, M.B.; Lamkin, D.M.; Suls, J. Associations of depression with C-reactive protein, IL-1, and IL-6: A meta-analysis. *Psychosom. Med.* **2009**, *71*, 171–186. [CrossRef] [PubMed]
53. Dowlati, Y.; Herrmann, N.; Swardfager, W.; Liu, H.; Sham, L.; Reim, E.K.; Lanctôt, K.L. A Meta-Analysis of Cytokines in Major Depression. *Biol. Psychiatry* **2010**, *67*, 446–457. [CrossRef] [PubMed]
54. Valkanova, V.; Ebmeier, K.P.; Allan, C.L. CRP, IL-6 and depression: A systematic review and meta-analysis of longitudinal studies. *J. Affect. Disord.* **2013**, *150*, 736–744. [CrossRef]
55. Haapakoski, R.; Mathieu, J.; Ebmeier, K.P.; Alenius, H.; Kivimäki, M. Cumulative meta-analysis of interleukins 6 and 1β, tumour necrosis factor α and C-reactive protein in patients with major depressive disorder. *Brain Behav. Immun.* **2015**, *49*, 206–215. [CrossRef] [PubMed]
56. Felger, J.C.; Haroon, E.; Patel, T.A.; Goldsmith, D.R.; Wommack, E.C.; Woolwine, B.J.; Le, N.-A.; Feinberg, R.; Tansey, M.G.; Miller, A.H. What does plasma CRP tell us about peripheral and central inflammation in depression? *Mol. Psychiatry* **2020**, *25*, 1301–1311. [CrossRef] [PubMed]
57. Osimo, E.F.; Baxter, L.J.; Lewis, G.; Jones, P.B.; Khandaker, G.M. Prevalence of low-grade inflammation in depression: A systematic review and meta-analysis of CRP levels. *Psychol. Med.* **2019**, *49*, 1958–1970. [CrossRef] [PubMed]
58. Maes, M.; Carvalho, A.F. The Compensatory Immune-Regulatory Reflex System (CIRS) in Depression and Bipolar Disorder. *Mol. Neurobiol.* **2018**, *55*, 8885–8903. [CrossRef] [PubMed]
59. Siwek, M.; Dudek, D.; Schlegel-Zawadzka, M.; Morawska, A.; Piekoszewski, W.; Opoka, W.; Zieba, A.; Pilc, A.; Popik, P.; Nowak, G. Serum zinc level in depressed patients during zinc supplementation of imipramine treatment. *J. Affect. Disord.* **2010**, *126*, 447–452. [CrossRef]
60. Jonsson, B.H.; Orhan, F.; Bruno, S.; Oliveira, A.O.; Sparding, T.; Landen, M.; Sellgren, C.M. Serum concentration of zinc is elevated in clinically stable bipolar disorder patients. *Brain Behav.* **2022**, *12*, e2472. [CrossRef]
61. Baldessarini, R.J. Bipolar Depression: An Orphan Syndrome? *Dusunen Adam J. Psychiatry Neurol. Sci.* **2015**, *28*, 89–95. [CrossRef]
62. McIntyre, R.S.; Calabrese, J.R. Bipolar depression: The clinical characteristics and unmet needs of a complex disorder. *Curr. Med. Res. Opin.* **2019**, *35*, 1993–2005. [CrossRef] [PubMed]
63. Johnson, S.L.; Morriss, R.; Scott, J.; Paykel, E.; Kinderman, P.; Kolamunnage-Dona, R.; Bentall, R.P. Depressive and manic symptoms are not opposite poles in bipolar disorder. *Acta Psychiatr. Scand.* **2011**, *123*, 206–210. [CrossRef] [PubMed]
64. Li, X. Bipolar Disorder and Antidepressant Associated Hypomania. *Lect. Notes Educ. Psychol. Public Media* **2023**, *12*, 68–74. [CrossRef]
65. Colpo, G.D.; Leboyer, M.; Dantzer, R.; Trivedi, M.H.; Teixeira, A.L. Immune-based strategies for mood disorders: Facts and challenges. *Expert Rev. Neurother.* **2018**, *18*, 139–152. [CrossRef] [PubMed]
66. Bauer, M.E.; Teixeira, A.L. Inflammation in psychiatric disorders: What comes first? *Ann. N. Y. Acad. Sci.* **2019**, *1437*, 57–67. [CrossRef]
67. Chang, H.H.; Chen, P.S. Inflammatory Biomarkers for Mood Disorders—A Brief Narrative Review. *Curr. Pharm. Des.* **2020**, *26*, 236–243. [CrossRef]
68. Tanaka, M.; Kinney, D.K. Does the Immune System Regulate Mood to Defend against Infection? Evidence from Studies of Immune Factors, Depression, and Antidepressants. *Curr. Psychiatry Rev.* **2011**, *7*, 57–66. [CrossRef]
69. Huang, T.-L. Lower Serum Albumin Levels in Patients with Mood Disorders. *Chang Gung Med. J.* **2002**, *25*, 509–513. [PubMed]
70. Forty, L.; Smith, D.; Jones, L.; Jones, I.; Caesar, S.; Cooper, C.; Fraser, C.; Gordon-Smith, K.; Hyde, S.; Farmer, A.; et al. Clinical differences between bipolar and unipolar depression. *Br. J. Psychiatry* **2008**, *192*, 388–389. [CrossRef] [PubMed]
71. Coryell, W.; Solomon, D.A.; Fiedorowicz, J.G.; Endicott, J.; Schettler, P.J.; Judd, L.L. Anxiety and Outcome in Bipolar Disorder. *Am. J. Psychiatry* **2009**, *166*, 1238–1243. [CrossRef]
72. Otto, M.W.; Simon, N.M.; Wisniewski, S.R.; Miklowitz, D.J.; Kogan, J.N.; Reilly-Harrington, N.A.; Frank, E.; Nierenberg, A.A.; Marangell, L.B.; Sagduyu, K.; et al. Prospective 12-month course of bipolar disorder in out-patients with and without comorbid anxiety disorders. *Br. J. Psychiatry* **2006**, *189*, 20–25. [CrossRef] [PubMed]
73. Phillips, M.L. The neural basis of mood dysregulation in bipolar disorder. *Cogn. Neuropsychiatry* **2006**, *11*, 233–249. [CrossRef] [PubMed]
74. Fountoulakis, K.N. The emerging modern face of mood disorders: A didactic editorial with a detailed presentation of data and definitions. *Ann. Gen. Psychiatry* **2010**, *9*, 14. [CrossRef]
75. Rybakowski, J.K. Factors Associated with Lithium Efficacy in Bipolar Disorder. *Harv. Rev. Psychiatry* **2014**, *22*, 353–357. [CrossRef] [PubMed]
76. Turkheimer, F.E.; Veronese, M.; Mondelli, V.; Cash, D.; Pariante, C.M. Sickness behaviour and depression: An updated model of peripheral-central immunity interactions. *Brain Behav. Immun.* **2023**, *111*, 202–210. [CrossRef]
77. Dantzer, R.; O'Connor, J.C.; Freund, G.G.; Johnson, R.W.; Kelley, K.W. From inflammation to sickness and depression: When the immune system subjugates the brain. *Nat. Rev. Neurosci.* **2008**, *9*, 46–56. [CrossRef] [PubMed]

78. Miller, A.H.; Raison, C.L. The role of inflammation in depression: From evolutionary imperative to modern treatment target. *Nat. Rev. Immunol.* **2016**, *16*, 22–34. [CrossRef] [PubMed]
79. Chasapis, C.T.; Loutsidou, A.C.; Spiliopoulou, C.A.; Stefanidou, M.E. Zinc and human health: An update. *Arch. Toxicol.* **2012**, *86*, 521–534. [CrossRef] [PubMed]

current issues in molecular biology

MDPI

Article

Testing Protein Stress Signals in Peripheral Immunocytes Under the Same Treatment Capable of Decreasing the Incidence of Alzheimer's Disease in Bladder Cancer Patients

Benjamin Y. Klein [1,*], Ofer N. Gofrit [2] and Charles L. Greenblatt [1]

[1] Department of Microbiology and Molecular Genetics, Hebrew University Medical School, Jerusalem 91120, Israel; charlesg@ekmd.huji.ac.il
[2] Department of Urology, Hadassah University Medical School, Ein-Karem, Jerusalem 91120, Israel; ogofrit@gmail.com
* Correspondence: byklein@mail.huji.ac.il or byklein@yahoo.com

Abstract: Several studies showed that the incidence of Alzheimer's disease (AD) is significantly lower in patients with non-muscle invasive bladder cancer (NMIBC) treated with intravesical bacillus Calmette–Guérin (BCG) instillations compared to treatment by alternative methods. Hypothetically, failure to clear misfolded and aggregated proteins (i.e., beta-amyloid) in AD brains and peripheral blood mononuclear cells (PBMCs) implicates BCG in upgrading the unfolded protein response (UPR). To test this hypothesis, pre- versus post-BCG PBMC proteins of the UPR pathway were compared in six NMIBC patients by capillary immunoelectrophoresis on an Abby instrument. PERK, the endoplasmic reticulum (ER) resident kinase, a stress-activated sensor, and its substrate alpha component of the eIF2 translation factor (eIF2a) complex inactivation were considered as potentially proapoptotic via a downstream proapoptotic transcription factor only if persistently high. GAPDH, a glycolytic marker of innate immunocyte training by BCG, and eight other UPR proteins were considered antiapoptotic. Summation of antiapoptotic %change scores per patient showed that the older the age, the lower the antiapoptotic %change. Higher antiapoptotic scores were observed upon a longer time from BCG treatment (with the exception of the patient in her ninth decade of life). Studies with more individuals could substantiate that BCG enhances the antiapoptotic aggregate-clearance effect of the UPR in PBMCs of NMIBC patients, which hypothetically protects brain cells against AD.

Keywords: BCG vaccine; peripheral blood mononuclear cells; unfolded protein response; endoplasmic reticulum stress; cell signaling; immunoelectrophoretic

1. Introduction

1.1. Alzheimer's Disease Prevention by Bacillus Calmette–Guérin

High-grade superficial or recurrent low-grade bladder cancer is treated by transurethral tumor resection and adjuvant intravesical instillations of the bacillus Calmette–Guérin (BCG) vaccine. This treatment effectively reduces tumor relapse compared with tumor resection only [1]. The sequence of the immunological events that follow BCG instillations has not been completely deciphered yet, but a general scheme of participating immunocytes has been described [2], where the primary responding cells are granulocytes, monocytes, macrophages, and natural killer cells. Subsets of T cells are subsequently recruited by various cytokines secreted mainly by the initial polymorphonuclear neutrophil responders, and the T cells are stimulated by antigen-presenting cells to recognize tumor-specific antigens [3]. Neutrophils have also been shown to accumulate in the bladder urine following BCG instillation and are responsible for the effective anti-tumor activity of BCG [4]. This connects to the ability of BCG to induce innate immune cell "training", a phenomenon that epigenetically generates a non-specific memory, upgrading the cytokine response to subsequent encounters with BCG (and other pathogens) of these innate immunocytes [5,6]. BCG is an attenuated live bovine tuberculosis mycobacterium used globally since 1921 as an anti-tuberculosis vaccine [7]. As newborns have not been BCG-vaccinated prophylactically against tuberculosis in the USA, as opposed to Sweden, we were impressed by the low incidence of Alzheimer's disease (AD) in Sweden compared to the USA and hypothesized that BCG vaccination may be one factor responsible for this difference [8]. The long-lasting practice for decades of treatment of non-muscle invasive bladder cancer (NMIBC) by BCG instillations was employed to analyze the incidence of AD during the recent decades in BCG-treated versus other treatments of NMIBC patients. The results indicated that intravesical BCG treatment reduced the incidence of AD by up to fourfold relative to control patients [9]. Since then, variable levels of effectiveness of BCG against AD in NMIBC patients have been demonstrated [10]. However, vaccinations against other pathogens have also been shown to reduce the incidence of AD [11,12]. This indicates that the prevention of AD by BCG does not depend on immunity against specific antigens as in the case of NMIBC but is due to biochemical changes that immunocytes undergo through immunization stimulus, for example, the epigenetic "training" of innate immunocytes [13,14]. A significant feature of AD is the failure to control the misfolding and aggregation of newly synthesized proteins such as beta-amyloid and its derivatives [15–17]. The successful clearance of beta-amyloid plaques by designated antibodies is not always beneficial to the patient's clinical status [18–20], indicating that factors upstream to the normal biochemical clearance are responsible for plaque accumulation. This implies that the unfolded protein response (UPR) in the brain, the immediate upstream responding pathway to endoplasmic reticulum (ER) stress, is chronically less efficient than normal [21].

1.2. Involvement of the Unfolded Protein Response in Alzheimer's Disease

We raised the question of whether BCG treatment can significantly influence the signaling proteins of the UPR in peripheral blood mononuclear cells (PBMCs), influencing brain tissue and postponing or protecting against AD. The UPR pathway consists of ER stress-sensing proteins that transduce cap-dependent translation shutdown, i.e., for most cellular mRNA. A minority of cap-independent mRNA translation uses internal ribosome entry sites (IRESs). During translation shutdown, activation of transcription factors that activate the expression of chaperones and aggregate clearance factors correct misfolded proteins and degrade the aggregates [22–24]. The UPR signaling pathway has been reviewed in general [25] and is related to AD pathology [26,27] and can be briefly summarized. Newly synthesized proteins translocate into the ER for quality control of their proper and functional folding by chaperones such as the immunoglobulin binding protein (BiP). Upon ER overflow with new translation products, the free excess proteins unmatched by chaperones cause ER stress, sensed by stress sensors on the ER membrane. One of these ER stress sensors, the protein kinase R (PKR)-like ER-resident kinase (PERK), causes PERK monomers to dimerize and undergo phosphorylation that opens a kinase domain at the cytosolic face of the ER membrane [24,28]. This kinase domain specifically phosphorylates the eIF2a component of the eIF2 translation factor complex on its Ser51, and this inhibits all cap-dependent mRNA translation until ER stress is resolved [25]. ER stress also activates the transcription factor 6 (ATF6). This stress sensor migrates laterally in the membrane towards the Golgi apparatus [25]. It then undergoes an intramembranous cleavage [29] in which the cytosol-facing N-terminal fragment becomes a transcription factor (ATF6[N]). Its nuclear transcription program includes activation of the BiP and the X-Box protein 1 (XBP1) genes and ER stress-associated degradation (ERAD) factors that remove misfolded proteins from the ER for degradation at the proteasome [30]. Old astrocyte-specifically induced substance (OASIS) is cleaved similarly to ATF6 and is synergistic with it [31]. Inositol-requiring enzyme 1 (IRE1a) dimerizes or oligomerizes and becomes phosphorylated in response to ER stress to uncover an RNA endonuclease at its cytosolic face that excises 26 nucleotides of the XBP1 mRNA [25]. This unconventional mRNA splicing translates into the spliced XBP1 variant (XBPs), which acts as a transcription factor activating the expression of the BiP gene [29,30,32]. These are the major components of the UPR cycle of protein overload that activate the ER stress sensors. The stress-induced expression of ER chaperones controls the folding of proteins and removes misfolded proteins from the ER until the next ER stress cycle. In case of failure to clear misfolded proteins from the ER, the activated PERK (p-PERK) and its phosphorylated substrate (p-eIF2a) increase chronically to stimulate the activated transcription factor 4 (ATF4) expression [33]. The C/EBP homolog protein (CHOP) activation by ATF4 inhibits the expression of cell survival proteins; therefore, CHOP promotes the expression of cell death proteins (Figure 1). Thus, chronic UPR failure may cause apoptosis of brain glia and astroglia on which neuron energy metabolism depends [34–36]. An interesting question is how peripheral immunocytes react to the two divergent targets, AD versus NMIBC pre- and post-BCG therapy. Here, we focus mainly on AD. The brain is infiltrated by immunocytes, which may contribute to dementia during aging [37–39]. We hypothesize that PBMCs with enhanced UPR induced by BCG can replace pre-BCG brain-infiltrating immunocytes and, in this way, protect against AD. The accumulation of neutrophils in the urine of NMIBC patients treated with BCG, as described above, may reflect granulopoiesis whose results should be detectable in the PBMCs. The task of proving this hypothesis is formidable; we thus undertook a simple pilot study to reveal the impact of BCG intravesical instillations on the UPR in PBMCs.

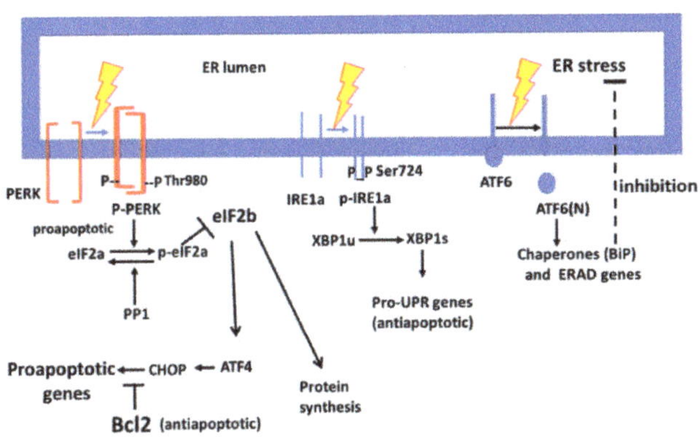

Figure 1. The response of ER stress of three ER membrane resident stress sensors and downstream responses. The designation of p-PERK, p-eIF2a, and CHOP as proapoptotic relates to prolonged ER stress.

2. Materials and Methods

2.1. Treatment Protocol

Patients with high-grade NMIBC were considered candidates for BCG therapy by six weekly intravesical instillations of OncoTICE BCG (Merck, Kirkland, QC, Canada) in

50 cubic centimeters (cc) of normal saline (0.9% NaCl), following peripheral blood sampling for PBMC isolation. For age, gender, and time of blood sampling post-BCG therapy, see Table 1. This study was approved by the committee on research involving human subjects of the Hadassah Hebrew University Hospital (application 0798-21 HMO, 3rd year extension up to 27 February 2025). All patients provided informed consent.

Table 1. NMIBC patients treated with intravesical BCG instillations and their pre- and post-BCG PBMC samples.

	Patient Number					
	1	**2**	**3**	**4**	**5**	**6**
Gender	**Male**	**Male**	**Male**	**Male**	**Male**	**Female**
Age of pre-BCG sample donation	58	57	64	47	61	82
Age of bladder exposed to BCG	58	57	64	47	61	82
Age of post-BCG PBMC sample donation	60	60	66	50	65	86
Months from the start of BCG exposure to the PBMC sample donation	24	29	28	36	50	52
Diagnostic information	Heavy smoker	Heavy smoker	Heavy smoker	Seasonal allergy	Arthritis reactive to BCG	Crohn's disease

2.2. *Peripheral Blood Mononuclear Cell Sampling*

Before and after intravesical BCG instillation, venous blood was drawn and separated on Ficoll Histopaque-10771 (Sigma, Rehovot, Israel); centrifuged at 1200× *g* for 30 min. PBMCs at the interphase with dilute upper-phase plasma were aspirated, washed in RPMI-1640 (R8758, Sigma), suspended in cold DMSO (D2438, Sigma), and 20% cold fetal calf serum (FCS) (F9665, Sigma) and gradually frozen to −170 °C, to be kept in liquid nitrogen until further use.

2.3. *Thawing of Peripheral Blood Mononuclear Cells and Protein Extraction*

PBMCs in frozen vials were rapidly thawed in a water bath at room temperature until the frozen suspension reached 0 °C. Cells were diluted in 20 volumes of RPMI, spun for 10 min, 300× *g* at 4 °C, and washed twice in cold plain Dulbecco's phosphate-buffered saline (D8537, Sigma) to remove all cryopreservation solution and FCS traces. The cell pellets were suspended in a 0.2 mL ice-cold Bicine/CHAPS detergent lysis buffer kit containing inhibitors of proteases and phosphatases (CBS403, ProteinSimple, San Jose, CA, USA) designed to minimize nuclear lysis. The cell suspension was incubated on ice for 30 min and spun for 30 min at 10,000× *g* at 4 °C. Protein supernatants were frozen at −20 °C until further use.

2.4. *Preparation of Immune-Electrophoresis Samples*

Samples were prepared using a separation module kit for a molecular weight range of 12–230 kDa MW for a 25-capillary cartridge (SM-W004) compatible with an Abby instrument (see ProteinSimple website for the Abby instrument). A master-mix solution was prepared according to the producer's instructions using a standard pack from the kit that provides dithiothreitol, a proprietary master mix compound, and a 5× concentrated sample buffer. The ready-to-use master mix was prepared such that for one capillary, a 0.6 µL master mix was added to 2.4 µL of protein solution (total volume/sample = 3 µL, with 0.8 µg protein), boiled at 95 °C for 5 min and loaded on a producer-designed plate in a row of 24 wells for the samples, and 1 well for the supplied biotinylated molecular weight ladder. The kit's detection module (mostly anti-rabbit DM-001) contained the secondary antibody horse radish peroxidase (HRP) conjugate, the antibody diluent, which also serves as a blocking buffer, luminol, and hydrogen peroxide. The rest of the separation module of the kit contains a wash buffer, plates, and capillary cartridges. We also used a total-protein detection module (DM-TP01) in a Re-Plex format, in which, after the regular immune electrophoresis, the antibodies underwent in-capillary stripping and a catalytic reagent biotinylated the total in-capillary proteins detected by streptavidin. The primary antibodies were purchased separately from other suppliers. From the plate loading onto the instrument to the end of the procedure, all the described electrophoretic and catalytic steps were automatically performed and computer-recorded in run files, without human intervention. The run protocol included the following steps: a separation time of 25 min, 375 V, primary and secondary antibodies 30 min each and detection time of 30 min.

2.5. Antibodies

Anti-PERK rabbit monoclonal antibodies (R-mAb) from Cell Signaling Technology (CST) (Danvers, MA, USA), catalog number (#) 3192, included anti-phospho-PERK pThr980 R-mAb CST #3179, anti-IRE1a R-mAb CST #3294, anti-phospho-IRE1a p-S724 R-polyclonal Ab Novus Biologicals (NB) (Centennial, CO, USA) #NB100-2323, anti-BiP R-mAb CST #3177, anti-glyceraldehyde phosphate dehydrogenase (GAPDH) R-mAb XP CST #5174, anti eIF2a mouse-mAb CST #2103, anti-phospho-eIF2a Ser51 R-mAb CST #9721, anti ATF6 rabbit polyclonal Ab NB #NBP1-75478, anti-XBP1 R-polyclonal Ab NB #NBP1-77681, in addition to anti-OASIS R-polyclonal Ab NBP1-31017 NB, anti-GADD153/CHOP R-polyclonal Ab NBP2-13172 NB, anti-Bcl-2 mouse mAb #15071 CST, and anti-Bcl-2A1 mouse mAb NB100-58070 NB. Antibodies were diluted 1:100 in the diluent solution provided in the detection module of the electrophoresis kit (ProteinSimple).

2.6. Analysis of the Results

The Abby instrument provided results by presenting protein curve peaks (detected by antibodies), and the quantities of proteins under the curves were recorded in the run files. The arbitrary numbers of the relevant antigen sizes were copied from the original run files of the instrument and presented in the Supplementary Section (Table S1). The relevant protein peaks were expressed as arbitrary unit numbers per total protein values obtained by a designated kit for in-capillary protein quantitation (DM-TP01, ProteinSimple). The values of the total protein along each capillary were recorded by the instrument and were copied into an Excel file, to which the antigen density of peaks from respective capillaries is related.

2.7. Presentation of the Results

The arbitrary antigen densities are mostly presented as a fraction of the total protein density, obtained in arbitrary numbers of chemiluminescence, as detected by the Abby instrument. These relative antigen (signaling protein) densities are presented per patient, as pre- versus post-BCG treatment values. The illustration is either by comparative bar graphs or linear or other regression in which the regression lines contain pre-BCG results in blue versus post-BCG results in red. The correlation coefficients of each regression are provided using PowerPoint software, and their statistical significance is computed via the statistical package for the social sciences. The regression lines express the relation between enzymes on the x-axis and expected responding protein substrates on the y-axis. On top of some regression lines, the effect of the BCG-reinforced vaccine course is overlaid by an arrow pointing up or downwards for the substrate (y-axis) or the responding protein, and horizontally for the enzyme or activation protein (x-axis). Each pair of arrows represents a respective patient number. A summary table of positive or negative effects of BCG is presented separately for all detected antigens. A positive (+) or negative (−) score is added as a quantitative evaluation that indicates the potential survival or apoptotic direction of each patient's total UPR. The scores (total %changes) of each patient are recorded in the bottom rows.

2.8. Calculation of the Score

For each UPR protein factor per patient, the pre-BCG value is subtracted from the post-BCG value; thus, if BCG increases or decreases the protein/total protein ratio, the result is positive (gain) or negative (loss) of expression, respectively. The expression gain is presented as the percentage gain incurred in the post-BCG results, and the loss is expressed as the percentage of the loss incurred in the pre-BCG result. Phosphorylation of PERK and eIF2a leads to CHOP expression, which stimulates cell death-inducing protein genes. Therefore, p-PERK, p-eIF2a, and CHOP are proapoptotic because if their phosphorylation persists, the cell will undergo apoptosis. The total proapoptotic effect by the tested UPR proteins is the sum of these three results. If one of these showed a negative proapoptotic value, it is considered a reduction in the proapoptotic effect and subtracted from the positive proapoptotic total. The opposite practice is considered for the rest of the nine antiapoptotic effects of the UPR and cell survival proteins. A third scoring value is a balance between pro- and antiapoptotic scores. The calculations are presented in the Supplementary Material Section (Table S2).

3. Results

3.1. Presentation of the BCG Impact on the UPR

BCG-induced changes for each UPR signaling protein are illustrated separately for patients in a horizontal row (Table 2). A scheme of the UPR landscape is presented in Figure 1.

Table 2. Percent change of UPR signaling proteins in PBMCs before and after BCG bladder instillations.

Line No.	UPR Signals	Patients Number						
		1	2	3	4	5	6	
1	p-eIF2a	−61.1	−78.9	−83.3	−93.8	−8.66	−3.1	Pro-apoptotic
2	p-PERK	93.5	−89.86	−32.97	−61.9	23.59	−91.3	Pro-apoptotic
3	CHOP	58.3	62.3	64.4	93.96	81.6	12.86	Pro-apoptotic
4	BCL2	63	27.9	69.77	94.6	−96.87	−21.2	Anti-apoptotic
5	BCL2A1	58.3	-74	−58.7	59.4	18.8	−88.2	Anti-apoptotic
6	p-IRE1a	65.9	−50	84.6	99.99	58	−81.7	Anti-apoptotic
7	XBP1s	82	99.99	98.3	77.5	93	99.9	Anti-apoptotic
8	ATF6	−96.6	−98.4	−97.6	−80.6	51.3	−98.16	Anti-apoptotic
9	ATF6(N)	70.5	99.99	70.5	−13.5	−61	−65.5	Anti-apoptotic
10	OASIS	17.7	91.6	70.2	99	9.4	−50.3	Anti-apoptotic
11	BiP	20	36	−6.9	88	3.3	−49	Anti-apoptotic
12	GAPDH	5.9	93	27.3	94	56	95.8	Anti-apoptotic
13	Sum of lines 1–3	90.7	−106.46	−51.87	−61.74	96.53	−81.54	Pro-apoptotic
14	Sum of lines 4–12	286.7	226.48	257.47	518.89	131.93	−258.06	Anti-apoptotic
15	Balance between pro and anti-apoptotic effects.	196	332.94	309.34	580.13	35.4	−176.82	Balance

To deal with patient heterogeneity, BCG-induced changes for each UPR protein are expressed by a numbered value in Table 2.

3.2. PERK Response to Endoplasmic Reticulum Stress After Bacillus Calmette–Guérin Treatment

Figure 2A shows a high ratio of activated PERK (p-PERK, Thr980) relative to the total PERK before BCG treatment in patients 1, 2, and 4. BCG treatment has drastically decreased the p-PERK/PERK ratio due to increased denominator (total PERK, Table S1). When total PERK is replaced by total protein as the denominator (p-PERK/total protein, Figure 2B), BCG treatment increases the total protein-normalized p-PERK in patients 1, 2, 3, 5, and 6 compared to the respective untreated PBMC samples. The total eIF2a, an alpha component of the eIF2 translation factor complex, shows an inactivating phosphorylation of p-eIF2a relative to total eIF2a in untreated patients 2, 3, 4, and 6 (Figure 2A). When p-eIF2a is related to total protein, instead of total eIF2a protein levels, there is a higher abundance of inactivated eIF2a (p-eIF2a/total protein) in samples of BCG-treated patients 2, 3, 4, 5, and 6 (Figure 2B). These results indicate that BCG increases the total protein, but it increases p-PERK and p-eIF2a abundance more than the respective protein relative to most untreated patient samples (Table S1). Mean PERK is activated by BCG (to p-PERK), although insignificantly. Nevertheless, BCG significantly inactivates the PERK substrate p-eIF2a.

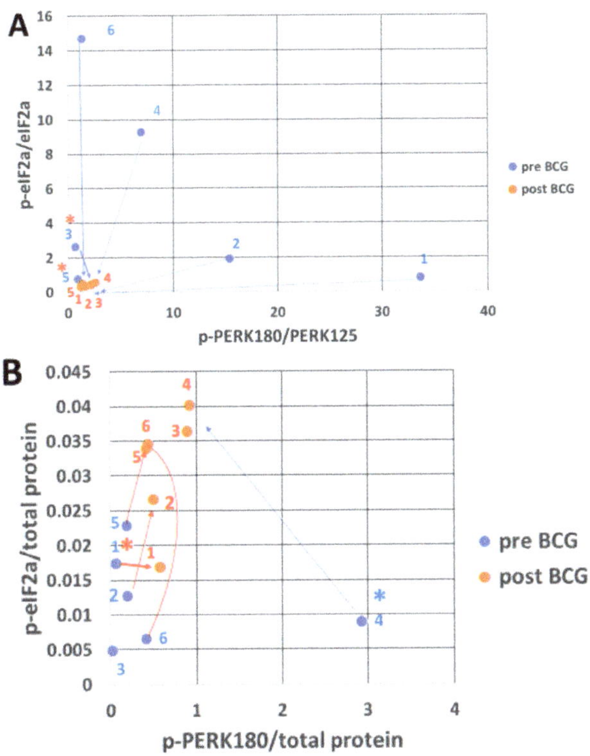

Figure 2. Inactivated eIF2a protein (p-eIF2a) abundance versus its activated kinase p-PERK abundance. Pre-BCG p-PERK (*x*-axis) is plotted against its responsive substrate pre-BCG p-eIF2a (*y*-axis, blue dots),

each relative to its total pre-BCG abundance (**A**). The same relation is depicted for each patient post-BCG treatment in red. (**A**) Note the drastic reduction in the post-BCG ratios and the restriction to the lower left corner. For patients 3 and 5, the red asterisk denotes a slight increase in p-PERK expression; the mean p-PERK activity pre-BCG is 9.9139 and post-BCG is 0.218 (p = 0.094, n = 6) according to the T-test. The parallel pre-BCG expression of the inactive p-eIF2a form is 5.042 and becomes 0.4437 post-BCG (p = 0.038, n = 6) by T-test. (**B**) p-PERK and p-eIF2a are related to the total cell protein for each patient pre- versus post-BCG treatment. The mean p-PERK/total protein ratio is 0.4107 pre and 0.6383 post-BCG (p = 0.459, n = 6) by T-test. In parallel, the pre-BCG mean p-eIF2a/total protein level is 0.0075 (high activity) versus 0.0213 post-BCG, demonstrating lower activity relative to the reduced protein translation (p = 0.019, n = 6) according to the T-test. Exceptional results shown by the blue and red asterisks indicate heterogeneity in patient response. See Table S1 for data.

3.3. *CHOP and BCL2 Expression After Bacillus Calmette–Guérin Treatment*

The CHOP, Bcl2A1, and Bcl2 response to BCG treatment is shown in Figure 3. The A1 variant of the cell survival protein Bcl2 shows a limited response to BCG (Figure 3A). Canonical Bcl2 responded positively to BCG at a variable range in patients 1, 2, 3, and 4, and decreased in patients 5 and 6. The response of CHOP to BCG showed a variable range, increasing in all patients as seen in Figure 3A,B. Thus, in patients 1, 2, 3, and 4, Bcl2 poses a counteracting challenge to the potential cell death inducer CHOP. CHOP expression is an event downstream of the activation of PERK (p-PERK) and inactivation of its substrate eIF2a (p-eIF2a).

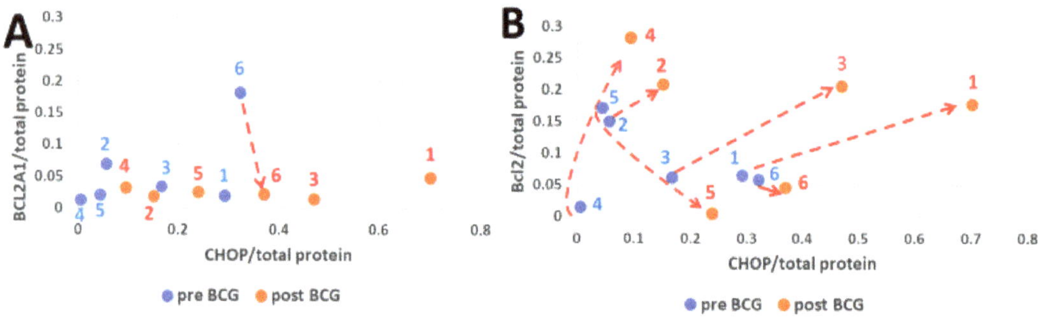

Figure 3. The impact of BCG on Bcl2A1 and Bcl2 cell survival proteins in parallel to the proapoptotic transcription factor CHOP. In all the patients, the CHOP/total protein abundance ratio increased by treatment with BCG (y-axis red versus blue dots (and red dashed arrows) panels **A** and **B**). The range of Bcl2A1 changes (x-axis, **A**) is small, except for patient 6. The range of Bcl2 changes is much more pronounced (**B**) than seen for Bcl2A1 (**A**). The mean activity of CHOP relative to total protein is 0.14796 pre- and 0.33726 post-BCG, which is significant (p = 0.0022, n = 6) according to a paired T-test. The mean Bcl2 activity is 0.08712 pre- and 0.15426 post-BCG, insignificant according to a T-test (p = 0.315, n = 6) as patients 5 and 6 have lost activity. By T-test, Bcl2A1 showed insignificant mean activity after BCG therapy (p = 0.342, n = 6).

3.4. *The Response of IRE1a and Its XBP1 Substrate to Bacillus Calmette–Guérin*

Phosphorylation of the ER stress sensor IRE1a is activated by ER stress to yield p-IRE1a (Figure 4A,B), which is followed by its downstream splicing effect on unspliced XBP1 (XBP1u) mRNA to obtain the spliced translation product XBP1s (Figure 4C). The low abundance of IRE1a corrected by total protein is congruent with the low abundance of p-IRE1a in patients 1, 3, 5, and 6 before BCG treatment, and so is the high abundance of IRE1a in patient 2. For patient 4 pre-BCG treatment, their low abundance resulted in a high activated p-IRE1a/total protein abundance ratio, lowering the correlation coefficient versus the BCG-treated patients, where r = 0.7575, p = 0.0405, versus r = 0.9357 and p = 0.003, respectively. Of note, the pre-BCG total p-PERK abundance was higher than that of post-BCG in patient 4 when normalized to total protein (Figure 2B), inversely to the IRE1a in which a relatively low total protein denominator leads to high p-IRE1a value on the y-axis (Figure 2A, see Discussion for a possible mechanism). The levels of IRE1a conversion to p-IRE1a at absolute abundance (Figure 4B) were roughly congruent in all patients for both the pre- and post-BCG treated groups (r = 0.8363, p = 0.019 and r = 0.8173, p = 0.023). The ratios of IRE1a to p-IRE1a conversion were similar, but the quantities were higher after BCG treatment for patients 1, 3, 4, 5, and 6. For patient 2, they were equal (Figure 4B). The mean pre-BCG was 0.1749 pre- and 0.6136 post-BCG (p = 0.016, n = 6). The abundance of XBP1s normalized to total protein has increased in patients 1, 2, 3, and 4 after BCG treatment, which was congruent with the levels of p-IRE1a only for patients 1, 3, and 5, while the increase in patients 2 and 4 was much less than expected from the high levels of the pre-BCG p-IRE1a (Figure 4C).

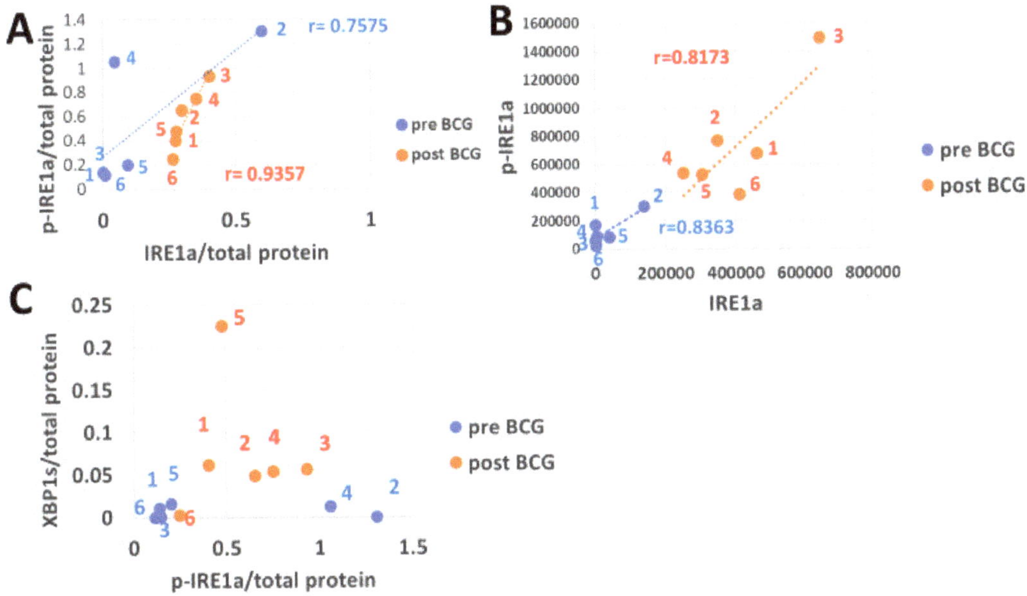

Figure 4. BCG activation of stress response via the IRE1a stress sensor. The abundance of IRE1a for six BCG-treated patients on the x-axis matched the resulting p-IRE1a depicted on the y-axis. P-IRE1a in patients 2 and 4 is downregulated (**A**). (**B**) Pre- and post-BCG dot scatter plots represent absolute values of p-IRE1a abundance (y-axis) matched with those of IRE1a abundance (x-axis). (**C**) The spliced XBP1 protein (XBP1s/total protein abundance ratio) on the y-axis is matched with p-IRE1a/total protein on the x-axis. The mean IRE1a/total protein pre-BCG increased significantly from 0.124 to 0.3099 post-BCG (p = 0.043, n = 6) according to the T-test, both on the x-axis (**A**). The mean p-IRE1a/total protein abundance ratio pre-BCG increased insignificantly from 0.492 pre-BCG to 0.575 post-BCG (p = 0.35, n = 6), both on the y-axis, (**A**). Responding to p-IRE1a, the XBP1/total protein mean value grew significantly from 0.00657 pre-BCG to 0.07435 post-BCG (p = 0.03445, n = 6, panel **C**) according to the T-test. Dashed lines indicate by color the regression lines.

3.5. The Impact of Bacillus Calmette–Guérin on BiP Expression in Response to Endoplasmic Reticulum Stress-Induced Transcription Factors

Figure 5 shows the pre- versus post-BCG levels of ATF6(N), XBP1s, and OASIS matched with levels of the BiP protein expression in response to these transcription factors. The pre-BCG abundance of ATF6(N) is substantially higher than that of XBP1s in patients 2, 3, 4, 5, and 6 by >10, >26, >21, >14, >2000 fold, respectively, and in patient 1, it is only >1.3 fold higher than the XBP1s. The pre-BCG abundance of OASIS was higher than that of XBP1s in patients 1, 2, 3, 5, and 6 by >6, >4800, >19, >5, and >2300 fold, respectively. Patient 4 was an exception in which OASIS abundance was 0.1 of that of XBP1s. These results are consistent with the delayed XBP1 protein expression compared with the faster expression of ATF6(N) [30], which is synergistic with OASIS. In all patients post-BCG treatment, XBP1 abundance was higher than that of the pre-BCG samples. The ATF6(N) abundance was reduced in patients 4, 5, and 6 and increased in 1, 2, and 3 after BCG treatment, indicating a BCG mitigating effect on ATF6(N). The abundance of OASIS increased after BCG treatment in all patients.

Expression of GAPDH, a representative enzyme of the glycolytic pathway, was variably upregulated in PBMCs of all patients by BCG therapy (Figure 6). This is consistent with converting anaerobic glycolysis to aerobic glycolysis by BCG, part of the innate immune training [40,41], and the metabolic change in activated adaptive immune cells [42]. GAPDH increased in PBMCs in response to intravesical BCG instillations. GAPDH, important for the glycolytic pathway, was elevated by BCG treatment in all patients. The variability of its increase reflects the heterogeneity between patients in converting from anaerobic to aerobic glycolysis in PBMCs.

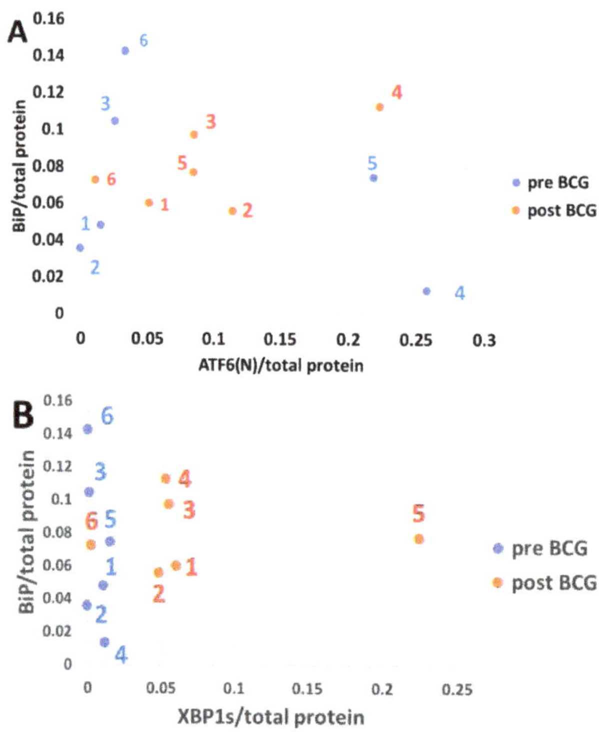

Figure 5. *Cont.*

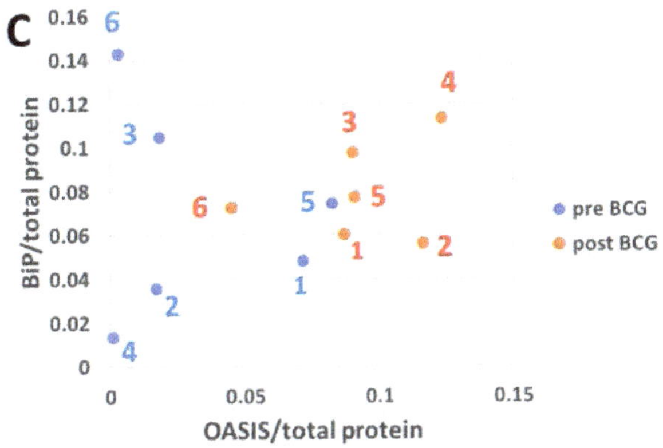

Figure 5. The effect of BCG on UPR transcription factor activation responding to ER stress sensors. BiP (*y*-axis) transcription target abundance plotted in comparison to that of ATF6(N) (**A**), XBP1s (**B**), and OASIS (**C**) (*x*-axis). Note the very low levels of pre-BCG XBP1s compared to ATF6(N). The mean ATF6(N)/total protein levels pre-BCG grew only slightly and insignificantly from 0.0917 to 0.0953 post-BCG ($p = 0.46$, n = 6, panel **A**) according to the *T*-test; only patients 1, 2, and 3 contributed to its growth. The mean BiP/total protein abundance ratio grew minimally from 0.0699 pre-BCG to 0.0794 post-BCG (by *T*-test, $p = 0.343$, n = 6, *y*-axis in panels **A**–**C**); only patients 1, 2, and 5 contributed to its growth. The mean OASIS/total protein grew significantly from 0.0353 pre-BCG to 0.0923 post-BCG (by *T*-test, $p = 0.012$, n = 6, *x*-axis panel **C**).

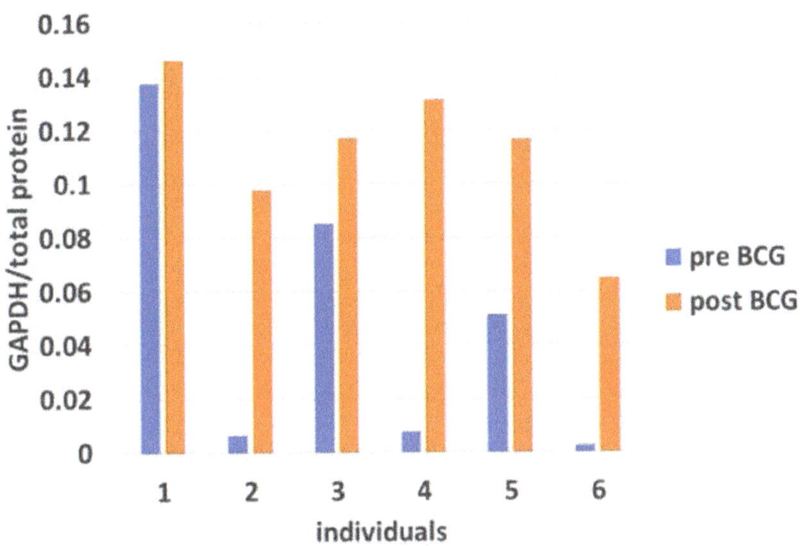

Figure 6. GAPDH levels increase in PBMCs in response to intravesical BCG instillations. GAPDH expression was elevated by BCG treatment in all patients. The mean GAPDH/total protein abundance ratio grew significantly from 0.04854 pre-BCG to 0.11238 post-BCG ($p = 0.0061$, n = 6, by *T*-test).

3.6. Combining the Bacillus Calmette–Guérin Apoptotic and Antiapoptotic Effects

The BCG antiapoptotic effect is a combination of %gain/loss of p-eIF2a, p-PERK, and CHOP depicted in Table 2, in which p-eIF2a is related to total eIF2a and p-PERK to total PERK as shown in Figure 2A and not when related to total protein (Figure 2B). Figure 7A shows that the antiapoptotic effect of BCG (combining the rest of UPR proteins in Table 2, line 14, related to the time elapsed from the start of BCG treatment shown in Table 1) decreases with age and stays above the *y*-axis 0-line until the 8th decade and falls below it for one patient in the 9th decade. In contrast, the proapoptotic line stays stable as a flat line close to the 0 line. Figure 7B shows the effect of BCG on the anti- and proapoptotic scores as a measure of time elapsed from the post-BCG harvest of PBMCs, along the *x*-axis of the short time scale (month intervals in Figure 7B versus age in years in Figure 7A). The time-dependent impact of BCG on the antiapoptotic effect is reminiscent of the time required for BCG to convert anaerobic to aerobic glycolysis in type 1 diabetics [41]. Yet, for the oldest patient (86 years old), 52 months of BCG treatment were insufficient to raise the BCG-induced antiapoptotic effect above the *y*-axis 0 line. These results may indicate that the younger the patient, the higher the BCG-induced antiapoptotic score, as its level requires about 3 years to show the full BCG impact. Unlike in Table 2, the p-PERK and p-eIF2a abundances are expressed per total protein, in Table 3. This brings the proapoptotic curve (Figure 8A) to a higher level about the *y*-axis than in Figure 7A while maintaining its flatness as in Figure 7A. These results indicate that in the present experiment, the proapoptotic potential with BCG treatment does not change with advancing age as the antiapoptotic score does.

Table 3. Percent change of UPR signaling proteins/total protein abundance ratio in PBMCs before versus after BCG bladder instillations.

Line No.	UPR Signals	Patients Number						
		1	2	3	4	5	6	
1	p-eIF2a	−3	52	86.5	76.6	32	80.6	Pro-apoptotic
2	p-PERK	94.7	99.99	94.98	−54.7	99.99	43.4	Pro-apoptotic
3	CHOP	58.3	62.3	64.4	93.96	81.6	12.86	Pro-apoptotic
4	BCL2	63	27.9	69.77	94.6	−96.87	−21.2	Anti-apoptotic
5	BCL2A1	58.3	−74	−58.7	59.4	18.8	−88.2	Anti-apoptotic
6	p-IRE1a	65.9	−50	84.6	99.99	58	−81.7	Anti-apoptotic
7	XBP1s	82	99.99	98.3	77.5	93	99.9	Anti-apoptotic
8	ATF6	−96.6	−98.4	−97.6	−80.6	51.3	−98.16	Anti-apoptotic
9	ATF6(N)	70.5	99.99	70.5	−13.5	−61	−65.5	Anti-apoptotic
10	OASIS	17.7	91.6	70.2	99	9.4	−50.3	Anti-apoptotic
11	BiP	20	36	−6.9	88	3.3	−49	Anti-apoptotic
12	GAPDH	5.9	93	27.3	94	56	95.8	Anti-apoptotic
13	Sum of lines 1–3	150	214.29	245.88	115.59	181.59	136.86	Pro-apoptotic
14	Sum of lines 4–12	286.7	226.48	257.47	518.89	131.93	−258.06	Anti-apoptotic
15	Balance between pro- and anti-apoptotic effects.	136.7	12.19	11.59	403.03	−49.66	−394.92	Balance

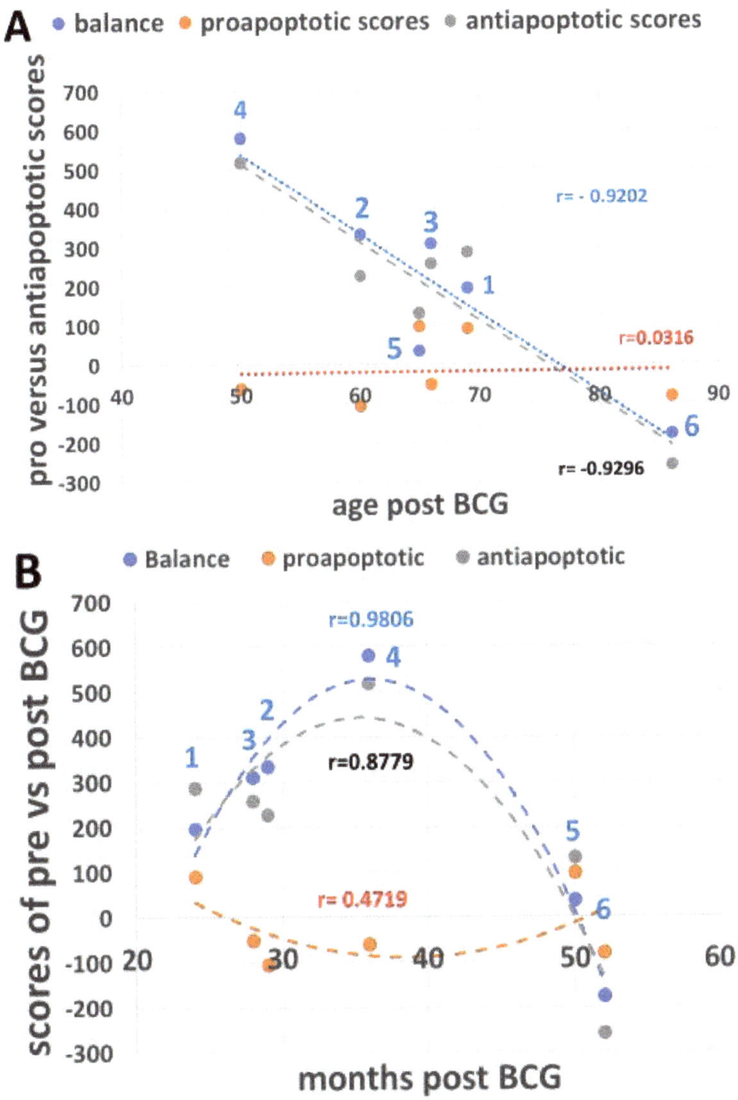

Figure 7. UPR signaling scores of BCG-induced percent changes versus patient age and months post-BCG treatment (Table 1). (**A**) The effect of age on the scores post-BCG treatment (from Table 2) resulting from the sum of percent changes of pro- versus antiapoptotic UPR signals and the balance between them (antiapoptotic r = −0.9296, proapoptotic r = 0.03162, for the balance between them r = −0.9202). The proapoptotic scores result from p-PERK and p-eIF2a related to total PERK and eIF2a, respectively. The difference between pro- and antiapoptotic correlations and between the balance and the proapoptotic correlation, according to Fisher's r-to-z transformation test, is significant ($p = 0.0388$ and $p = 0.0400$, respectively). (**B**) The effect of time elapsed from BCG treatment (Table 1) to signaling score differences in PBMCs (Table 2) shows differences between the proapoptotic versus antiapoptotic values, with the best fit being a binomial correlation (proapoptotic r = −0.4719 versus antiapoptotic r = 0.8779, correlation difference $p = 0.0213$). The difference in apoptotic regression (r = −0.4719) from the regression of balance (r = 0.9806) is significant ($p = 0.0005$) in Fisher's transformation. Dashed red, gray, and blue lines denote proapoptotic, antiapoptotic, and the balance between them, respectively.

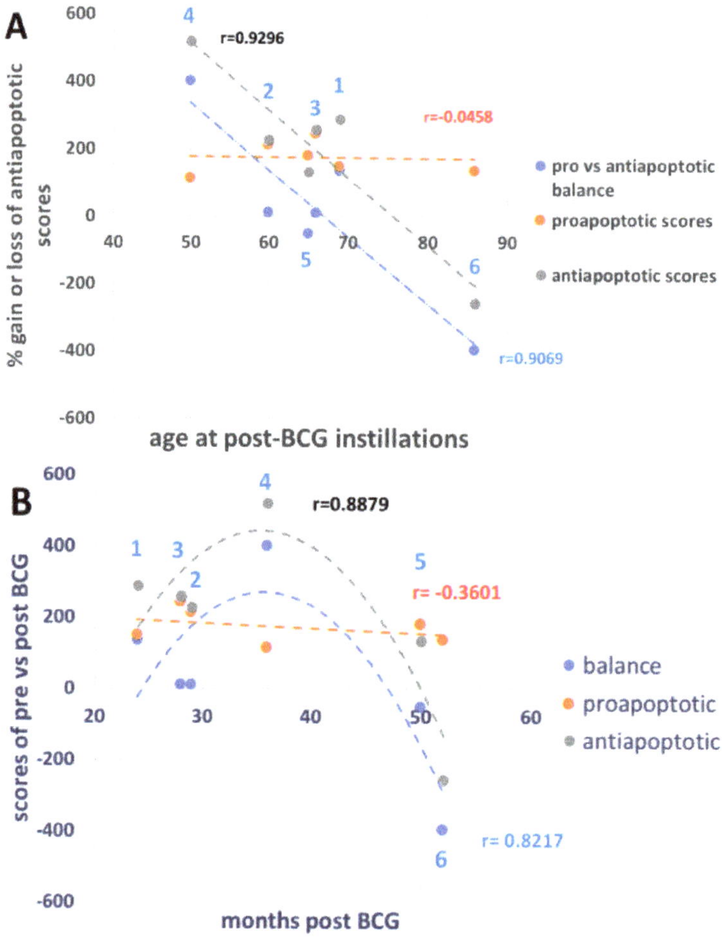

Figure 8. UPR signaling scores of BCG-induced percent changes versus patient age and months post-BCG treatment (Table 1). (**A**) Age post-BCG treatment effect on the scores taken from Table 3, in which the UPR proapoptotic signals are expressed as abundance relative to total cell protein. Note the elevation of the linear proapoptotic scores is still almost parallel to the *x*-axis, indicating that the proapoptotic scores are not affected by age or time post-BCG treatments. (**B**) The effect of the time interval between BCG therapy and the post-BCG treatment antiapoptotic scores. Note that the longer the interval, the higher the antiapoptotic scores of patients 1, 2, 3, and 4. The proapoptotic scores are less affected by the elapsed time. The antiapoptotic best fit regression is binomial, and the proapoptotic regression is linear. Dashed red, gray, and blue lines denote proapoptotic, antiapoptotic, and the balance between them, respectively.

4. Discussion

The rationale for examining the impact of BCG on the signaling cascade of UPR, which responds to ER stress, is that we found that extensive exposure to BCG via intravesical treatment lowered the incidence of AD compared to alternative therapies for the same diagnosis [9]. NMIBC is the only diagnosis where patients undergo such a course of BCG, and their PBMCs may be repurposed for analysis of the UPR concerning AD. PBMC analysis has merit because peripheral immunocytes are present in the brain [37,38] and may support the protection of the aging brain [43,44], separately from their involvement in NMIBC therapy. ER stress, and consequently the UPR activation, is an early event in AD [17,45]. Therapeutic clearance of beta-amyloid aggregates with no benefit to the patients [18–20] indicates dysfunction in the UPR cascade or even more upstream, in the PBMCs or brain cells. The fact that numerous publications implicate the UPR in AD pathology [15–17,21,26,27,45–49] is compelling, and the fact that BCG reduces AD incidence in NMIBC makes it obvious that PBMCs should be analyzed for BCG impact on the UPR. The fate of the donors of pre- and post-BCG PBMCs to develop AD is not known, and yet the BCG impact on PBMCs is important as these immunocytes potentially support brain wellness if and when needed [43,44].

Patients suffering from NMIBC may benefit from intravesical BCG instillations and are expected to show variability in their responses corresponding to the variability of their immunogenetic gestalt, age, health factors (Table 1), and other factors that we still cannot predict. Therefore, we have compared PBMC features of ER stress response to BCG on a longitudinal basis to remove part of the individual variability from the analysis of the results. Another factor responsible for the heterogeneity of the NMIBC patients is the reported correlation of the tumor cells and their infiltrated immunocytes to express checkpoint ligands (PD-L1) of their receptor (PD-1), which raises the chance of the anti-tumor immunological therapy [50,51]. BCG has upregulated PD-L1 expression in PBMCs of melanoma patients, which raises the question of what kind of therapeutic effect PD-L1 expression in PBMCs has versus bladder tumors and versus brain cells in preventing AD, which must be investigated in the future. It should be stressed that the recruitment of controls of individuals not diagnosed as NMIBC receiving the same BCG treatment is unachievable.

PERK protein is one of the ER membrane resident stress sensors; PERK becomes p-PERK upon its activation, which converts its cytosol-facing domain into a protein kinase that specifically targets Ser51 of the alpha component (eIF2a) of the translation factor 2 into p-eIF2a [24,28]. The p-PERK and p-eIF2a in PBMCs of pre-BCG patients were highly abundant when expressed per total (deficient levels) PERK and eIF2a denominators, respectively (Figure 2A). In contrast, BCG treatment pushed the ratios (p-PERK/PERK and p-eIF2a/eIF2a) down and shifted them to the left by strongly increasing total PERK and eIF2a. A possible reason is that PERK and eIF2a mRNAs may translate cap-independently (which has not been shown yet in the literature). The cap-independent translation enables mRNAs to use IRES instead of the cap, which has been best studied in yeast [52,53]. The high total PERK and eIF2a is consistent with their IRES-dependent translation, ignoring the p-eIF2a-imposed limitation on cap-dependent translation, which is expected to affect the majority of cap-dependent cellular mRNA translations. Both p-PERK and p-eIF2a determine the rate of cellular protein synthesis, and their expression should not be normalized by total cellular protein to avoid the erroneous picture seen in Figure 2B versus Figure 2A. Instead, both p-PERK and p-eIF2a should be normalized by PERK and eIF2a, respectively, as normalization by total protein levels, which they determine, posits them in a "conflict of function", so to speak. Activated p-PERK that increases p-eIF2a may cause increased expression of ATF4 that leads to increased CHOP expression [54], a dominant-negative competitor against CREB transcription factors, and thus may upregulate the expression of proapoptotic proteins [33,54,55]. BCG treatment increases Bcl2 expression, a cell survival protein [56,57], pari passu with the increased CHOP as preemptive antiapoptotic protection (Figure 3B, Table S2). Interestingly, Bcl2A1 was much lower than the canonical Bcl2 (Figure 3A), which was the opposite of the case in BCG-vaccinated melanoma patients [58]. This might be ascribed to several differences in BCG strains and administration modes. In the melanoma patients, the BCG strain obtained from the Danish Statens Serum Institute was injected intradermally, and the time interval between pre-BCG and post-BCG sampling was only 4 months. Contrarily, for the NMIBC patients, the Tice strain was used, the exposure was via the bladder, and the interval between pre- and post-BCG sampling was up to several years. The total IRE1a (Figure 4B pre-BCG) is almost zero in patient 4 because most of it is phosphorylated (activated by stress), while in patient 2 (also under ER stress), there is sufficient IRE1a and therefore also more p-IRE1a than in patient 4. After BCG treatment, IRE1a increases in both patients by a similar ratio, and so does the increase in p-IRE1a. Figure 4A (pre-BCG) shows the same dot scatter (for patients 4 and 2) as in Figure 4B, only that here the figures are related to the total protein. This leaves the IRE1a/total protein abundance ratio in a similar relative position for patients 4 and 2; patient 2 is related to less total protein than patient 4, which spans the distance between them but less so on the *y*-axis. In the post-BCG state, patient 2 has gained total protein, and patient 4 lost total protein, such that, versus IRE1a/total protein (*x*-axis, Figure 4A), they fall between the pre-BCG state, as if BCG mitigates them. They also lose height versus the p-IRE1a/total protein abundance ratio (*y*-axis, Figure 4A), which relates them to the increased total protein denominator. In Figure 4C, the post-BCG p-IRE1a values of patients 4 and 2 (red dots) are depicted on the *x*-axis to the left (reduced abundance ratio), versus the pre-BCG of patients 2 and 4, outlined by blue dots. BCG increased the activated stress sensor p-IRE1a (although it virtually decreased it relative to a higher normalizing total protein). P-IRE1a activated the XBP1 transcription factor, whose increase can be seen on the *y*-axis (Figure 4C) in response to the post-BCG p-IRE1a of patients 2 and 4 and also patients 1, 3, and 5. This is consistent with the ability of BCG to activate XBP1 splicing via p-IRE1a, which elicits part of the UPR protein recruitment [54] and helps clear misfolded proteins in PBMCs. XBP1s, in turn, increased BiP expression (Figure 5B) in patients 2 and 4. Interestingly, patient 4 had a full 3 years to express the BCG impact, followed by patient 2, with 2.5 years to express the BCG impact on the anti-apoptotic score (Figures 7B and 8B).

ATF6(N) and its cooperating protein OASIS act as transcription factors shortly after their stress-sensing precursors undergo intramembranous cleavage [54], whereas XBP1 has to first undergo splicing into XBP1s at the mRNA stage by the stress sensor p-IRE1a on the XBP1u (unspliced) mRNA, before being translated. This was shown to cause a delay in XBP1s versus ATF6(N) protein expression [54] and may partially explain the low abundance of XBP1s versus ATF6(N) and OASIS, comparing Figure 4B to Figure 4A,C. In patients 1, 2, and 3, ATF6 (the precursor of ATF6(N) is maximally cleaved/consumed for the generation of the UPR proteins important for the clearance of misfolded and aggregated ER proteins. This could occur in association with heavy smoking by patients 1, 2, and 3 (Table 1). Heavy smoking causes oxidative stress in lung tissue that causes ER stress and activation of the UPR [59]. The results show that PBMCs may also react to smoking by increasing the UPR, including ATF6 precursor expression and consumption by its conversion to ATF6(N). Contrarily, in patients 4, 5, and 6 (not recorded as heavy smokers), the ATF6 cleavage is only partial; this results in lower survival odds for the PBMCs of these patients and requires a compensatory activity for lower ATF6(N) expression. There is potential evidence of this compensatory activity in patient 4 (compare line 10 to line 9 of patient 4 in Table 2).

GAPDH upregulation by BCG, other than being part of the characteristics of innate immunity against bladder cancer, might reflect the expedited glycolytic pathway [40,60] for the benefit of brain tissue. If the hypothesis that BCG-induced PBMC aerobic glycolysis means that it may sustain astroglia, then more of the lactate end product could perhaps boost the ability of neurons to maintain their oxidative phosphorylation [61]. The missing part is the documentation of PBMCs approaching the brain from the periphery, enacting the transfer, or instructing glia to transfer lactate to neurons.

The response diversity of patients to BCG treatment is reflected in the diverse responses of the UPR proteins. One of the contributing factors to this heterogeneity seems to be the patient age during BCG therapy, their health status, and also environmental effects such as smoking. The relationship between the UPR and the patient age is observed by matching it with the score summary of UPR proteins that reflect expected cell survival (antiapoptotic) effects separated from potential cell death (proapoptotic) effects. Based on the results of Figures 7A and 8A, it can be hypothesized that the benefit of BCG for resolving ER stress is maintained up to the 7th decade. This is consistent with diminishing cognition test scores with advancing age in NMIBC patients on the one hand and corrected cognition scores by BCG on the other hand [62]. The time it takes for adults to complete the full BCG treatment course (induction and maintenance) is 3 years (36 months, Figure 7B) from the treatment course, which is consistent with the peak response of GAPDH reinforced by BiP, OASIS, p-IRE1a, and Bcl2 in patient 4 (Table 2). BCG-induced activation of the glycolytic enzyme GAPDH may relate to the conversion of anaerobic to aerobic glycolysis demonstrated in type 1 diabetic patients vaccinated with BCG that showed glycemic relief only 3 years [63,64] after vaccination. The UPR protein expression changes by BCG in six patients presented here are compelling because retrospective studies show that BCG protects against AD in NMIBC patients [10,65,66]. Studies of the impact of BCG on the UPR should be expanded in more patients, including additional proteins commonly diagnostic for AD and NMIBC, which are the checkpoint receptor and ligand in PBMCs. For AD specifically, the beta-amyloid and Tau proteins and their response to BCG treatment may add to the value of BCG therapy. The limitation of this study is the lack of human brain tissue analysis, which prevented bridging the gap between the peripheral immunocytes and the changes that occur in the glia and neurons under the effect of BCG therapy.

Supplementary Materials: The following supporting information can be downloaded at https://www.mdpi.com/article/10.3390/cimb47060392/s1.

Author Contributions: Conceptualization, B.Y.K. and C.L.G. Formal analysis, B.Y.K. and C.L.G.; Investigation, B.Y.K. and O.N.G.; Methodology, B.Y.K. and O.N.G.; Project administration, C.L.G.; Resources, O.N.G. and C.L.G.; Validation, O.N.G. and C.L.G.; Writing—original draft, B.Y.K.; Writing—review and editing, O.N.G. All authors have read and agreed to the published version of the manuscript.

Funding: This work was supported by the Cure Alzheimer's Disease Fund. This funding source did not provide award numbers.

Institutional Review Board Statement: The Committee on Research Involving Human Subjects of the Hebrew University-Hadassah Medical School Jerusalem, Israel. The committee on research involving Human Subjects reviewed the research application 0798-21 HMO of Prof Ofer Gofrit on Deciphering the mechanism by which BCG decreases the risk of Alzheimer's disease. After reviewing the report on the progress of the research, continuation is hereby authorized until 27 February 2025.

Informed Consent Statement: Informed consent was obtained from all subjects involved in the study.

Data Availability Statement: The data used in this study are available in Tables S1 and S2 of the Supplementary Section.

Conflicts of Interest: The authors declare no conflicts of interest of the study; in the collection, analysis, or interpretation of data; in the writing of the manuscript; or in the decision to publish the results.

References

1. Milosevic, R.; Milovic, N.; Aleksic, P.; Lazic, M.; Cerovic, S.; Bancevic, V.; Kosevic, B.; Maric, P.; Spasic, A.; Simic, D.; et al. Difference in recurrence frequencies of non-muscle-invasive-bladder tumors depending on optimal usage of intravesical immunotherapy of bacillus Calmette-Guerin. *Vojnosanit. Pregl.* **2015**, *72*, 241–246. [CrossRef] [PubMed]
2. Jiang, S.; Redelman-Sidi, G. BCG in Bladder Cancer Immunotherapy. *Cancers* **2022**, *14*, 3073. [CrossRef]
3. Beatty, J.D.; Islam, S.; North, M.E.; Knight, S.C.; Ogden, C.W. Urine dendritic cells: A noninvasive probe for immune activity in bladder cancer? *BJU Int.* **2004**, *94*, 1377–1383. [CrossRef]
4. Suttmann, H.; Riemensberger, J.; Bentien, G.; Schmaltz, D.; Stöckle, M.; Jocham, D.; Böhle, A.; Brandau, S. Neutrophil granulocytes are required for effective Bacillus Calmette-Guerin immunotherapy of bladder cancer and orchestrate local immune responses. *Cancer Res.* **2006**, *66*, 8250–8257. [CrossRef]
5. Moorlag, S.J.; Rodriguez-Rosales, Y.A.; Gillard, J.; Fanucchi, S.; Theunissen, K.; Novakovic, B.; de Bont, C.M.; Negishi, Y.; Fok, E.T.; Kalafati, L.; et al. BCG Vaccination Induces Long-Term Functional Reprogramming of Human Neutrophils. *Cell Rep.* **2020**, *33*, 108387. [CrossRef] [PubMed]
6. Benn, C.S.; Fisker, A.B.; Rieckmann, A.; Sorup, S.; Aaby, P. Vaccinology: Time to change the paradigm? *Lancet Infect. Dis.* **2020**, *20*, e274–e283. [CrossRef]
7. Lange, C.; Aaby, P.; Behr, M.A.; Donald, P.R.; Kaufmann, S.H.E.; Netea, M.G.; Mandalakas, A.M. 100 years of *Mycobacterium bovis bacille* Calmette-Guerin. *Lancet Infect. Dis.* **2022**, *22*, e2–e12. [CrossRef]
8. Gofrit, O.N.; Bercovier, H.; Klein, B.Y.; Cohen, I.R.; Ben-Hur, T.; Greenblatt, C.L. Can immunization with Bacillus Calmette-Guerin (BCG) protect against Alzheimer's disease? *Med. Hypotheses* **2019**, *123*, 95–97. [CrossRef] [PubMed]
9. Gofrit, O.N.; Klein, B.Y.; Cohen, I.R.; Ben-Hur, T.; Greenblatt, C.L.; Bercovier, H. Bacillus Calmette-Guerin (BCG) therapy lowers the incidence of Alzheimer's disease in bladder cancer patients. *PLoS ONE* **2019**, *14*, e0224433. [CrossRef]
10. Gofrit, O.N.; Greenblatt, C.L.; Klein, B.Y.; Ben-Hur, T.; Bercovier, H. Can immunization with BCG delay the onset of Alzheimer's disease? *Geriatr. Gerontol. Int.* **2023**, *23*, 889–890. [CrossRef]
11. Scherrer, J.F.; Salas, J.; Wiemken, T.L.; Hoft, D.F.; Jacobs, C.; Morley, J.E. Impact of herpes zoster vaccination on incident dementia: A retrospective study in two patient cohorts. *PLoS ONE* **2021**, *16*, e0257405. [CrossRef] [PubMed]
12. Poynton-Smith, E.; Orrell, M.; Morley, J.E.; Scherrer, J.F. Could routine vaccinations prevent dementia? *Int. J. Geriatr. Psychiatry* **2023**, *38*, e5978. [CrossRef]
13. Adams, K.; Weber, K.S.; Johnson, S.M. Exposome and Immunity Training: How Pathogen Exposure Order Influences Innate Immune Cell Lineage Commitment and Function. *Int. J. Mol. Sci.* **2020**, *21*, 8462. [CrossRef] [PubMed]
14. Kalafati, L.; Kourtzelis, I.; Schulte-Schrepping, J.; Li, X.; Hatzioannou, A.; Grinenko, T.; Hagag, E.; Sinha, A.; Has, C.; Dietz, S.; et al. Innate Immune Training of Granulopoiesis Promotes Anti-tumor Activity. *Cell* **2020**, *183*, 771–785.e12. [CrossRef]
15. Ansari, N.; Khodagholi, F. Molecular mechanism aspect of ER stress in Alzheimer's disease: Current approaches and future strategies. *Curr. Drug Targets.* **2013**, *14*, 114–122. [CrossRef]
16. Cornejo, V.H.; Hetz, C. The unfolded protein response in Alzheimer's disease. *Semin. Immunopathol.* **2013**, *35*, 277–292. [CrossRef]
17. Di Domenico, F.; Coccia, R.; Cocciolo, A.; Murphy, M.P.; Cenini, G.; Head, E.; Butterfield, D.A.; Giorgi, A.; Schinina, M.E.; Mancuso, C.; et al. Impairment of proteostasis network in Down syndrome prior to the development of Alzheimer's disease neuropathology: Redox proteomics analysis of human brain. *Biochim. Biophys. Acta.* **2013**, *1832*, 1249–1259. [CrossRef] [PubMed]
18. Doody, R.S.; Thomas, R.G.; Farlow, M.; Iwatsubo, T.; Vellas, B.; Joffe, S.; Kieburtz, K.; Raman, R.; Sun, X.; Aisen, P.S.; et al. Phase 3 trials of solanezumab for mild-to-moderate Alzheimer's disease. *N. Engl. J. Med.* **2014**, *370*, 311–321. [CrossRef]
19. Karran, E.; De Strooper, B. The amyloid cascade hypothesis: Are we poised for success or failure? *J. Neurochem.* **2016**, *139* (Suppl. 2), 237–252. [CrossRef]
20. van Dyck, C.H.; Swanson, C.J.; Aisen, P.; Bateman, R.J.; Chen, C.; Gee, M.; Kanekiyo, M.; Li, D.; Reyderman, L.; Cohen, S.; et al. Lecanemab in Early Alzheimer's Disease. *N. Engl. J. Med.* **2023**, *388*, 9–21. [CrossRef]
21. Endres, K.; Reinhardt, S. ER-stress in Alzheimer's disease: Turning the scale? *Am. J. Neurodegener. Dis.* **2013**, *2*, 247–265. [PubMed]
22. Calfon, M.; Zeng, H.; Urano, F.; Till, J.H.; Hubbard, S.R.; Harding, H.P.; Clark, S.G.; Ron, D. IRE1 couples endoplasmic reticulum load to secretory capacity by processing the XBP-1 mRNA. *Nature* **2002**, *415*, 92–96. [CrossRef] [PubMed]
23. Kim, J.I.; Kaufman, R.J.; Back, S.H.; Moon, J.Y. Development of a Reporter System Monitoring Regulated Intramembrane Proteolysis of the Transmembrane bZIP Transcription Factor ATF6alpha. *Mol. Cells* **2019**, *42*, 783–793.
24. Urra, H.; Hetz, C. Fine-tuning PERK signaling to control cell fate under stress. *Nat. Struct. Mol. Biol.* **2017**, *24*, 789–790. [CrossRef]
25. Hetz, C.; Martinon, F.; Rodriguez, D.; Glimcher, L.H. The unfolded protein response: Integrating stress signals through the stress sensor IRE1alpha. *Physiol. Rev.* **2011**, *91*, 1219–1243. [CrossRef] [PubMed]
26. Gerakis, Y.; Hetz, C. Emerging roles of ER stress in the etiology and pathogenesis of Alzheimer's disease. *FEBS J.* **2018**, *285*, 995–1011. [CrossRef]

27. Ghemrawi, R.; Khair, M. Endoplasmic Reticulum Stress and Unfolded Protein Response in Neurodegenerative Diseases. *Int. J. Mol. Sci.* **2020**, *21*, 6127. [CrossRef]
28. Hong, F.; Liu, B.; Wu, B.X.; Morreall, J.; Roth, B.; Davies, C.; Sun, S.; Diehl, J.A.; Li, Z. CNPY2 is a key initiator of the PERK-CHOP pathway of the unfolded protein response. *Nat. Struct. Mol. Biol.* **2017**, *24*, 834–839. [CrossRef] [PubMed]
29. Yoshida, H.; Matsui, T.; Yamamoto, A.; Okada, T.; Mori, K. XBP1 mRNA is induced by ATF6 and spliced by IRE1 in response to ER stress to produce a highly active transcription factor. *Cell* **2001**, *107*, 881–891. [CrossRef]
30. Yamamoto, K.; Sato, T.; Matsui, T.; Sato, M.; Okada, T.; Yoshida, H.; Harada, A.; Mori, K. Transcriptional induction of mammalian ER quality control proteins is mediated by single or combined action of ATF6alpha and XBP1. *Dev. Cell* **2007**, *13*, 365–376. [CrossRef]
31. Vellanki, R.N.; Zhang, L.; Volchuk, A. OASIS/CREB3L1 is induced by endoplasmic reticulum stress in human glioma cell lines and contributes to the unfolded protein response, extracellular matrix production, and cell migration. *PLoS ONE* **2013**, *8*, e54060. [CrossRef] [PubMed]
32. Lee, K.; Tirasophon, W.; Shen, X.; Michalak, M.; Prywes, R.; Okada, T.; Yoshida, H.; Mori, K.; Kaufman, R.J. IRE1-mediated unconventional mRNA splicing and S2P-mediated ATF6 cleavage merge to regulate XBP1 in signaling the unfolded protein response. *Genes Dev.* **2002**, *16*, 452–466. [CrossRef] [PubMed]
33. Rozpedek, W.; Pytel, D.; Mucha, B.; Leszczynska, H.; Diehl, J.A.; Majsterek, I. The Role of the PERK/eIF2alpha/ATF4/CHOP Signaling Pathway in Tumor Progression During Endoplasmic Reticulum Stress. *Curr. Mol. Med.* **2016**, *16*, 533–544. [CrossRef] [PubMed]
34. Herrero-Mendez, A.; Almeida, A.; Fernandez, E.; Maestre, C.; Moncada, S.; Bolanos, J.P. The bioenergetic and antioxidant status of neurons is controlled by continuous degradation of a key glycolytic enzyme by APC/C-Cdh1. *Nat. Cell Biol.* **2009**, *11*, 747–752. [CrossRef]
35. Allaman, I.; Belanger, M.; Magistretti, P.J. Astrocyte-neuron metabolic relationships: For better and for worse. *Trends Neurosci.* **2011**, *34*, 76–87. [CrossRef]
36. Belanger, M.; Allaman, I.; Magistretti, P.J. Brain energy metabolism: Focus on astrocyte-neuron metabolic cooperation. *Cell Metab.* **2011**, *14*, 724–738. [CrossRef] [PubMed]
37. Berry, K.; Farias-Itao, D.S.; Grinberg, L.T.; Plowey, E.D.; Schneider, J.A.; Rodriguez, R.D.; Suemoto, C.K.; Buckwalter, M.S. B and T Lymphocyte Densities Remain Stable with Age in Human Cortex. *ASN Neuro* **2021**, *13*, 17590914211018117. [CrossRef]
38. Medina-Rodriguez, E.M.; Han, D.; Lowell, J.; Beurel, E. Stress promotes the infiltration of peripheral immune cells to the brain. *Brain Behav. Immun.* **2023**, *111*, 412–423. [CrossRef]
39. Nguyen, J.N.; Chauhan, A. Bystanders or not? Microglia and lymphocytes in aging and stroke. *Neural Regen. Res.* **2023**, *18*, 1397–1403.
40. van der Meer, J.W.; Joosten, L.A.; Riksen, N.; Netea, M.G. Trained immunity: A smart way to enhance innate immune defence. *Mol. Immunol.* **2015**, *68*, 40–44. [CrossRef]
41. Kuhtreiber, W.M.; Faustman, D.L. BCG Therapy for Type 1 Diabetes: Restoration of Balanced Immunity and Metabolism. *Trends Endocrinol. Metab.* **2019**, *30*, 80–92. [CrossRef] [PubMed]
42. Kühtreiber, W.M.; Takahashi, H.; Keefe, R.C.; Song, Y.; Tran, L.; Luck, T.G.; Shpilsky, G.; Moore, L.; Sinton, S.M.; Graham, J.C.; et al. BCG Vaccinations Upregulate Myc, a Central Switch for Improved Glucose Metabolism in Diabetes. *iScience* **2020**, *23*, 101085. [CrossRef] [PubMed]
43. Schwartz, M. Can immunotherapy treat neurodegeneration? Cancer Immunotherapy could guide treatment for Alzheimer's disease. *Science* **2017**, *357*, 254–255. [CrossRef] [PubMed]
44. Abellanas, M.A.; Purnapatre, M.; Burgaletto, C.; Schwartz, M. Monocyte-derived macrophages act as reinforcements when microglia fall short in Alzheimer's disease. *Nat. Neurosci.* **2025**, *28*, 436–445. [CrossRef]
45. Hoozemans, J.J.; van Haastert, E.S.; Nijholt, D.A.; Rozemuller, A.J.; Scheper, W. Activation of the unfolded protein response is an early event in Alzheimer's and Parkinson's disease. *Neurodegener. Dis.* **2012**, *10*, 212–215. [CrossRef]
46. Hoozemans, J.J.M.; Veerhuis, R.; Van Haastert, E.S.; Rozemuller, J.M.; Baas, F.; Eikelenboom, P.; Scheper, W. The unfolded protein response is activated in Alzheimer's disease. *Acta Neuropathol.* **2005**, *110*, 165–172. [CrossRef]
47. Nijholt, D.A.; van Haastert, E.S.; Rozemuller, A.J.; Scheper, W.; Hoozemans, J.J. The unfolded protein response is associated with early tau pathology in the hippocampus of tauopathies. *J. Pathol.* **2012**, *226*, 693–702. [CrossRef]
48. Doody, R.S.; Farlow, M.; Aisen, P.S. Alzheimer's Disease Cooperative Study Data Analysis and Publication Committee Phase 3 Trials of Solanezumab and Bapineuzumab for Alzheimer's Disease. *N. Engl. J. Med.* **2014**, *370*, 1460.
49. Abisambra, J.F.; Jinwal, U.K.; Blair, L.J.; O'Leary, J.C., 3rd; Li, Q.; Brady, S.; Wang, L.; Guidi, C.E.; Zhang, B.; Nordhues, B.A.; et al. Tau accumulation activates the unfolded protein response by impairing endoplasmic reticulum-associated degradation. *J. Neurosci.* **2013**, *33*, 9498–9507. [CrossRef]

50. Kates, M.; Matoso, A.; Choi, W.; Baras, A.S.; Daniels, M.J.; Lombardo, K.; Brant, A.; Mikkilineni, N.; McConkey, D.J.; Kamat, A.M.; et al. Adaptive Immune Resistance to Intravesical BCG in Non-Muscle Invasive Bladder Cancer: Implications for Prospective BCG-Unresponsive Trials. *Clin. Cancer Res.* **2020**, *26*, 882–891. [CrossRef]
51. Bedke, J.; Black, P.C.; Szabados, B.; Guerrero-Ramos, F.; Shariat, S.F.; Xylinas, E.; Brinkmann, J.; Blake-Haskins, J.A.; Cesari, R.; Redorta, J.P. Optimizing outcomes for high-risk, non-muscle-invasive bladder cancer: The evolving role of PD-(L)1 inhibition. *Urol. Oncol.* **2023**, *41*, 461–475. [CrossRef] [PubMed]
52. Reineke, L.C.; Komar, A.A.; Caprara, M.G.; Merrick, W.C. A small stem loop element directs internal initiation of the URE2 internal ribosome entry site in *Saccharomyces cerevisiae*. *J. Biol. Chem.* **2008**, *283*, 19011–19025. [CrossRef]
53. Reineke, L.C.; Cao, Y.; Baus, D.; Hossain, N.M.; Merrick, W.C. Insights into the role of yeast eIF2A in IRES-mediated translation. *PLoS ONE* **2011**, *6*, e24492. [CrossRef] [PubMed]
54. Wen, L.; Xiao, B.; Shi, Y.; Han, F. PERK signalling pathway mediates single prolonged stress-induced dysfunction of medial prefrontal cortex neurons. *Apoptosis* **2017**, *22*, 753–768. [CrossRef] [PubMed]
55. Gow, A.; Wrabetz, L. CHOP and the endoplasmic reticulum stress response in myelinating glia. *Curr. Opin. Neurobiol.* **2009**, *19*, 505–510. [CrossRef]
56. Hetz, C.A. ER stress signaling and the BCL-2 family of proteins: From adaptation to irreversible cellular damage. *Antioxid. Redox Signal.* **2007**, *9*, 2345–2355. [CrossRef]
57. Wang, X.; Olberding, K.E.; White, C.; Li, C. Bcl-2 proteins regulate ER membrane permeability to luminal proteins during ER stress-induced apoptosis. *Cell Death Differ.* **2011**, *18*, 38–47. [CrossRef]
58. Klein, B.Y.; Ben-David, I.; Gofrit, O.N.; Greenblatt, C.L. Repurposing peripheral immunocytes of Bacillus Calmette-Guérin-vaccinated melanoma patients to reveal Alzheimer's disease mechanisms, possibly via the unfolded protein response. *J. Alzheimer's Dis. Rep.* **2025**, *9*, 25424823241309664. [CrossRef]
59. Martin, R.; Nora, M.; Anna, L.; Olivia, P.; Leif, B.; Gunilla, W.-T.; Ellen, T.; Anna-Karin, L.-C. Altered hypoxia-induced cellular responses and inflammatory profile in lung fibroblasts from COPD patients compared to control subjects. *Respir. Res.* **2024**, *25*, 282. [CrossRef]
60. Angelidou, A.; Diray-Arce, J.; Conti, M.-G.; Netea, M.G.; Blok, B.A.; Liu, M.; Sanchez-Schmitz, G.; Ozonoff, A.; van Haren, S.D.; Levy, O. Human Newborn Monocytes Demonstrate Distinct BCG-Induced Primary and Trained Innate Cytokine Production and Metabolic Activation In Vitro. *Front. Immunol.* **2021**, *12*, 674334. [CrossRef]
61. Dias, C.; Fernandes, E.; Barbosa, R.M.; Laranjinha, J.; Ledo, A. Astrocytic aerobic glycolysis provides lactate to support neuronal oxidative metabolism in the hippocampus. *Biofactors* **2023**, *49*, 875–886. [CrossRef] [PubMed]
62. Greenblatt, C.L.; Bercovier, H.; Klein, B.Y.; Gofrit, O.N. Intravesical Bacille Calmette-Guerin (BCG) Vaccine Affects Cognition. *J. Alzheimers Dis.* **2024**, *100*, 771–774. [CrossRef] [PubMed]
63. Kühtreiber, W.M.; Tran, L.; Kim, T.; Dybala, M.; Nguyen, B.; Plager, S.; Huang, D.; Janes, S.; Defusco, A.; Baum, D.; et al. Long-term reduction in hyperglycemia in advanced type 1 diabetes: The value of induced aerobic glycolysis with BCG vaccinations. *Npj Vaccines* **2018**, *3*, 23. [CrossRef] [PubMed]
64. Dias, H.F.; Kuhtreiber, W.M.; Nelson, K.J.; Ng, N.C.; Zheng, H.; Faustman, D.L. Epigenetic changes related to glucose metabolism in type 1 diabetes after BCG vaccinations: A vital role for KDM2B. *Vaccine* **2022**, *40*, 1540–1554. [CrossRef]
65. Klinger, D.; Hill, B.L.; Barda, N.; Halperin, E.; Gofrit, O.N.; Greenblatt, C.L.; Rappoport, N.; Linial, M.; Bercovier, H. Bladder Cancer Immunotherapy by BCG Is Associated with a Significantly Reduced Risk of Alzheimer's Disease and Parkinson's Disease. *Vaccines* **2021**, *9*, 491. [CrossRef]
66. Weinberg, M.S.; Zafar, A.; Magdamo, C.; Chung, S.Y.; Chou, W.H.; Nayan, M.; Deodhar, M.; Frendl, D.M.; Feldman, A.S.; Faustman, D.L.; et al. Association of BCG Vaccine Treatment with Death and Dementia in Patients with Non-Muscle-Invasive Bladder Cancer. *JAMA Netw. Open.* **2023**, *6*, e2314336. [CrossRef]

current issues in molecular biology

MDPI

Article

Assessment of the Concentration of Transforming Growth Factor Beta 1–3 in Degenerated Intervertebral Discs of the Lumbosacral Region of the Spine

Rafał Staszkiewicz [1,2,3,*], Dorian Gładysz [2,3], Dawid Sobański [1,4], Filip Bolechała [5], Edward Golec [6], Małgorzata Sobańska [1,4], Damian Strojny [1,7,8], Artur Turek [9] and Beniamin Oskar Grabarek [1,10]

1 Collegium Medicum, WSB University, 41-300 Dabrowa Gornicza, Poland; drdsobanski@gmail.com (D.S.); sobanskamalgorzata05@gmail.com (M.S.); strojny.ds@gmail.com (D.S.); bgrabarek7@gmail.com (B.O.G.)
2 Department of Neurosurgery, 5th Military Clinical Hospital with the SP ZOZ Polyclinic in Krakow, 30-901 Cracow, Poland; gladyszdorian875@gmail.com
3 Department of Neurosurgery, Faculty of Medicine in Zabrze, Academy of Silesia, 40-555 Katowice, Poland
4 Department of Neurosurgery, Szpital sw. Rafala in Cracow, 30-693 Cracow, Poland
5 Department of Forensic Medicine, Jagiellonian University Medical College, 31-531 Cracow, Poland; filip.bolechala@uj.edu.pl
6 Department of Rehabilitation in Orthopaedics, Faculty of Motor Rehabilitation, Bronisław Czech University of Physical Education, 31-571 Krakow, Poland; bgolec@poczta.onet.pl
7 Institute of Health Care, National Academy of Applied Sciences in Przemyśl, 37-700 Przemyśl, Poland
8 New Medical Techniques Specjalist Hospital of St. Family in Rudna Mała, 36-060 Rzeszów, Poland
9 Chair and Department of Biopharmacy, Faculty of Pharmaceutical Sciences in Sosnowiec, Medical University of Silesia, Katowice, 41-200 Sosnowiec, Poland; a.turek75@gmail.com
10 Department of Molecular Biology, Gyncentrum, Laboratory of Molecular Biology and Virology, 40-851 Katowice, Poland
* Correspondence: rafalstaszkiewicz830@gmail.com

Abstract: The purpose of this study was to evaluate the feasibility of using the expression profile of transforming growth factor beta (TGF-β-1-3) to assess the progression of L/S spine degenerative disease. The study group consisted of 113 lumbosacral (L/S) intervertebral disc (IVD) degenerative disease patients from whom IVDs were collected during a microdiscectomy, whereas the control group consisted of 81 participants from whom IVDs were collected during a forensic autopsy or organ harvesting. Hematoxylin and eosin staining was performed to exclude degenerative changes in the IVDs collected from the control group. The molecular analysis consisted of reverse-transcription real-time quantitative polymerase chain reaction (RT-qPCR), an enzyme-linked immunosorbent assay (ELISA), Western blotting, and an immunohistochemical analysis (IHC). In degenerated IVDs, we noted an overexpression of all TGF-β-1-3 mRNA isoforms with the largest changes observed for TGF-β3 isoforms (fold change (FC) = 19.52 ± 2.87) and the smallest for TGF-β2 (FC = 2.26 ± 0.16). Changes in the transcriptional activity of TGF-β-1-3 were statistically significant ($p < 0.05$). Significantly higher concentrations of TGF-β1 (2797 ± 132 pg/mL vs. 276 ± 19 pg/mL; $p < 0.05$), TGF-β2 (1918 ± 176 pg/mL vs. 159 ± 17 pg/mL; $p < 0.05$), and TGF-β3 (2573 ± 102 pg/mL vs. 152 ± 11 pg/mL) were observed in degenerative IVDs compared with the control samples. Determining the concentration profiles of TGF-β1-3 appears to be a promising monitoring tool for the progression of degenerative disease as well as for evaluating its treatment or developing new treatment strategies with molecular targets.

Keywords: intervertebral disc; intervertebral disc degeneration; transforming growth factor beta

1. Introduction

Degenerative disease of the intervertebral disc (IVD) of the lumbosacral (L/S) spine is a common spinal ailment that is affecting increasingly younger people [1–3]. It is estimated that 60–90% of the population will experience pain symptoms of the L/S spine as a result of degenerative disease at least once in their lifetime [1,2].

The IVD is divided into two main parts, the AF and the nucleus pulposus (NP) [4–7]. The determining factor for the occurrence of spinal pain over the course of the degenerative disease of IVD is the penetration of free nerve endings deep into the annulus fibrosus (AF) of the IVD from the surrounding environment [8–12]. Repeated damage to the connections between the vertebral endplates and the IVD leads to a reduction in hydration and the ability of nutrients to permeate into the IVD, creating conditions for neoinversion [8–12].

From a molecular aspect, in the etiology of the induction and development of pain complaints resulting from L/S spine IVD degenerative disease, it is indicated that a significant role is played by neurotrophic factors, which are primarily secreted by nervous system cells and immune system cells [13–15].

Among the transforming growth factor beta (TGF-β) superfamily proteins involved in the induction and progression of L/S spine IVD degenerative disease are the TGF-β family and the glial-cell-derived neurotrophic factor family [16–19]. Nonetheless, knowledge regarding the induction and development of degenerative spine disease on the molecular level, including the role of TGF-β superfamily molecules, remains fragmented [20]. Hence, TGF-β signalization is required for normal development and IVD growth and may be involved in IVD degeneration [20].

The NP typically exhibits a higher concentration of TGF-β due to its role in promoting extracellular matrix (ECM) production and especially high concentrations of proteoglycans and collagen type II, which are critical for the NP's function as a load-bearing, compressive structure. TGF-β signaling in the NP supports matrix synthesis and cell survival, helping to maintain disc hydration and prevent degeneration. On the other hand, the AF has a lower concentration of TGF-β compared to the NP. This difference is consistent with the AF's composition, which is more focused on producing collagen type I for tensile strength rather than proteoglycans for compression resistance. While TGF-β is still involved in ECM synthesis in the AF, particularly in response to injury or stress, its expression and activity are less prominent compared to that in the NP [4–7,21,22].

Chen et al. found that TGF-β expression changes with age and degeneration progression, though studies in human IVD models have yielded inconclusive results [20]. Nerlich et al. reported elevated TGF-β1 expression in degenerative IVDs with further studies linking TGF-β1 upregulation to degeneration severity [23–25]. Schroeder et al. observed decreased TGF-β in NP tissues but increased expression in AF tissues [26], while Abbott et al. found lower TbRI expression in severely degenerated NPCs [27]. Tsarouhas et al. noted no significant differences in TGF-β1 mRNA expression between herniated and control IVD tissues [28]. Tolonen et al. demonstrated increased TGF-β expression in osteoarthritic IVD samples, underscoring its role in spinal osteoarthritis [29]. Additionally, studies showed that TGF-β concentration rises with the radiological progression of IVD degeneration [30].

TGF-β1 accounts for over 90% of TGF-β activity and is crucial in various biological processes, including angiogenesis and ECM regulation in intervertebral disc (IVD) degeneration [20]. TGF-β1 promotes endothelial cell proliferation and adhesion, contributing to angiogenesis and inflammation during fibrosis [30,31]. TGF-β1 supports ECM synthesis and reduces apoptosis in early degeneration stages but also drives angiogenesis and fibrosis as degeneration progresses, particularly through VEGF expression in response to hypoxia [20,32–35].

Therefore, the aim of this study was to assess changes in the concentration profile of TGF-β-1-3 mRNA and proteins in degenerated IVDs of the lumbosacral (L/S) spine, depending on the degree of degeneration.

2. Materials and Methods

2.1. Ethical Considerations

This study was performed according to the 2013 Declaration of Helsinki guidelines on human experimentation. Data confidentiality and patient anonymity were maintained at all times. Patient-identifying information was deleted before the database was analyzed. Identifying patients individually in this article or in the database is impossible. Informed consent was obtained from all the patients. Approval from the bioethical committee operating at the Regional Medical Chamber in Krakow (No. 162/KBL/OIL/2021) was obtained for this study. The issue of obtaining post-mortem material for research is regulated by the Act of 1 July 2005, on the collection, storage, and transplantation of cells, tissues, and organs (Journal of Laws of 2020, Item 2134) [36].

Written informed consent was obtained from all the patients involved in the study, including consent to publish this paper. Each participant was fully informed of the nature of the study, and their rights were thoroughly protected throughout the process.

2.2. Study Group

The study group comprised 113 patients (55 women, 49%; 58 men, 51%; mean age of 45.5 ± 1.5 years) diagnosed with IVD disease of the L/S spine, who met the criteria for microdiscectomy surgery. The diagnosis process involved a comprehensive assessment, including magnetic resonance imaging (MRI), clinical symptom evaluation, neurological and physical examinations, and a detailed patient interview. Patients included in the study had IVD degeneration characterized by prolapse or extrusion and experienced persistent discogenic pain or symptomatic sciatica that had not improved after at least six weeks of non-surgical treatment. Due to the lack of symptom relief or worsening of their condition, these patients were scheduled for surgical intervention. This selection ensured that the study group represented individuals with confirmed, isolated degeneration of the L/S spine IVD, which was consistent with criteria established for surgical intervention. Specific criteria for the inclusion and exclusion of patients in the study group were presented in previous publications [37,38]. The study applied specific inclusion and exclusion criteria to ensure a consistent sample within the study group of patients with isolated intervertebral disc (IVD) degeneration in the lumbosacral spine. Eligible participants were adults over 18 years old who demonstrated lumbosacral spine IVD degeneration characterized by disc prolapse or extrusion on MRI. Inclusion also required patients to have experienced discogenic pain or symptomatic sciatica that had not responded to non-surgical treatment for at least six weeks. Additionally, participants had to have no other coexisting spinal pathologies, and the disease duration needed to be between six and twelve weeks to align with the study's focus on recent, isolated degeneration cases. Conversely, patients under 18 years old were excluded, as were those with MRI findings of protrusion or sequestration-type disc degeneration. Individuals with prior surgical interventions for lumbosacral spine degeneration, spine-related inflammatory or autoimmune diseases, or a history of trauma were also excluded. Other exclusion criteria for the study group included mental disorders such as dementia, polyneuropathy, pregnancy, and the presence of significant coexisting diseases, various types of cancers (e.g., metastatic tumors, leukemia, and spinal cord tumors), osteoporosis, and active spinal infections. Patients with less than six weeks or more than twelve weeks of disease duration were also excluded to ensure uniformity in the timeframe of disease progression under investigation [37,38].

The degree of advancement of the L/S spine IVD degenerative disease was defined using the Pfirrmann scale [22]. Pfirrmann developed a five-stage radiological classification system to evaluate the severity of IVD degeneration using MRI [39–41].

In 27 patients, the advancement of degenerative changes corresponded to grade 2 on the Pfirrmann scale; 43 patients had grade 3 advancement of changes according to the Pfirrmann scale; in 32 patients, the changes corresponded to grade 4 according to the Pfirrmann scale; and in 11 patients, the changes corresponded to grade 5 on the Pfirrmann scale. Specifically, 18 IVDs (15.93%) were taken from the L1/L2 segment, 26 cases (23%)

from the L2/L3 segment, 27 cases (23.89%) from the L3/L4 segment, 32 cases (28.32%) from the L4/L5 segment, and 10 cases (8.86%) from the L5/S1 segment [38].

2.3. Control Group

The control group consisted of 81 participants (43 women, 53%; 38 men, 47%; a mean age of 31.5 ± 1.5 years old) from whom L/S spine IVD samples were collected post-mortem during a forensic autopsy or organ collection no more than 48 h after death. IVDs were removed from the L1/L2 segment in 12 cases (14.81%), the L2/L3 segment in 16 cases (19.75%), the L3/L4 segment in 18 cases (22.22%), the L4/L5 segment in 27 cases (33.33%), and the L5/S1 segment in 8 cases (9.89%) [38].

Specific criteria for the inclusion and exclusion of patients in the control group were presented in previous publications. The control group participants were selected based on specific inclusion and exclusion criteria to ensure a comparison group without signs of IVDs degeneration. Participants in the control group were required to be up to 45 years of age and show no signs of degeneration in the collected tissue samples, as confirmed by microscopic examination with hematoxylin and eosin staining (H&E). Additionally, eligible participants had no history of neoplastic diseases or inflammatory conditions affecting the spine or surrounding tissues. Participants were excluded from the control group if they were over 45 years old or if microscopic examination revealed any degenerative features in the collected material. A history of neoplastic disease or inflammatory spinal conditions also led to exclusion, including conditions such as osteomyelitis, IVD inflammation, epidural empyema, shingles, arthritis, inflammatory infiltrates of the rectum, Scheuermann's disease, and Paget's disease. Those with a general history of spinal or inflammatory disease were not eligible for the control group, ensuring that participants represented a non-degenerated baseline [37,38].

The confirmation of the absence of degenerative changes in the collected IVD samples was performed using H&E staining in accordance with the study protocol. An example of H&E staining is shown in our previous publication [38].

2.4. Securing the Extracted Material for Molecular Examination

The clinical materials (IVDs) were extracted from patients in the study group during a microdiscectomy using the en bloc method as well as from deceased patients. After the IVDs were thoroughly washed to remove blood, they were placed into sterile Eppendorf tubes pre-filled with TRIzol reagent (Invitrogen Life Technologies, Carlsbad, CA, USA) and stored at −80 °C until the molecular section of the experiment commenced (RT-qPCR, ELISA, Western blot analysis) or embedded in paraffin (POL-AURA, Dywity, Poland) for the immunohistochemical (IHC) analysis. Storing samples at low temperatures effectively minimizes endogenous RNase activity, which is a critical precaution for ensuring successful RNA extraction [42–44]. The tissue samples were generally small and consistent with the needs of histological and biochemical analyses. The typical size of the samples ranged from [insert specific dimensions, e.g., 1–2 cm in diameter and 0.5 cm in thickness], allowing for both immediate study and long-term storage.

The molecular analysis was performed on 113 degenerated IVD samples and 81 control samples.

2.5. Extraction of Whole Ribonucleic Acid (RNA)

First, the study and control samples were homogenized using a hand-held homogenizer (T18 Digital Ultra-Turrax, IKA Polska Sp. z o.o., Warsaw, Poland) until no solid fragments were visible [42,44,45].

The extraction of whole RNA from the study and control samples was conducted using a modified Chomczyński–Sacchi method with the use of TRIzol reagent (Invitrogen Life Technologies, Carlsbad, CA, USA), as recommended by the manufacturer. After this procedure, the extracts were dried and stored in this form at a temperature of −80 °C until the next stage of the molecular analysis. An assessment of the RNA extract quality was conducted using electrophoretic separation in a 1% agarose gel stained with ethidium bromide at a concentration of 0.5 mg/mL (SigmaAldrich, St. Louis, MO, USA), and a quantitative assessment was performed through a spectrophotometric measurement (Nanodrop®, Thermo Fisher Scientific, Waltham, MA, USA).

2.6. Determination of Changes in the Expression Profile of TGF-β-1-3 mRNA in Degenerated and Control IVDs Using RT-qPCR

The RT-qPCR reaction was performed using a set of Sensi-Fast™ One-Step Probe Assay reagents (Bioline, London, UK). RT-qPCR was conducted in 50 μL of reaction mixture with the following thermal profile: reverse transcription (45 °C, 10 min); polymerase activation (95 °C, 2 min); and 40 three-step cycles consisting of denaturation (95 °C, 5 s), hybridization (60 °C, 10 s), and annealing (72 °C, 5 s). The RT-qPCR primers were purchased from Genomed (Gdańsk, Poland), and their nucleotide sequence is provided in Table 1. Glyceraldehyde 3-phosphate dehydrogenase (GAPDH) was used as an endogenous control for RT-qPCR. For each biological repeat, three technical repeats were conducted.

Table 1. Nucleotide sequence of the primers used in RT-qPCR for TGF-β-1-3 and GAPDH.

mRNA	Oligonucleotide Sequence	Tm (°C)
TGF-β1	Forward: 5′-GGCCAGATCCTGTCCAAGC-3′ Reverse: 5′-GTGGGTTTCCACCATTAGCAC-3′	85.4
TGF-β2	Forward: 5′-CAGCACACTCGATATGGACCA-3′ Reverse: 5′-CCTCGGGCTCAGGATAGTCT-3′	88.7
TGF-β3	Forward: 5′-CTGGATTGTGGTTCCATGCA-3′ Reverse: 5′-TCCCCGAATGCCTCACAT-3′	86.6
GAPDH	Forward: 5′-GGTGAAGGTCGGAGTCAACGGA-3′ Reverse: 5′-GAGGGATCTCGCTCCTGGAAGA-3′	86.4

Forward, sense primer; reverse, antisense primer; Tm, melting temperature; GAPDH, glyceraldehyde 3-phosphate dehydrogenase; TGF-β-1-3, transforming growth factor beta 1-3. The specificity of RT-qPCR was confirmed by determining the melting temperature for each amplimer.

Because the PCR efficiency ranged from 90% to 110% and GAPDH had stable expression across all samples (both healthy and diseased), changes in gene expression were presented as the normalized relative mRNA expression ($2^{-\Delta\Delta Ct}$ method), where 1 corresponded to an equal expression of the given gene in the study and control samples; a result below 1 corresponded to the decreased expression of the gene in the study samples compared with the control; and a result above 1 indicated an overexpression of the given gene in the study samples compared to the control.

2.7. Determination of the Profile of TGF-β-1-3 Proteins Through ELISA and Western Blot Separation Procedures in Degenerated and Healthy IVDs

Changes in the concentration profile of TGF-β-1-3 in normal and degenerated IVDs were determined using ELISA and electrophoretic separation in a polyacrylamide gel (Western blot), using the following antibodies: polyclonal anti-TGF-β1 antibody bs-0086R (STI, Poznan, Poland; 1:1000 dilution), polyclonal anti-TGF-β2 antibody bs-20412R (STI, Poznan, Poland; 1:1000 dilution), and polyclonal anti-TGF-β3 antibody bs-0099R (STI, Poznan, Poland; 1:1000 dilution), according to the manufacturer's recommendations.

GAPDH sc-47724 (GAPDH; Santa Cruz Biotech, Dallas, TX, USA; 1:500 dilution) was used as the endogenous control protein. The secondary antibody used was HRP-conjugated goat anti-rabbit IgG (BioRad, Milan, Italy; catalog number 1706515; 1:3000 dilution). The absorbance at 540 nm was measured using an M200PRO plate reader (Tecan, Männedorf, Switzerland).

A detailed protocol for conducting the ELISA and Western blot procedures is provided in previous papers [37,38].

2.8. IHC Analysis

The specimens were sectioned on a microtome (Leica Microsystems, Wetzlar, Germany) into 8.0 μm thick serial slices. The subsequent preparation steps of the tissue sections, such as dehydration, antigen retrieval, antibody incubations, and staining, were performed according to the manufacturer's instruction manuals (DAB Substrate Kit, Peroxidase (HRP), Vector Laboratories, Newark, California, USA, and IHC-Paraffin Protocol (IHC-P), Abcam plc, Cambridge, UK). The obtained immunohistochemical reactions were examined and captured on a Nikon Coolpix fluorescent optic system. Both the cellular location of the selected proteins and their quantity were assessed through a computer image analysis using the ImageJ software [46]. A total of 15 photographs were taken from three slides of each patient under 200× magnification. Using the ImageJ software with the IHC-Profiler plug-in [47], the optical density of the DAB reaction products was evaluated in the fields where the immunohistochemical reaction occurred in response to the presence of the selected proteins. An average percentage of the DAB-stained area was also calculated in relation to the background values in each field. An example of H&E staining is shown in our previous work [38].

2.9. Statistical Analysis

The statistical analysis of the results was performed by assuming a statistical significance threshold (p) of <0.05 in Statistica 13 PL software (Statsoft, Krakow, Poland). The Shapiro–Wilk test was used to assess the conformity of the data distribution with a normal distribution, which was confirmed. Accordingly, the next statistical analysis stage used parametric methods, i.e., Student's t-test for independent groups or a one-way ANOVA and Tukey's post hoc test. The homogeneity of variance was checked using Levene's test.

3. Results

3.1. Changes in the Expression Profile of TGF-β-1-3 mRNA in Degenerated and Control IVDs

In degenerated IVDs, we noted an overexpression of all TGF-β-1-3 mRNA isoforms with the largest changes observed for *TGF-β3* isoforms (fold change (FC) = 19.52 ± 2.87) and the smallest for TGF-β2 (FC = 2.26 ± 0.16). Changes in the transcriptional activity of TGF-β-1-3 were statistically significant ($p < 0.05$).

3.2. TGF-β-1-3 Protein Expression Profile Determined Through the Enzyme-Linked Immunosorbent Assay (ELISA) Technique

The expression levels of the TGF-β1, TGF-β2, and TGF-β3 isoforms were assessed in both the study group (patients with degenerated IVDs) and the control group (participants with non-degenerated IVDs) using the ELISA technique. The results revealed significantly elevated concentrations of all three TGF-β isoforms in the degenerated IVDs when compared to the control group (Table 2; $p < 0.05$).

In the study group, TGF-β1 and TGF-β3 were expressed at comparable levels, while TGF-β2 exhibited the lowest concentration among the three isoforms. On the other hand, in the control group, TGF-β1 was the most abundantly expressed isoform with TGF-β3 being the least expressed (Table 2; $p < 0.05$).

A further analysis of the study group, stratified according to the severity of disc degeneration using the Pfirrmann grading system (grades 2 to 5), revealed a dynamic pattern in the concentration of the TGF-β isoforms. The concentrations of all three isoforms progressively increased with the advancement of degenerative changes from Pfirrmann grade 2 through grade 4 (Table 2; $p < 0.05$). Specifically, the concentration of TGF-β1 increased from 2876 ± 123 pg/mL in grades 2 and 3 to 198 ± 176 pg/mL in grade 4. Similarly, TGF-β2 increased from 1834 ± 201 pg/mL in grade 2 to 2043 ± 156 pg/mL in grade 4, and TGF-β3 increased from 2545 ± 165 pg/mL in grade 2 to 2761 ± 209 pg/mL in grade 4 (Table 2).

Table 2. Concentration of TGF-β-1-3 in L/S spine IVDs collected from the study and control groups, determined using ELISA.

Isoform of TGF-β	Group	Concentration (pg/mL)	95% CI
TGF-β1 [a,b,d,e]	Control	276 ± 19	210–345
	Study	2797 ± 132	2541–3098
	Pfirrmann 2	2876 ± 123	2456–3087
	Pfirrmann 3	3127 ± 165	2987–3456
	Pfirrmann 4	3198 ± 176	2898–3298
	Pfirrmann 5	1987 ± 156	1765–2321
TGF-β2 [a,b,e]	Control	159 ± 17	140–198
	Study	1918 ± 176	1561–2198
	Pfirrmann 2	1834 ± 201	1656–2098
	Pfirrmann 3	2034 ± 165	1871–2198
	Pfirrmann 4	2043 ± 156	1876–2198
	Pfirrmann 5	1761 ± 198	1456–2001
TGF-β3 [a,b,c,d,e]	Control	152 ± 11	134–189
	Study	2573 ± 102	2345–2761
	Pfirrmann 2	2545 ± 165	2456–2671
	Pfirrmann 3	2767 ± 187	2571–2981
	Pfirrmann 4	2761 ± 209	2671–2891
	Pfirrmann 5	2219 ± 187	2091–2348

TGF-β-1-3, transforming growth factor beta isoforms; 95% CI, 95% confidence interval; a, statistically significant difference in protein concentration between study and control groups ($p < 0.05$); b, statistically significant difference in protein concentration between Pfirrmann 4 and Pfirrmann 5 groups ($p < 0.05$); c, statistically significant difference in protein concentration between Pfirrmann 2 and Pfirrmann 4 groups ($p < 0.05$); d, statistically significant difference in protein concentration between Pfirrmann 2 and Pfirrmann 5 groups ($p < 0.05$); e, statistically significant difference in protein concentration between Pfirrmann 3 and Pfirrmann 5 groups ($p < 0.05$). Results are presented as mean ± standard deviation.

However, in the most advanced stage of degeneration (Pfirrmann grade 5), a decline in the concentrations of all three TGF-β isoforms was observed. The TGF-β1 levels decreased to 1987 ± 156 pg/mL, the TGF-β2 levels decreased to 1761 ± 198 pg/mL, and the TGF-β3 levels decreased to 2219 ± 187 pg/mL (Table 2; $p < 0.05$). These findings suggest that while the TGF-β expression is initially upregulated in response to disc degeneration, there may be a threshold at which further degeneration results in a decrease in these cytokine levels.

3.3. TGF-β-1-3 Concentration Profile in Degenerated and Control IVDs Determined Using the Western Blot Technique

The expression profile of TGF-β-1-3 in degenerated and control IVDs, determined using the Western blot technique, was the same as that noted in the ELISA procedure. Figure 1 presents an example electropherogram that confirms the specificity of the reaction as well as the nativity of the samples (based on the GAPDH result; molecular mass of 36 kDa). Normalized relative to GAPDH, the band optical density for TGF-β1 (molecular weight of 44 kDa) in the study samples was 9.87 ± 4.31, and it was 0.67 ± 0.12 in the control samples ($p < 0.05$). Normalized relative to GAPDH, the band optical density for TGF-β2 (molecular weight of 50 kDa) in the study samples was 3.29 ± 0.98, and it was 0.91 ± 0.28 in the control samples ($p < 0.05$). Normalized relative to GAPDH, the band optical density for TGF-β3 (molecular weight of 47 kDa) in the study samples was 5.98 ± 1.09, and in the control samples, it was 0.18 ± 0.07 ($p < 0.05$).

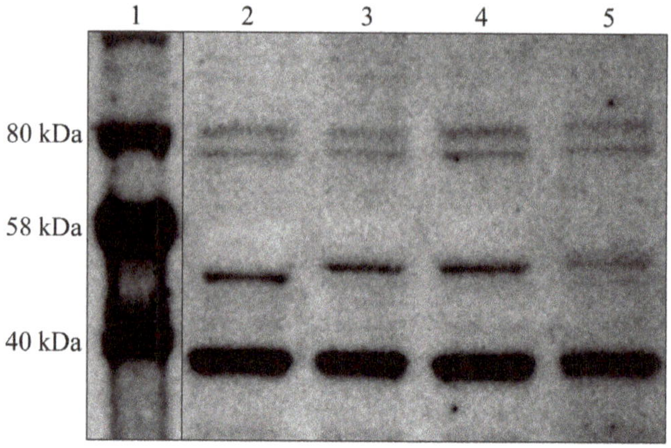

Figure 1. Normalized expression of TGF-β-1-3 in IVDs normalized against GAPDH expression. Track 1, molecular weight marker; Track 2, TGF-β-1;Track 3, TGF-β-2; Track 4;, TGF-β-3, Track 5, GAPDH.

The normalized band optical density of TGF-β-1-3 in degenerated and control IVDs is presented in Figure 2.

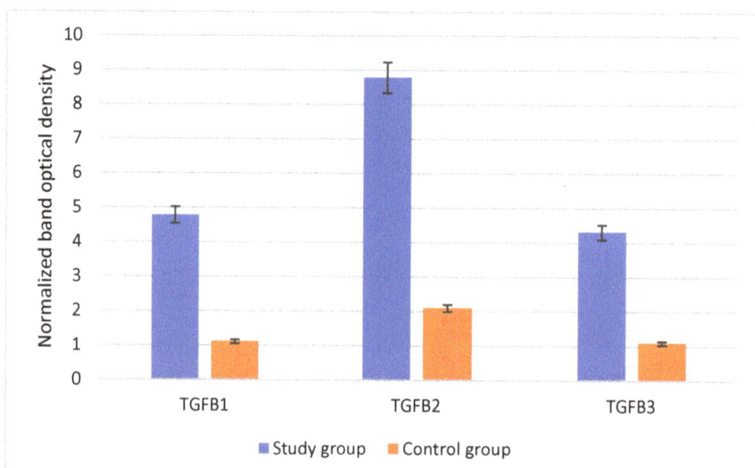

Figure 2. Band optical density of TGF-β-1-3 in L/S spine IVDs collected from the study and control groups determined using Western blotting. TGF-β-1-3, transforming growth factor beta isoforms.

3.4. TGF-β-1-3 Expression in IVDs Collected from Patients in the Study Group and Control Group Participants, Determined Through the IHC Technique

The expression of TGF-β1, TGF-β2, and TGF-β3 was visualized in both degenerated and non-degenerated (control) intervertebral discs (IVDs) using the IHC technique.

Quantitatively, the optical density of the IHC reaction product revealed a significantly higher expression of the TGF-β isoforms in the degenerated IVDs compared to the control group. For TGF-β1, the optical density in the degenerated IVDs was 430.63% of the control group ($p < 0.05$), showing a marked upregulation in degenerated tissues (Table 3). Similarly, the optical densities for TGF-β2 and TGF-β3 in the study group were 418.10% and 395.41% of the control, respectively ($p < 0.05$), reflecting substantial increases in these isoforms in degenerated IVDs as well.

Table 3. The optical density of the reaction product for selected proteins in IVDs obtained from the study and control groups.

Isoform of TGF-β	Group	Optical Density	95% CI
TGF-β1 [a,b,c,e,f]	Control	1.11 ± 0.13	1.04–1.18
	Study	4.78 ± 0.65	4.45–5.11
	Pfirrmann 2	3.29 ± 0.91	2.83–3.75
	Pfirrmann 3	6.42 ± 1.23	5.79–7.04
	Pfirrmann 4	7.29 ± 1.87	6.34–8.24
	Pfirrmann 5	2.09 ± 0.54	1.82–2.36
TGF-β2 [a,c,f]	Control	2.10 ± 0.32	1.93–2.26
	Study	8.78 ± 0.18	8.69–8.87
	Pfirrmann 2	5.44 ± 0.23	5.33–5.56
	Pfirrmann 3	7.01 ± 0.55	6.73–7.28
	Pfirrmann 4	12.11 ± 2.32	10.94–13.28
	Pfirrmann 5	10.57 ± 1.98	9.57–11.57
TGF-β3 [a,c,d,e,f]	Control	1.09 ± 0.18	0.99–1.18
	Study	4.31 ± 0.98	3.81–4.81
	Pfirrmann 2	2.00 ± 0.14	1.93–2.07
	Pfirrmann 3	4.34 ± 0.71	3.98–4.70
	Pfirrmann 4	5.21 ± 0.56	4.93–5.49
	Pfirrmann 5	5.68 ± 0.34	5.51–5.85

TGF-β-1-3, transforming growth factor beta 1-3. Data are presented as mean ± standard deviation. a, statistically significant difference in protein concentration between study and control groups ($p < 0.05$); b, statistically significant difference in protein concentration between Pfirrmann 4 and Pfirrmann 5 groups ($p < 0.05$); c, statistically significant difference in protein concentration between Pfirrmann 2 and Pfirrmann 4 groups ($p < 0.05$); d, statistically significant difference in protein concentration between Pfirrmann 2 and Pfirrmann 5 groups ($p < 0.05$); e, statistically significant difference in protein concentration between Pfirrmann 3 and Pfirrmann 5 groups ($p < 0.05$). Results are presented as mean ± standard deviation. f, statistically significant difference in protein concentration between Pfirrmann 3 and Pfirrmann 4 groups ($p < 0.05$).

The study group also showed variations in TGF-β expression across different stages of degeneration, as classified by the Pfirrmann grading system. For TGF-β1, the optical density increased progressively from Pfirrmann grade 2 (3.29 ± 0.91) to grade 4 (7.29 ± 1.87) before decreasing in grade 5 (2.09 ± 0.54). A similar trend was observed for TGF-β2, with the highest optical density observed in Pfirrmann grade 4 (12.11 ± 2.32), which was followed by a decrease in grade 5 (10.57 ± 1.98). TGF-β3 also exhibited progressive increases from Pfirrmann grade 2 (2.00 ± 0.14) to grade 5 (5.68 ± 0.34), though this pattern was less pronounced than for TGF-β1 and TGF-β2 (Table 3).

These findings suggest that the expression of TGF-β isoforms is significantly upregulated in degenerated discs and varies according to the stage of degeneration. The highest expression levels are generally observed in mid-level degenerative stages (Pfirrmann 3 and 4), followed by a decline in the most advanced degenerative stage (Pfirrmann 5), indicating a potential complex role for TGF-β in the pathophysiology of disc degeneration. Examples of the immunochemical expression of TGF-β-1-3 in the study and control samples are presented in Figure 3.

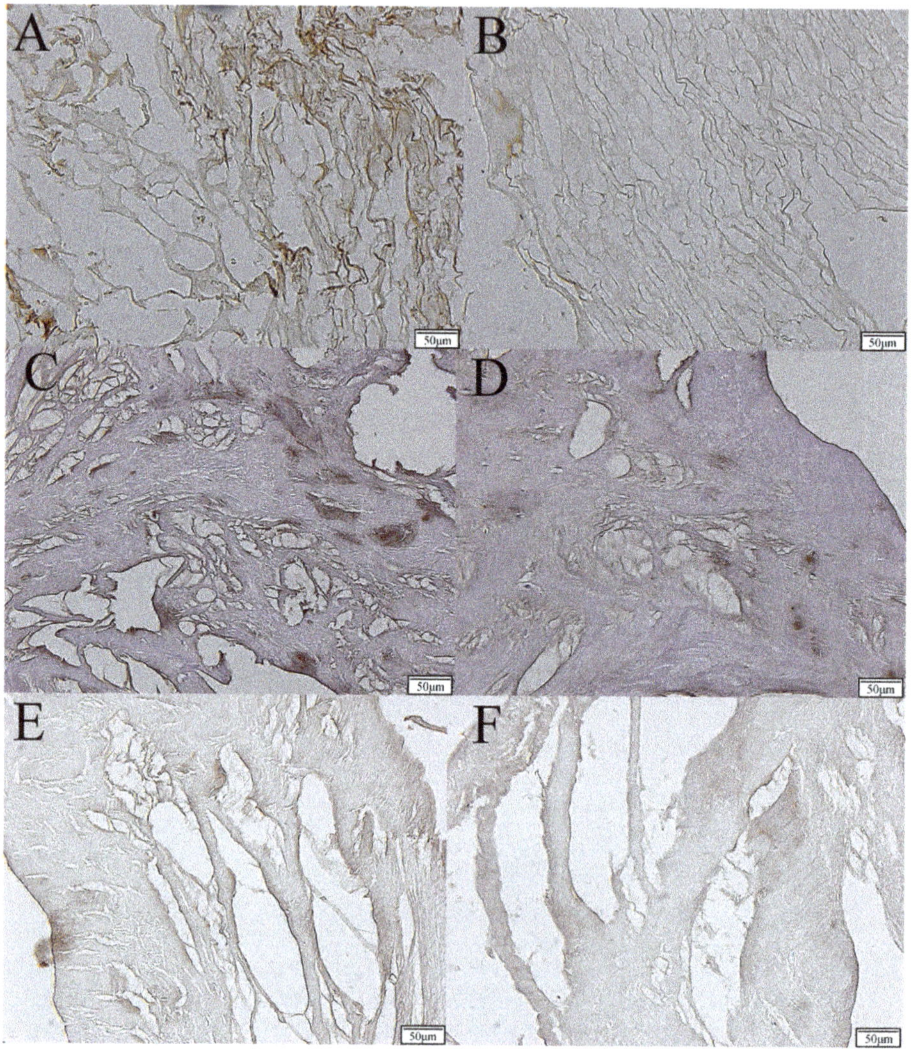

Figure 3. The immunochemical expression of TGF-β-1-3 in the study and control samples. TGF-β-1-3, transforming growth factor beta 1-3. (**A**)—expression of TGF-β-1 in the study group; (**B**)—expression of TGF-β-1 in the control group; (**C**)—expression of TGF-β-2 in the study group; (**D**)—expression of TGF-β-2 in the control group; (**E**)—expression of TGF-β-3 in the study group; (**F**)—expression of TGF-β-3 in the control group.

4. Discussion

The TGF-β family plays a very important role in homeostatic behavior over the course of spinal osteoarthritis [48–50]. In mammals, three TGF-β isoforms have been identified, namely TGF-β1, TGF-β2, and TGF-β3 [51].

It seems that TGF-β fulfills a protective function in the development of IVD degenerative disease through the activation of extracellular matrix synthesis or through the inhibition of catabolic processes occurring in the cell [52]. Nonetheless, the overexpression of TGF-β family members is considered a promoting factor for IVD degenerative changes, namely by contributing to an increase in the nerve growth factor (NGF) concentration, which is considered a significant factor in the etiopathogenesis of pain over the course of IVD degeneration [20,53]. It seems that the duality of TGF-β's action may be related to the pathways activated by this cytokine [49,54]. In joints not affected by the degenerative process, the TGF-β expressed by chondrocytes exerts a protective effect through the SMAD2/3 pathway, whereas during the degenerative process, the SMAD1/5/8 pathway is activated [55]. Bian et al. [52,56] noted in a mouse model of IVD degeneration that the administration of a TGF-βR1 receptor inhibitor inhibited the signalization of R-SMAD, contributing to a decrease in the grade of IVD degeneration [52,56]. However, Kwon et al. [57] noted an increase in the concentration of TGF-β1 and the activation of the SMAD2/3 and SMAD1/5/8 pathways in bovine IVDs, whereby the SMAD1/5/8 cascade may contribute to the inhibition of the SMAD2/3 pathway, the result of which was an advancement in IVD degeneration [57]. Nevertheless, it should be noted that the vast majority of the studies regarding the role of TGF-β in IVD degenerative disease were conducted on animal models and lasted a few days or weeks, whereas in the case of human tissues and cells, there exists a tendency for aging and the degeneration of material. Therefore, further analyses are necessary [49].

Previous studies have indicated that the concentration of some pro-inflammatory cytokines, such as tumor necrosis factor (TNF) and interleukin (IL)-1β, increases over the course of the IVD degeneration process, promoting the degradation of the ECM. This is mediated by an increased expression of catabolic enzymes, including matrix metalloproteinases (MMPs) and a disintegrin and metalloproteinase with thrombospondin motifs (ADAMTS) [58,59]. Therefore, it is suggested that TGF-β may exert a regulatory effect on the expression of genes encoding proteins responsible for ECM degradation [60–63]. On the other hand, observations conducted regarding signalization dependent on TGF-β indicate that it may exert not only a destructive but also a protective effect on the ECM [60–63].

It seems that TGF-β actively participates in the synthesis of glycosaminoglycans (GAG) through the SMAD-dependent pathway, the Ras homolog gene family member A (RHOA)/Rho-associated protein kinase (ROCK) pathway, and the mitogen-activated protein kinase (MAPK) pathway [64–68]. Furthermore, TGF-β induces the expression of aggrecan, proteoglycans, and type II collagen [64–68]. This confirms the duality of TGF-β's action and the signaling cascades activated by it, while the biological effect exerted by TGF-β is dependent on age [64–68].

In vivo research regarding the expression pattern of TGF-β in the context of IVD degenerative disease was conducted on both animal and human models.

Nagano et al. [69] determined the expression of TGF-β-1-3 and its receptors (TGF-βRI-III) through immunohistochemical staining using IVDs obtained from 10 mice at the ages of 8, 24, and 50 weeks after birth as a research model [69]. These authors demonstrated the expression of TGF-β-1-3 and TGF-βRI-III in 8-week-old mice, noting a decrease in the concentration together with the age of the mice. This observation confirmed the involvement of TGF-β-1-3 in postnatal IVD development and the degeneration process [69].

The same observations as those of Nagano et al. [54] were noted in a study conducted by Matsunaga et al. [70]. Additionally, Zhang et al. [71] determined a decrease in the SMAD2 and SMAD3 protein concentrations in C57BL/6 mice at 2 and 18 months old [71].

In this article, the expression profile of TGF-β-1-3 was determined in the whole IVD, not separately in the NP and AF. Therefore, a valuable addition to this study would be to determine the TGF-β-1-3 expression in the NP and AF. However, during the collection of IVDs from study group participants, the en bloc technique was used, which makes it difficult to separate the two compartments of the IVD structure. This technique involves the removal of a herniated disc in one single, intact piece (en bloc) rather than in fragments, as is typical in a traditional microdiscectomy. As a result, the anatomical boundaries between the AF, NP, and CEP may be preserved as they are extracted together, potentially complicating the post-operative separation of these components for further study or analysis.

In turn, Murakami et al. [72] indicated an increased expression of TGF-β1 mRNA in the NP and AF of rabbits at 6 months and 3 years of age [72]. Moreover, Hiyama et al. [73]

determined the overexpression of TGF-β2, TGF-β3, SMAD3, and SMAD5 in rat NPs, while SMAD3 expression decreased in the AF [73]. Changes in the expression profile of TGF-β-1-3 at the MRNA and protein levels in an animal model suggest that its expression is not only dependent on the IVD compartment but can also be regulated by microRNA (miRNA) [74,75].

The significant costs, pain, and disability associated with degenerative disc disease (DDD) highlight the critical need for a biological agent capable of mitigating the progression of this condition [76].

Additionally, reports indicating the use of TGF-β-dependent signaling as a potential target in IVD degenerative disease therapy, using molecular targets, are worthy of attention. Yang et al. indicated an overexpression of TGF-β1 in a coculture model of NP cells with bone marrow mesenchymal cells compared to cultures containing NP cells alone, which was associated with the inhibition of nuclear factor kappa B (NF-κB)-dependent signaling [32,33]. Additionally, Xiong et al. [77] compared the concentration of TGF-β1 and proteins dependent on signalization activated by this cytokine in cervical spine IVDs in a group of patients with cervical osteoarthritis in relation to the co-occurrence of osteophytes or ossifications around the IVD [77]. Additionally, emerging treatments for IVD degeneration involve the use of platelet-rich plasma (PRP), which contains a platelet-derived growth factor, TGF-β, an epidermal growth factor, insulin-like growth factor 1, and VEGF. These components exhibit potent anti-inflammatory and regenerative properties that promote the repair of damaged tissue [78]. A 2016 prospective randomized controlled trial enrolled 47 patients to evaluate the PRP treatment for IDD. Of these, 29 received PRP injections, while the remaining 18 were administered only contrast agents. The group treated with PRP injections demonstrated pain relief and improved functionality as early as eight weeks post-treatment with benefits persisting for at least one year and no reported adverse events [79].

In vivo experiments have demonstrated that the transfection of TGF-β1 in rabbit NP cells led to increased proteoglycan synthesis [80]. Similarly, the transfection of TGF-β1 in aged human NP cells promoted the production of both proteoglycans and collagen [22]. In turn, Matta et al. found a decrease in the expression of TGF-β1, connective tissue growth factor (CTGF), and WNT1-inducible signaling pathway protein 2 (WISP2) in degenerative disc NPs, suggesting a link to the loss of notochordal cells (NCs). Notably, in their pre-clinical models, treatment with a combination of TGF-β1 and CTGF successfully restored a healthy, cellular NP rich in NCs and stem cells compared to the sham control discs. Furthermore, their findings showed that the TGF-β1 and CTGF treatment enhanced cell viability, deoxyribonucleic acid (DNA) synthesis, and the expression of healthy ECM genes in NP cells derived from degenerative human discs [81]. In their review report, Hodgkinson et al. also evaluated the therapeutic potential of TGF-β in IVD degeneration. They found that GDF (100 ng/mL) with TGF-β1 had a synergic effect on promotor chondrogenic differentiation [82]. Previous research has identified that a single injection of a combination of recombinant human (rh) TGF-β1 and CTGF proteins into the NP of an injured intervertebral disc (IVD) can effectively mediate IVD degeneration in pre-clinical rodent models. In this study, a novel molecular therapy, NTG-101, containing rhTGF-β1 and rhCTGF proteins suspended in an excipient solution was developed, and its efficacy was evaluated using in vivo models of DDD, including the rat-tail model and chondrodystrophic (CD) canines. The findings demonstrated that a single intra-discal injection of NTG-101 produced anti-degenerative effects, leading to a reduction in the expression of pro-inflammatory cytokines such as IL-1β, IL-6, and IL-8, as well as ECM-degrading enzymes such as MMP-13 and cyclooxygenase-2 (Cox-2). Furthermore, the treatment induced pro-anabolic effects in the IVD-NP, restoring the expression of healthy extracellular matrix (ECM) proteins, including aggrecan and collagen 2A1 [83]. In turn, Risbud et al. demonstrated that TGF-β3 can enhance the structure and function of the NP and AF by increasing the levels of activated ERK1/2, which in turn regulates TGF-β receptors I and II (TGF-β-RI and TGF-β-RII) [84]. Hegewald et al. confirmed this finding and suggested that the administration of TGF-β3 could be a potential candidate for the biological treatment of AF degeneration. They showed that AF stimulation with TGF-β3 was associated with an increased production of type X collagen [85]. Given the results proposed for the potential use of TGF-β in IVD degeneration [22,79–84], along with the dual nature of TGF-β's role in the disease [31,86,87], it appears that administering TGF-β within the IVD is justified in the early and late stages of degenerative disc disease (Pfirrmann grades 2 and 5). However, greater therapeutic success in treating IVD degeneration would likely be observed in the early stages of degeneration. On the other hand, in the intermediate stages of IVD degeneration, it seems that molecular treatments should focus on inhibiting the expression of TGF-β and its related pathways. Nevertheless, further research is necessary.

The safety concerns surrounding gene therapy pose challenges for its clinical use. Specifically, the potential risk of tumor formation associated with high-dose exposure and prolonged application in treating chronic IVD degeneration has emerged as a significant issue. Advancements in the reliability of viral vector designs and better control over transgene expression could pave the way for safer and more effective clinical applications of gene therapy [88,89].

The current study, while providing valuable insights into the role of TGF-β isoforms in IVDs degeneration, has several limitations that future research could address to deepen understanding. Notably, investigating the methylation status of TGF-β-1-3 genes in both degenerated and healthy disc tissues could reveal epigenetic regulation in response to degeneration, potentially indicating reversible pathways. Additionally, miRNAs may modulate TGF-β-1-3 expression in disc tissues with specific miRNAs potentially acting as regulators or biomarkers for early-stage degeneration. Employing a microarray analysis could expand understanding by identifying co-expressed genes and pathways that interact with TGF-β, including those involved in inflammation and extracellular matrix degradation. Moreover, assessing the prevalence of polymorphic variants within TGF-β1-3 genes may reveal genetic predispositions, guiding personalized interventions targeting specific isoforms. Finally, next-generation sequencing (NGS) could provide a more comprehensive view of the genomic landscape, identifying novel mutations, rare variants, and alternative splicing events affecting TGF-β and related pathways.

For similar studies, it is important to consider limitations in sample inclusion criteria. Cases with coexisting spinal diseases, history of spine-related inflammatory or neoplastic diseases, or those with past spinal surgeries should generally be excluded to maintain focus on isolated degeneration. Similarly, age restrictions may be necessary, as degeneration rates and TGF-β expression vary with age, potentially impacting results. Including or excluding these groups can influence findings, so future studies should tailor selection criteria based on specific study aims, ensuring uniformity and reducing confounding factors.

5. Conclusions

This study underscores the central role of TGF-β signaling in L/S IVDs degeneration with TGF-β-1 emerging as the most impactful isoform. Notably, all TGF-β isoforms (TGF-β-1, TGF-β-2, and TGF-β-3) were overexpressed during the early stages of degeneration, which was likely as a response to shifting microenvironmental conditions within the discs. As degeneration advanced from grades 2 to 4 on the Pfirrmann scale, the concentrations of these isoforms steadily rose, indicating an active role of TGF-β signaling in the progression of degeneration. However, in the most advanced degeneration stage (grade 5), the isoform levels dropped, suggesting that TGF-β's influence wanes as degeneration becomes more severe, highlighting its potential as a therapeutic target during earlier stages. Comparative findings from prior studies suggest that the effects of TGF-β are shaped by patient age, species, detection methods, and tissue type—factors that future research should consider refining therapeutic strategies. These results advocate for an in-depth exploration of TGF-β signaling, including its epigenetic regulation via methylation, miRNA interactions, and genetic variations. Advanced tools such as NGS could further illuminate the genetic landscape of TGF-β in IVD degeneration, offering a foundation for precise diagnostic markers and targeted therapies.

Author Contributions: Conceptualization, R.S.; methodology, R.S., D.G., D.S. (Dawid Sobański) and B.O.G.; software, B.O.G. and D.S. (Damian Strojny); investigation, R.S., D.G., D.S. (Dawid Sobański), B.O.G., F.B. and E.G.; resources, M.S. and A.T.; data curation, B.O.G. and D.S. (Damian Strojny); writing—original draft preparation, R.S., D.G., D.S. (Dawid Sobański) and B.O.G.; writing—review and editing, R.S., D.G., and B.O.G.; supervision, B.O.G.; project administration, B.O.G. All authors have read and agreed to the published version of the manuscript.

Funding: This research received no external funding.

Institutional Review Board Statement: Approval from the bioethical committee operating at the Regional Medical Chamber in Krakow (No. 162/KBL/OIL/2021) was obtained for this study.

Informed Consent Statement: Written informed consent was obtained from the patients (study group) involved in this study. Written informed consent was also obtained from the patients to publish this paper.

Data Availability Statement: The data used to support the findings of this study are included in the article. The data cannot be shared due to third-party rights and commercial confidentiality.

Acknowledgments: We would like to thank Nikola Zmarazly for their assistance with the preparation of the figures.

Conflicts of Interest: The authors declare no conflicts of interest.

References

1. Oichi, T.; Taniguchi, Y.; Oshima, Y.; Tanaka, S.; Saito, T. Pathomechanism of Intervertebral Disc Degeneration. *JOR SPINE* **2020**, *3*, e1076. [CrossRef] [PubMed]
2. Lyu, F.-J.; Cui, H.; Pan, H.; MC Cheung, K.; Cao, X.; Iatridis, J.C.; Zheng, Z. Painful Intervertebral Disc Degeneration and Inflammation: From Laboratory Evidence to Clinical Interventions. *Bone Res.* **2021**, *9*, 1–14. [CrossRef] [PubMed]
3. Kirnaz, S.; Capadona, C.; Wong, T.; Goldberg, J.L.; Medary, B.; Sommer, F.; McGrath Jr, L.B.; Härtl, R. Fundamentals of Intervertebral Disc Degeneration. *World Neurosurg.* **2022**, *157*, 264–273. [CrossRef]
4. Ciapetti, G.; Granchi, D.; Devescovi, V.; Leonardi, E.; Greggi, T.; Di Silvestre, M.; Baldini, N. Ex Vivo Observation of Human Intervertebral Disc Tissue and Cells Isolated from Degenerated Intervertebral Discs. *Eur. Spine. J.* **2012**, *21*, 10–19. [CrossRef]
5. Yamabe, D.; Murakami, H.; Chokan, K.; Endo, H.; Oikawa, R.; Sawamura, S.; Doita, M. Evaluation of Water Content in Lumbar Intervertebral Discs and Facet Joints Before and After Physiological Loading Using T2 Mapping MRI. *Spine* **2017**, *42*, E1423–E1428. [CrossRef]
6. Abu-Awwad, A.; Folescu, R.; Pop, D.L.; Motoc, A.G.M.; Oprea, D.M.; Tudoran, M.; Zamfir, C.L.; Faur, C.I.; Vermesan, D.; Deleanu, B.N. Morphometric Characteristics of Fibrocartilaginous Tissue in the Herniated Intervertebral Disc. *Rom. J. Morphol. Embryol* **2019**, *60*, 629–634.
7. Adams, M.A.; Roughley, P.J. What Is Intervertebral Disc Degeneration, and What Causes It? *Spine* **2006**, *31*, 2151–2161. [CrossRef]
8. Groen, G.J.; Baljet, B.; Drukker, J. Nerves and Nerve Plexuses of the Human Vertebral Column. *Am. J. Anat.* **1990**, *188*, 282–296. [CrossRef] [PubMed]
9. Chapman, K.B.; Groenen, P.S.; Vissers, K.C.; van Helmond, N.; Stanton-Hicks, M.D. The Pathways and Processes Underlying Spinal Transmission of Low Back Pain: Observations From Dorsal Root Ganglion Stimulation Treatment. *Neuromodulation* **2021**, *24*, 610–621. [CrossRef]
10. Yoshimura, N.; Dennison, E.; Wilman, C.; Hashimoto, T.; Cooper, C. Epidemiology of Chronic Disc Degeneration and Osteoarthritis of the Lumbar Spine in Britain and Japan: A Comparative Study. *J. Rheumatol.* **2000**, *27*, 429–433.
11. Kettler, A.; Wilke, H.-J. Review of Existing Grading Systems for Cervical or Lumbar Disc and Facet Joint Degeneration. *Eur. Spine J.* **2006**, *15*, 705–718. [CrossRef] [PubMed]
12. Brazill, J.M.; Beeve, A.T.; Craft, C.S.; Ivanusic, J.J.; Scheller, E.L. Nerves in Bone: Evolving Concepts in Pain and Anabolism. *J. Bone Miner. Res.* **2019**, *34*, 1393–1406. [CrossRef] [PubMed]
13. Kennon, J.C.; Awad, M.E.; Chutkan, N.; DeVine, J.; Fulzele, S. Current Insights on Use of Growth Factors as Therapy for Intervertebral Disc Degeneration. *Biomol. Concepts* **2018**, *9*, 43–52. [CrossRef]
14. Mahyudin, F.; Prakoeswa, C.R.S.; Notobroto, H.B.; Tinduh, D.; Ausrin, R.; Rantam, F.A.; Suroto, H.; Utomo, D.N.; Rhatomy, S. An Update of Current Therapeutic Approach for Intervertebral Disc Degeneration: A Review Article. *Ann. Med. Surg.* **2022**, *77*, 103619.
15. Skaper, S.D. Neurotrophic Factors: An Overview. In *Neurotrophic Factors: Methods and Protocols*; Skaper, S.D., Ed.; Methods in Molecular Biology; Springer: New York, NY, USA, 2018; pp. 1–17. ISBN 978-1-4939-7571-6.

16. Sahay, A.S.; Jadhav, A.T.; Sundrani, D.P.; Wagh, G.N.; Joshi, S.R. Differential Expression of Nerve Growth Factor (NGF) and Brain Derived Neurotrophic Factor (BDNF) in Different Regions of Normal and Preeclampsia Placentae. *Clin. Exp. Hypertens* **2020**, *42*, 360–364. [CrossRef]
17. Hsiao, S.J.; Zehir, A.; Sireci, A.N.; Aisner, D.L. Detection of Tumor NTRK Gene Fusions to Identify Patients Who May Benefit from Tyrosine Kinase (TRK) Inhibitor Therapy. *J. Mol. Diagn.* **2019**, *21*, 553–571. [CrossRef]
18. Kirkeby, A.; Barker, R.A. Parkinson Disease and Growth Factors - Is GDNF Good Enough? *Nat. Rev. Neurol.* **2019**, *15*, 312–314. [CrossRef]
19. Cintrón-Colón, A.F.; Almeida-Alves, G.; Boynton, A.M.; Spitsbergen, J.M. GDNF Synthesis, Signaling, and Retrograde Transport in Motor Neurons. *Cell Tissue Res.* **2020**, *382*, 47–56. [CrossRef]
20. Chen, S.; Liu, S.; Ma, K.; Zhao, L.; Lin, H.; Shao, Z. TGF-β Signaling in Intervertebral Disc Health and Disease. *Osteoarthr. Cartil.* **2019**, *27*, 1109–1117. [CrossRef]
21. Cui, L.; Wei, H.; Li, Z.-M.; Dong, X.-B.; Wang, P.-Y. TGF-B1 Aggravates Degenerative Nucleus Pulposus Cells Inflammation and Fibrosis through the Upregulation of Angiopoietin-like Protein 2 Expression. *Eur. Rev. Med. Pharmacol. Sci.* **2020**, *24*, 12025–12033.
22. Lee, Y.-J.; Kong, M.-H.; Song, K.-Y.; Lee, K.-H.; Heo, S.-H. The Relation Between Sox9, TGF-B1, and Proteoglycan in Human Intervertebral Disc Cells. *J. Korean Neurosurg. Soc.* **2008**, *43*, 149–154. [CrossRef] [PubMed]
23. Nerlich, A.; Bachmeier, B.; Boos, N. Expression of Fibronectin and TGF-SS1 mRNA and Protein Suggest Altered Regulation of Extracellular Matrix in Degenerated Disc Tissue. *Eur. Spine J.* **2005**, *14*, 17–26. [CrossRef] [PubMed]
24. Tolonen, J.; Grönblad, M.; Virri, J.; Seitsalo, S.; Rytömaa, T.; Karaharju, E. Transforming Growth Factor Beta Receptor Induction in Herniated Intervertebral Disc Tissue: An Immunohistochemical Study. *Eur. Spine J.* **2001**, *10*, 172–176. [CrossRef] [PubMed]
25. Wu, Q.; Wang, J.; Skubutyte, R.; Kepler, C.K.; Huang, Z.; Anderson, D.G.; Shapiro, I.M.; Risbud, M.V. Smad3 Controls β-1,3-Glucuronosyltransferase 1 Expression in Rat Nucleus Pulposus Cells: Implications of Dysregulated Expression in Disc Disease. *Arthritis Rheum.* **2012**, *64*, 3324–3333. [CrossRef]
26. Schroeder, M.; Viezens, L.; Schaefer, C.; Friedrichs, B.; Algenstaedt, P.; Rüther, W.; Wiesner, L.; Hansen-Algenstaedt, N. Chemokine Profile of Disc Degeneration with Acute or Chronic Pain: Laboratory Investigation. *J. Neurosurg. Spine* **2013**, *18*, 496–503. [CrossRef]
27. Abbott, R.D.; Purmessur, D.; Monsey, R.D.; Brigstock, D.R.; Laudier, D.M.; Iatridis, J.C. Degenerative Grade Affects the Responses of Human Nucleus Pulposus Cells to Link-N, CTGF, and TGFβ3. *J. Spinal Disord. Tech.* **2013**, *26*, E86–E94. [CrossRef]
28. Tsarouhas, A.; Soufla, G.; Tsarouhas, K.; Katonis, P.; Pasku, D.; Vakis, A.; Tsatsakis, A.M.; Spandidos, D.A. Molecular Profile of Major Growth Factors in Lumbar Intervertebral Disc Herniation: Correlation with Patient Clinical and Epidemiological Characteristics. *Mol. Med. Rep.* **2017**, *15*, 2195–2203. [CrossRef]
29. Wan, Z.Y.; Shan, H.; Liu, T.F.; Song, F.; Zhang, J.; Liu, Z.H.; Ma, K.L.; Wang, H.Q. Emerging Issues Questioning the Current Treatment Strategies for Lumbar Disc Herniation. *Front. Surg.* **2022**, *9*, 814531. [CrossRef]
30. Yang, Y.; He, X.; Li, Y.; Feng, J.; Pang, H.; Wang, J.; Liu, Q. Association of transforming growth factor-β1 with pathological grading of intervertebral disc degeneration. *Nan Fang Yi Ke Da Xue Xue Bao* **2012**, *32*, 897–900.
31. Koroth, J.; Buko, E.O.; Abbott, R.; Johnson, C.P.; Ogle, B.M.; Stone, L.S.; Ellingson, A.M.; Bradley, E.W. Macrophages and Intervertebral Disc Degeneration. *Int. J. Mol. Sci.* **2023**, *24*, 1367. [CrossRef]
32. Yang, H.; Cao, C.; Wu, C.; Yuan, C.; Gu, Q.; Shi, Q.; Zou, J. TGF-Bl Suppresses Inflammation in Cell Therapy for Intervertebral Disc Degeneration. *Sci. Rep.* **2015**, *5*, 13254. [CrossRef] [PubMed]
33. Yang, H.; Yuan, C.; Wu, C.; Qian, J.; Shi, Q.; Li, X.; Zhu, X.; Zou, J. The Role of TGF-β1/Smad2/3 Pathway in Platelet-rich Plasma in Retarding Intervertebral Disc Degeneration. *J. Cell Mol. Med.* **2016**, *20*, 1542–1549. [CrossRef] [PubMed]
34. Stich, S.; Jagielski, M.; Fleischmann, A.; Meier, C.; Bussmann, P.; Kohl, B.; Schmidt, J.; Krüger, J.-P.; Endres, M.; Cabraja, M. Degeneration of Lumbar Intervertebral Discs: Characterization of Anulus Fibrosus Tissue and Cells of Different Degeneration Grades. *Int. J. Mol. Sci.* **2020**, *21*, 2165. [CrossRef]
35. An, H.S.; Masuda, K.; Inoue, N. Intervertebral Disc Degeneration: Biological Biomechanical Factors. *J. Orthop. Sci.* **2006**, *11*, 541–552. [CrossRef]
36. Ustawa z Dnia 1 Lipca 2005 r. o Pobieraniu, Przechowywaniu i Przeszczepianiu Komórek, Tkanek i Narządów. Available online: https://isap.sejm.gov.pl/isap.nsf/DocDetails.xsp?id=wdu20051691411 (accessed on 13 February 2024).
37. Staszkiewicz, R.; Gralewski, M.; Gładysz, D.; Bryś, K.; Garczarek, M.; Gadzieliński, M.; Marcol, W.; Sobański, D.; Grabarek, B.O. Evaluation of the Concentration of Growth Associated Protein-43 and Glial Cell-Derived Neurotrophic Factor in Degenerated Intervertebral Discs of the Lumbosacral Region of the Spine. *Mol. Pain* **2023**, *19*, 17448069231158287. [CrossRef] [PubMed]
38. Staszkiewicz, R.; Gładysz, D.; Bryś, K.; Garczarek, M.; Gadzieliński, M.; Marcol, W.; Sobański, D.; Grabarek, B.O. Usefulness of Detecting Brain-Derived Neurotrophic Factor in Intervertebral Disc Degeneration of the Lumbosacral Spine. *Med. Sci. Monit. Int. Med. J. Exp. Clin. Res.* **2023**, *29*, e938663. [CrossRef]
39. Pfirrmann, C.W.; Metzdorf, A.; Zanetti, M.; Hodler, J.; Boos, N. Magnetic Resonance Classification of Lumbar Intervertebral Disc Degeneration. *Spine* **2001**, *26*, 1873–1878. [CrossRef]
40. Yu, L.-P.; Qian, W.-W.; Yin, G.-Y.; Ren, Y.-X.; Hu, Z.-Y. MRI Assessment of Lumbar Intervertebral Disc Degeneration with Lumbar Degenerative Disease Using the Pfirrmann Grading Systems. *PLoS ONE* **2012**, *7*, e48074. [CrossRef]

41. Hasanović-Vučković, S.; Jusufbegović, M.; Vegar-Zubović, S.; Milišić, L.; Šehić, A.; Hasanbegović, I.; Beganović, A. Assessment of Lumbar Spine Disc Degeneration in Coherence to Pfirrman Grades and Oswestry Disability Index. *J. Health Sci.* **2020**, *10*, 191–195. [CrossRef]
42. Pagani, S.; Maglio, M.; Sicuro, L.; Fini, M.; Giavaresi, G.; Brogini, S. RNA Extraction from Cartilage: Issues, Methods, Tips. *Int. J. Mol. Sci.* **2023**, *24*, 2120. [CrossRef]
43. Peirson, S.N.; Butler, J.N. RNA Extraction From Mammalian Tissues. In *Circadian Rhythms: Methods and Protocols*; Rosato, E., Ed.; Humana Press: Totowa, NJ, USA, 2007; ISBN 978-1-59745-257-1.
44. Leonova, O.N.; Elgaeva, E.E.; Golubeva, T.S.; Peleganchuk, A.V.; Krutko, A.V.; Aulchenko, Y.S.; Tsepilov, Y.A. A Protocol for Recruiting and Analyzing the Disease-Oriented Russian Disc Degeneration Study (RuDDS) Biobank for Functional Omics Studies of Lumbar Disc Degeneration. *PLoS ONE* **2022**, *17*, e0267384. Available online: https://journals.plos.org/plosone/article?id=10.1371/journal.pone.0267384 (accessed on 22 August 2024). [CrossRef]
45. Ruettger, A.; Neumann, S.; Wiederanders, B.; Huber, R. Comparison of Different Methods for Preparation and Characterization of Total RNA from Cartilage Samples to Uncover Osteoarthritis in Vivo. *BMC Res. Notes* **2010**, *3*, 7. [CrossRef] [PubMed]
46. Schroeder, A.B.; Dobson, E.T.A.; Rueden, C.T.; Tomancak, P.; Jug, F.; Eliceiri, K.W. The ImageJ Ecosystem: Open-source Software for Image Visualization, Processing, and Analysis. *Protein Sci.* **2021**, *30*, 234–249. [CrossRef] [PubMed]
47. Varghese, F.; Bukhari, A.B.; Malhotra, R.; De, A. IHC Profiler: An Open Source Plugin for the Quantitative Evaluation and Automated Scoring of Immunohistochemistry Images of Human Tissue Samples. *PLoS ONE* **2014**, *9*, e96801. [CrossRef] [PubMed]
48. Tzavlaki, K.; Moustakas, A. TGF-β Signaling. *Biomolecules* **2020**, *10*, 487. [CrossRef]
49. Rudnik-Jansen, I.; van Kruining Kodele, S.; Creemers, L.; Joosten, B. Biomolecular therapies for chronic dis-cogenic low back pain: A narrative review. *JOR Spine* **2024**, *7*, e1345. [CrossRef]
50. Kos, N.; Gradisnik, L.; Velnar, T. A Brief Review of the Degenerative Intervertebral Disc Disease. *Med. Arch.* **2019**, *73*, 421. [CrossRef]
51. Voisin, A.; Damon-Soubeyrand, C.; Bravard, S.; Saez, F.; Drevet, J.R.; Guiton, R. Differential Expression and Localisation of TGF-β Isoforms and Receptors in the Murine Epididymis. *Sci. Rep.* **2020**, *10*, 995. [CrossRef]
52. Bian, Q.; Ma, L.; Jain, A.; Crane, J.L.; Kebaish, K.; Wan, M.; Zhang, Z.; Edward Guo, X.; Sponseller, P.D.; Séguin, C.A. Mechanosignaling Activation of TGFβ Maintains Intervertebral Disc Homeostasis. *Bone Res.* **2017**, *5*, 1–14. [CrossRef]
53. Nakawaki, M.; Uchida, K.; Miyagi, M.; Inoue, G.; Kawakubo, A.; Satoh, M.; Takaso, M. Changes in Nerve Growth Factor Expression and Macrophage Phenotype Following Intervertebral Disc Injury in Mice. *J. Orthop. Res.* **2019**, *37*, 1798–1804. [CrossRef]
54. Zhang, G.-Z.; Liu, M.-Q.; Chen, H.-W.; Wu, Z.-L.; Gao, Y.-C.; Ma, Z.-J.; He, X.-G.; Kang, X.-W. NF-κB Signalling Pathways in Nucleus Pulposus Cell Function and Intervertebral Disc Degeneration. *Cell Prolif.* **2021**, *54*, e13057. [CrossRef]
55. Van Der Kraan, P.M. The Changing Role of TGFβ in Healthy, Ageing and Osteoarthritic Joints. *Nat. Rev. Rheumatol.* **2017**, *13*, 155–163. [CrossRef] [PubMed]
56. Bian, Q.; Jain, A.; Xu, X.; Kebaish, K.; Crane, J.L.; Zhang, Z.; Wan, M.; Ma, L.; Riley, L.H.; Sponseller, P.D. Excessive Activation of TGFβ by Spinal Instability Causes Vertebral Endplate Sclerosis. *Sci. Rep.* **2016**, *6*, 27093. [CrossRef] [PubMed]
57. Kwon, Y.-J.; Lee, J.-W.; Moon, E.-J.; Chung, Y.G.; Kim, O.-S.; Kim, H.-J. Anabolic Effects of Peniel 2000, a Peptide That Regulates TGF-B1 Signaling on Intervertebral Disc Degeneration. *Spine* **2013**, *38*, E49–E58. [CrossRef]
58. Ni, L.; Zheng, Y.; Gong, T.; Xiu, C.; Li, K.; Saijilafu; Li, B.; Yang, H.; Chen, J. Proinflammatory Macrophages Promote Degenerative Phenotypes in Rat Nucleus Pulpous Cells Partly through ERK and JNK Signaling. *J. Cell. Physiol.* **2019**, *234*, 5362–5371. [CrossRef]
59. Li, W.; Liu, T.; Wu, L.; Chen, C.; Jia, Z.; Bai, X.; Ruan, D. Blocking the Function of Inflammatory Cytokines and Mediators by Using IL-10 and TGF-β: A Potential Biological Immunotherapy for Intervertebral Disc Degeneration in a Beagle Model. *Int. J. Mol. Sci.* **2014**, *15*, 17270–17283. [CrossRef]
60. Najafi, M.; Farhood, B.; Mortezaee, K. Extracellular Matrix (ECM) Stiffness and Degradation as Cancer Drivers. *J. Cell. Biochem.* **2019**, *120*, 2782–2790. [CrossRef]
61. Guo, Z.; Su, W.; Zhou, R.; Zhang, G.; Yang, S.; Wu, X.; Qiu, C.; Cong, W.; Shen, N.; Guo, J. Exosomal MATN3 of Urine-Derived Stem Cells Ameliorates Intervertebral Disc Degeneration by Antisenescence Effects and Promotes NPC Proliferation and ECM Synthesis by Activating TGF-β. *Oxidative Med. Cell. Longev.* **2021**, *2021*, 5542241. [CrossRef]
62. Stich, S.; Möller, A.; Cabraja, M.; Krüger, J.P.; Hondke, S.; Endres, M.; Ringe, J.; Sittinger, M. Chemokine CCL25 Induces Migration and Extracellular Matrix Production of Anulus Fibrosus-Derived Cells. *Int. J. Mol. Sci.* **2018**, *19*, 2207. [CrossRef] [PubMed]
63. Hondke, S.; Cabraja, M.; Krüger, J.P.; Stich, S.; Hartwig, T.; Sittinger, M.; Endres, M. Proliferation, Migration, and ECM Formation Potential of Human Annulus Fibrosus Cells Is Independent of Degeneration Status. *CARTILAGE* **2020**, *11*, 192–202. [CrossRef]
64. Hu, B.; Shi, C.; Tian, Y.; Zhang, Y.; Xu, C.; Chen, H.; Cao, P.; Yuan, W. TGF-β Induces up-Regulation of Chondroitin Sulfate Synthase 1 (CHSY1) in Nucleus Pulposus Cells through MAPK Signaling. *Cell Physiol. Biochem.* **2015**, *37*, 793–804. [CrossRef]
65. Hu, B.; Xu, C.; Cao, P.; Tian, Y.; Zhang, Y.; Shi, C.; Xu, J.; Yuan, W.; Chen, H. TGF-β Stimulates Expression of Chondroitin Polymerizing Factor in Nucleus Pulposus Cells through the Smad3, RhoA/ROCK1, and MAPK Signaling Pathways. *J. Cell Biochem.* **2018**, *119*, 566–579. [CrossRef] [PubMed]
66. Bowles, R.D.; Setton, L.A. Biomaterials for Intervertebral Disc Regeneration and Repair. *Biomaterials* **2017**, *129*, 54–67. [CrossRef] [PubMed]

67. Chen, S.; Zhao, L.; Deng, X.; Shi, D.; Wu, F.; Liang, H.; Huang, D.; Shao, Z. Mesenchymal Stem Cells Protect Nucleus Pulposus Cells from Compression-Induced Apoptosis by Inhibiting the Mitochondrial Pathway. *Stem Cells Int.* **2017**, *2017*, 984312. [CrossRef]
68. Fontana, G.; See, E.; Pandit, A. Current Trends in Biologics Delivery to Restore Intervertebral Disc Anabolism. *Adv. Drug Deliv. Rev.* **2015**, *84*, 146–158. [CrossRef]
69. Nagano, S.; Matsunaga, S.; Takae, R.; Morimoto, N.; Suzuki, S.; Yoshida, H. Immunolocalization of Transforming Growth Factor-Betas and Their Receptors in the Intervertebral Disk of Senescence-Accelerated Mouse. *Int. J. Oncol.* **2000**, *17*, 461–467. [CrossRef]
70. Matsunaga, S.; Nagano, S.; Onishi, T.; Motimoto, N.; Suzuki, S. kOMIYA, s Age-Related Changes in Expression of Transforming Growth Factor-β and Receptors in Cells of Intervertebral Discs. *J. Neurosurg. Spine* **2003**, *98*, 63–67.
71. Zheng, L.; Cao, Y.; Ni, S.; Qi, H.; Ling, Z.; Xu, X.; Zou, X.; Wu, T.; Deng, R.; Hu, B.; et al. Ciliary Parathyroid Hormone Signaling Activates Transforming Growth Factor-β to Maintain Intervertebral Disc Homeostasis during Aging. *Bone Res.* **2018**, *6*, 21. [CrossRef] [PubMed]
72. Murakami, H.; Yoon, S.; Attallah-Wasif, E.; Tsai, K.; Fei, Q.; Hutton, W. The Expression of Anabolic Cytokines in Intervertebral Discs. *Spine* **2006**, *31*, 1770–1774. [CrossRef]
73. Hiyama, A.; Mochida, J.; Omi, H.; Serigano, K.; Sakai, D. Cross Talk between Smad Transcription Factors and TNF-α in Intervertebral Disc Degeneration. *Biochem. Biophys. Res. Commun.* **2008**, *369*, 679–685. [CrossRef]
74. Wu, M.; Chen, G.; Li, Y.-P. TGF-β and BMP Signaling in Osteoblast, Skeletal Development, and Bone Formation, Homeostasis and Disease. *Bone Res.* **2016**, *4*, 16009. [CrossRef]
75. Guo, H.-Y.; Guo, M.-K.; Wan, Z.-Y.; Song, F.; Wang, H.-Q. Emerging Evidence on Noncoding-RNA Regulatory Machinery in Intervertebral Disc Degeneration: A Narrative Review. *Arthritis Res. Ther.* **2020**, *22*, 270. [CrossRef] [PubMed]
76. James, S.L.; Abate, D.; Abate, K.H.; Abay, S.M.; Abbafati, C.; Abbasi, N.; Abbastabar, H.; Abd-Allah, F.; Abdela, J.; Abdelalim, A.; et al. Global, Regional, and National Incidence, Prevalence, and Years Lived with Disability for 354 Diseases and Injuries for 195 Countries and Territories, 1990–2017: A Systematic Analysis for the Global Burden of Disease Study 2017. *Lancet* **2018**, *392*, 1789–1858. [CrossRef] [PubMed]
77. Xiong, Y.; Yang, Y.-L.; Gao, Y.-S.; Wang, X.-M.; Yu, X. Histological Changes of Cervical Disc Tissue in Patients with Degenerative Ossification. *J. Korean Neurosurg. Soc.* **2022**, *65*, 186–195. [CrossRef] [PubMed]
78. Chen, X.; Wang, Z.; Deng, R.; Yan, H.; Liu, X.; Kang, R. Intervertebral Disc Degeneration and Inflammatory Microenvironment: Expression, Pathology, and Therapeutic Strategies. *Inflamm. Res.* **2023**, *72*, 1811–1828. [CrossRef] [PubMed]
79. Tuakli-Wosornu, Y.A.; Terry, A.; Boachie-Adjei, K.; Harrison, J.R.; Gribbin, C.K.; LaSalle, E.E.; Nguyen, J.T.; Solomon, J.L.; Lutz, G.E. Lumbar Intradiskal Platelet-Rich Plasma (PRP) Injections: A Prospective, Double-Blind, Randomized Controlled Study. *PMR* **2016**, *8*, 1–10. [CrossRef]
80. Nishida, K.; Kang, J.D.; Gilbertson, L.G.; Moon, S.H.; Suh, J.K.; Vogt, M.T.; Robbins, P.D.; Evans, C.H. Modulation of the Biologic Activity of the Rabbit Intervertebral Disc by Gene Therapy: An in Vivo Study of Adenovirus-Mediated Transfer of the Human Transforming Growth Factor Beta 1 Encoding Gene. *Spine* **1999**, *24*, 2419–2425. [CrossRef]
81. Matta, A.; Karim, M.Z.; Isenman, D.E.; Erwin, W.M. Molecular Therapy for Degenerative Disc Disease: Clues from Secretome Analysis of the Notochordal Cell-Rich Nucleus Pulposus. *Sci. Rep.* **2017**, *7*, 45623. [CrossRef]
82. Hodgkinson, T.; Shen, B.; Diwan, A.; Hoyland, J.A.; Richardson, S.M. Therapeutic Potential of Growth Differentiation Factors in the Treatment of Degenerative Disc Diseases. *JOR Spine* **2019**, *2*, e1045. [CrossRef]
83. Matta, A.; Karim, M.Z.; Gerami, H.; Jun, P.; Funabashi, M.; Kawchuk, G.; Goldstein, A.; Foltz, W.; Sussman, M.; Eek, B.C.; et al. NTG-101: A Novel Molecular Therapy That Halts the Progression of Degenerative Disc Disease. *Sci. Rep.* **2018**, *8*, 16809. [CrossRef]
84. Risbud, M.V.; Di Martino, A.; Guttapalli, A.; Seghatoleslami, R.; Denaro, V.; Vaccaro, A.R.; Albert, T.J.; Shapiro, I.M. Toward an Optimum System for Intervertebral Disc Organ Culture: TGF-Beta 3 Enhances Nucleus Pulposus and Anulus Fibrosus Survival and Function through Modulation of TGF-Beta-R Expression and ERK Signaling. *Spine* **2006**, *31*, 884–890. [CrossRef]
85. Hegewald, A.A.; Zouhair, S.; Endres, M.; Cabraja, M.; Woiciechowsky, C.; Thomé, C.; Kaps, C. Towards Biological Anulus Repair: TGF-B3, FGF-2 and Human Serum Support Matrix Formation by Human Anulus Fibrosus Cells. *Tissue Cell* **2013**, *45*, 68–76. [CrossRef] [PubMed]
86. Murphy, K.; Lufkin, T.; Kraus, P. Development and Degeneration of the Intervertebral Disc—Insights from Across Species. *Vet. Sci.* **2023**, *10*, 540. [CrossRef] [PubMed]
87. Sun, Y.; Lyu, M.; Lu, Q.; Cheung, K.; Leung, V. Current Perspectives on Nucleus Pulposus Fibrosis in Disc Degeneration and Repair. *Int. J. Mol. Sci.* **2022**, *23*, 6612. [CrossRef] [PubMed]
88. Takeoka, Y.; Yurube, T.; Nishida, K. Gene Therapy Approach for Intervertebral Disc Degeneration: An Update. *Neurospine* **2020**, *17*, 3–14. [CrossRef]
89. Hou, Z.; Tan, R.; Zhang, Y. Snapshots of a Tiny Ancestral Nuclease of Cas9. *Trends Biochem. Sci* **2023**, *48*, 9–10. [CrossRef]

current issues in molecular biology

MDPI

Article

The ER Stress Induced in Human Neuroblastoma Cells Can Be Reverted by Lumacaftor, a CFTR Corrector

Michela Pecoraro [1], Adele Serra [1,2], Maria Pascale [1] and Silvia Franceschelli [1,*]

[1] Department of Pharmacy, University of Salerno, Via Giovanni Paolo II, 84084 Fisciano, Salerno, Italy; mipecoraro@unisa.it (M.P.); adserra@unisa.it (A.S.); pascale@unisa.it (M.P.)
[2] Ph.D. Program in Drug Discovery and Development, University of Salerno, 84084 Fisciano, Salerno, Italy
* Correspondence: sfranceschelli@unisa.it

Abstract: Most neurodegenerative diseases share a common etiopathogenesis, the accumulation of protein aggregates. An imbalance in homeostasis brought on by the buildup of misfolded proteins within the endoplasmic reticulum (ER) results in ER stress in the cell. Three distinct proteins found in the ER membrane—IRE1α, PERK, and ATF6—control the unfolded protein response (UPR), a signal transduction pathway that is triggered to restore normal physiological conditions. Buildup of misfolded proteins in ER lumen leads to a shunting of GRP78/BiP, thus triggering the UPR. PERK autophosphorylation leads to activation of ATF4, the transcription factor; finally, ATF6 activates the UPR's target genes, including GRP78/Bip. Accordingly, the UPR is a cellular reaction to an ER stress state that, if left unchecked for an extended period, results in apoptosis and irreversible damage. The identification of caspase 4, which is in the ER and is selectively activated by apoptotic stimuli caused by reticular stress, further demonstrated the connection between reticular stress and programed cell death. Moreover, oxidative stress and ER stress are linked. Oxidative stress is brought on by elevated quantities of radical oxygen species, both mitochondrial and cytosolic, that are not under the enzymatic regulation of superoxide dismutases, whose levels fall with increasing stress. Here, we evaluated the activity of Vx-809 (Lumacaftor), a drug used in cystic fibrosis, in SH-SY5Y neuronal cells, in which an ER stress condition was induced by Thapsigargin, to verify whether the drug could improve protein folding, suggesting its possible therapeutic use in proteinopathies, such as neurodegenerative diseases (NDs). Our data show that Vx-809 is involved in the significant reduction in protein produced under ER stress, particularly in the levels of Bip, ATF4, and ATF6 by Western blotting analysis, the reduction in ROS in the cytosol and mitochondria, and the reduction in the activation of the apoptotic pathway, measured by flow cytofluorimetry analysis and in restoring calcium homeostasis.

Keywords: neuroblastoma cells; ER stress; oxidative stress; protein misfolding; Lumacaftor

1. Introduction

NDs are characterized by a progressive loss of neuronal function in specific regions of the nervous system, culminating in severe dysfunction [1]. NDs include highly debilitating illnesses, such as Parkinson's disease (PD), characterized by ubiquitinated protein deposits called Lewy bodies (composed of α-synuclein) in the neuronal cytosol; Alzheimer's disease (AD) in which intracellular deposits of tau are observed in neurofibrillary tangles and in which extracellular aggregates of amyloid β are seen in senile plaques; Huntington's disease, due to an aggregate of mutant huntingtin proteins and prion diseases (PrDs), are well known to form protein aggregates and are causally involved in the pathogenesis of a group of transmissible spongiform encephalopathies, including Creutzfeldt–Jakob disease and kuru [1]. Despite significant variations in clinical presentation and prevalence, NDs share several characteristics, such as their chronic and progressive nature, age-related increase in prevalence, degeneration of neurons in particular regions of brain, damage to synaptic networks, and selective damage of brain tissue. NDs are also characterized by aggregation of intrinsically disordered proteins (IDPs) (also called natively unfolded proteins), which refers to proteins that do not have an independently folded state. In many circumstances, interactions between intrinsically disordered proteins and target proteins or nucleic acids result in folding of the binding domain; in other cases, binding causes merely local ordering of short, extended, or helical portions of polypeptides [2].

Proteins are chains of amino acids consisting of 20 different L-α-amino acids, which fold into unique three-dimensional structures. The form in which a protein naturally folds is called its 'native state', which is determined by its amino acid sequence. Their three-dimensional structure contributes greatly to the performance of biological processes by cells.

Even though the protein aggregates involved in distinct NDs are different, the process of protein misfolding, its intermediates, end-products, and main features are remarkably similar [3].

Neuronal cells are very sensitive to protein misfolding, therefore excessive misfolding and aggregation results in synaptic dysfunction, apoptosis, and selective neuronal death [4,5].

Misfolded proteins can have two harmful effects: either they cause a deleterious "gain of function", as seen in many neurodegenerative diseases like AD, PD, and HD, where the formation of harmful amyloid is the result of protein misfolding, or they cause loss of function, as seen in cystic fibrosis (CF) and α1-antitrypsin deficiency. In other instances, on the other hand, the changes are quite small, and the resultant proteins only exhibit a slight reduction in their typical activity [3]. Susan Lindquist, a prion researcher, states that "up to half of all human diseases could be caused by protein misfolding".

Since protein homeostasis stops aberrant protein aggregation, it is essential for maintaining cellular health and function. Under normal conditions, misfolded proteins are recognized and made more easily degradable by the proteasome, lysosome, and autophagy pathways, whereas chaperones found in the cytosol and endoplasmic reticulum (ER) guarantee clear folding of freshly generated native proteins [6].

More than one-third of all proteins produced by a cell are synthesized, folded, and structurally matured in the ER. In addition, the ER coordinates many cellular processes, such as the maintenance of intracellular calcium levels, synthesis of lipids, and the folding and processing of most polypeptides intended for secretion [7].

Proteins must be folded into their distinct three-dimensional structures and undergo various post-translational processes, such as N-glycosylation and disulfide bonds formation, in the ER lumen [8].

Degenerative disorders are caused by protein aggregation in neurons that stop functioning properly. Protein aggregation and accumulation of misfolded protein cause ER stress, which activates the unfolded protein response (UPR), a protection mechanism that, through several transcriptional and translational modifications, acts both to increase the folding capacity of the ER and to decrease the load of unfolded proteins. Protein kinase RNA (PKR)-like ER kinase (PERK), inositol-requiring enzyme 1 (IRE1), and activating transcription factor 6 (ATF6) are the three transmembrane ER proteins that constitute the UPR. Under resting conditions, all three proteins form a complex with the chaperone GRP78/BiP. In response to an accumulation of misfolded proteins in the ER, BiP dissociates and binds the misfolded proteins. PERK, IRE1, and ATF6 are activated when BiP dissociates [9,10].

In short, after detection of unfolded proteins, IRE1 is activated and triggers the regulated splicing of an unconventional 26 nt intron of X-box binding protein 1 (Xbp1). This results in a frameshift, producing the spliced Xbp1 isoform (XBP1s), which acts as a transcription factor [7]. PERK is a protein kinase that reacts to extracellular reticulum stress by homo-multimerization and autophosphorylation. When PERK is activated, it phosphorylates the α subunit of eIF2α, which inhibits translation and stops the cytoplasm from synthesizing new proteins. Nevertheless, the activation of transcription factor 4 (ATF4), which in turn stimulates the transcription of UPR and apoptotic genes, including the pro-apoptotic C/EBP protein homolog (CHOP), is preferentially induced by phospho-eIF2α [9,11].

ATF6 travels from the ER to the Golgi apparatus in response to ER stress, where it is cleaved, moved to the nucleus, and stimulates the production of Xbp-1 and genes needed for ER-associated protein degradation (ERAD). Proteins that are terminally unfolded or misfolded are taken out of the ER by ERAD so that proteasomes can break them down [12].

The precise association between misfolded proteins and the etiology of neurodegenerative disorders is still unknown. Moreover, there is ongoing debate on the potential essential role of endogenous stress in neurodegenerative disorders.

Neurons can be killed by the accumulation of toxic protein species, and increasing research indicates that ER stress is a key mechanism causing this neurotoxicity [5]. In postmortem brain and spinal cord tissues from various NDs, activation of IRE1α and induction of UPR have been identified [13,14]. Several scientists attempted to alter the UPR murine neurodegenerative models in vivo in light of this evidence. In prion-infected mice, for instance, Moreno and associates [15] discovered that oral treatment of a highly selective PERK inhibitor that successfully penetrates the blood–brain barrier dramatically reduced neurodegeneration and clinical illness. Given the strong evidence of UPR activation in human patients, studies like these are raising awareness of the possibility that pharmacological modulation of the UPR may have disease-modifying advantages for a variety of neurodegenerative illnesses. Since calcium is an essential component of many intracellular processes and serves as a second messenger, the cytoplasmic calcium is actively transported out of cells and stored in the ER or mitochondria, hence maintaining very low concentrations of the mineral. For instance, dysregulation of cytosolic Ca^{2+} is seen in AD, which leads to ER stress-mediated apoptosis and ER malfunction. Moreover, an elevated Ca^{2+} influx that results in cell death is also seen in PD [16,17]. The redox balance in the ER is related to both protein folding and cellular calcium homeostasis. In the ER, oxidation is also used in an oxidative protein folding process to promote disulfide bond formation. Chronic ER stress-related neurodegeneration can be caused by a synergistic combination of protein misfolding and reactive oxygen species (ROS) accumulation [18]. Common issues in several NDs include redox status, ER stress, and protein misfolding that results in neurodegeneration. Even though the molecular mechanisms underlying NDs are well understood, effective treatments or a cure is yet unknown for these conditions. Therapeutic intervention focuses mostly on misfolded protein aggregates. Several approaches are under development to prevent the formation of or to remove misfolded aggregates.

Protein misfolding-induced neurotoxicity can be inhibited by increased chaperone expression, indicating a potential utility for chaperones as therapeutic agents. Chaperones, whether natural, synthetic, or pharmaceutical, have demonstrated promise as therapeutics for the management of numerous protein conformational diseases [19].

Lumacaftor (Vx-809) is a CFTR corrector, and it was the second treatment to be approved for use in CF therapy, though it can only be used in conjunction with Ivacaftor, a potentiator that improves channel function; also, it has been shown to be safe with biological activity in a Phase IIa clinical trial [19]. The drug has been shown in vitro to correct p. Phe508del misprocessing of CFTR and increase the amount of protein localized on the cell surface [20]. This compound is based on a di-fluorobenzodioxolyl-cyclopropane linked to a substituted arylpyridine via an amide bond discovered by screening compounds that enhance Phe-508del-CFTR-mediated chloride transport [21].

Its mechanism of action and their binding sites are still incompletely understood, but several studies indicate that it may stabilize folding of the molecule through direct binding to the first nucleotide-binding domain (NBD1) or promoting interactions between the first cytoplasmic loop (CL1) of transmembrane domain 1 (TMD1) and NBD1 [21,22]. Furthermore, it is not CFTR-specific because it was demonstrated to stop the trafficking of another defective ABC transporter (ABCA4), which has significant similarity with CFTR NBDs [9].

The approval of Lumacaftor in therapy represents the genesis of a new era of medicine in the treatment of CF, with a positive impact on patients' lives [19,21].

In previous work Pecoraro and co-workers [9] demonstrated how the Vx-809 corrector counteracts the activation of the UPR pathway by acting on protein folding on adenocarcinomic human alveolar basal epithelial (A549) and malignant melanoma (A375) cells.

Therefore, in this study, we investigated if the off-label mechanism of Vx-809 is also confirmed in a neuroblastoma cell model, often used as in vitro models of neuronal function and differentiation, leading to the hypothesis that the drug interacts not only with the CFTR protein but, by an unknown mechanism, also on other misfolded proteins, demonstrating that it can also be used in other diseases, like NDs (Figure 1).

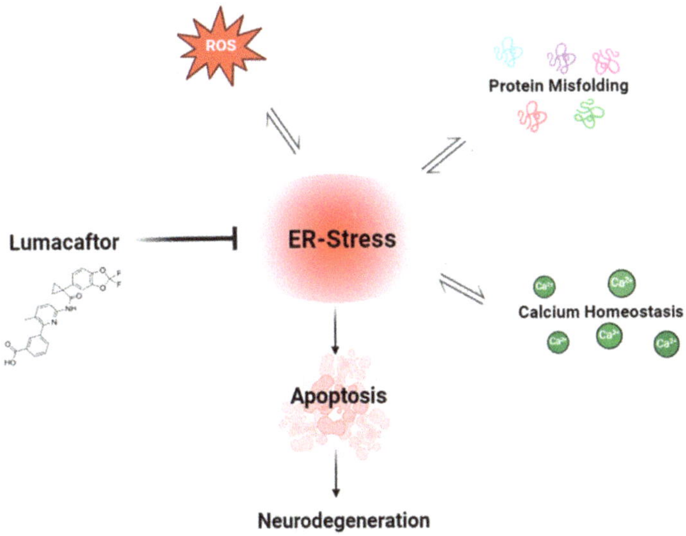

Figure 1. Schematic representation on the probable effect of Lumacaftor.

2. Materials and Methods

2.1. Reagents

Vx-809 (S1565) was acquired from Selleckchem (Houston, TX, USA). The monoclonal antibodies used included the following: anti-Grp78/BiP (3177, Cell Signaling, Danvers, MA, USA), anti-ATF6 (658805, Cell Signaling, Danvers, MA, USA), anti-ATF4 (10835-1-AP, Proteintech, San Diego, CA, USA), anti-PERK (3192, Cell Signaling), anti-MnSODIII (sc-271170), anti-actin (TA811000, OriGene, Rockville, MD, USA), anti-tubulin (sc-5286), anti-caspase 4 (sc-1229). Secondary antibodies (anti-rabbit, A120-101P, and anti-mouse, A90-137P) were bought from Bethyl Laboratories (Montgomery, TX, USA). The Texas red-conjugated secondary antibody (T6390 and PA1-28662) was procured from Thermo Fisher Scientific (Waltham, MA, USA). The mitochondrial superoxide indicator MitoSOX Red (M36008) was purchased from Invitrogen, ThermoFisher (Waltham, MA, USA). Thia-zolyl blue tetrazolium bromide, H_2DCF-DA, Thapsigargin, propidium iodide, FURA 2AM, and ionomycin were all purchased from Sigma-Aldrich (St. Louis, MO, USA).

2.2. Cell Culture

A human neuroblastoma cell line (SH-SY5Y, CL0208, Elabscience, Houston, TX, USA) was subcultured weekly in 75 cm^2 sterile culture flasks with Dulbecco's modified Eagle's Medium/F12 (DMEM/F12; Euroclone, Pero (Milan), Italy) containing 10% fetal bovine serum (FBS; Euroclone), 100 U/mL penicillin, and 100 µg/mL streptomycin in a humidified atmosphere of 5% CO_2 at 37 °C. The experiments were always performed at a confluence of less than 80% of the cells.

2.3. Experimental Protocol

The cells were seeded and, after 24 h of adhesion, were pretreated with 300 nM Thapsigargin (TG) for 30 min, 1 h, and 4 h, to induce an ER stress condition. Then, after the TG was removed, fresh media, with and without Vx, were added to cells. Corrector Vx-809 (2 μM) was administered for 24 h, and then, cell lysates were collected after 24 h of treatment for both the Vx- and TG-treated cells.

2.4. Cell Viability

The potential cytotoxic effects of Vx-809 and TG on neuroblastoma cells were investigated by MTT (3-[4,5-dimetiltiazol-2,5-diphenyl-2H-tetrazolium bromide]) assay, as reported in Pecoraro et al. 2018 [23]. In summary, cells (4.5×10^3/well) were seeded in 96-well plates, and after 24 h, they were treated as described above. Staurosporin (Sp) 0.2 μM was used as a positive control.

At the end of treatment, 25 μL of MTT (5 mg/mL) was added to each well, and the plates were incubated for other 1 h to allow the formation of formazan salt. After this, salt formazan was solubilized with 100 μL of a solution containing 20% (*w*/*v*) SDS, 50% (*v*/*v*) *N*, *N*-dimethylformamide, at pH 4.5. The absorbance at 620 nm was analyzed by a Multiskan Spectrum Thermo Electron Corporation Reader. Cell vitality was calculated as % vitality = $100 \times (OD_{treated}/OD_{DMSO})$.

2.5. Protein Extraction and Western Blotting Assay

The cells (1×10^6 cells/plate) were plated and processed as described in the experimental procedure. Proteins were extracted from the cells by incubation with lysis buffer (20 mM Tris-HCl pH 7.5, 1 mM EGTA, 150 mM NaCl, 1 mM Na_2EDTA, 1% sodium deoxycholate, 1× protease and phosphatase inhibitor cocktail, and 2% IGEPAL), for 30 min. Afterwards, the lysates were centrifuged at 14,000 rpm for 15 min at 4 °C. Protein content was determined by the Bradford protocol, and 60 μg of protein was loaded onto 8–10% acrylamide gels and separated by SDS-PAGE, in denaturing conditions, and transferred to nitrocellulose membranes by means of a minigel apparatus (Bio-Rad Laboratories, Richmond, BC, Canada). Next, the blots were blocked in 5% Tris-buffered saline in non-fat dry milk for 2 h at room temperature and treated with primary antibodies anti-BiP or anti-ATF4 or ATF6 or anti-PERK or anti-SODIII for an entire night at 4 °C. Actin or tubulin was used as loading control. After various washes with PBS/0.1% Tween, the appropriate secondary antibodies were also added for 1 h at room temperature. The immunoreactive protein bands were viewed with enhanced chemiluminescence (ECL) reagents and blot imaging (LAS 4000; GE Healthcare, Milan, Italy). Western blotting imaging data were quantified using ImageJ software Version 1.54j [9,20].

2.6. RNA Extraction and Real-Time RT-PCR Protocol

SH-SY5Y cells were seeded in 100 mm culture dishes and treated as above. RevertAid First Strand cDNA Synthesis Kit (K1622) was used to retrotranscribe 0.5 μg of total RNA that was extracted using TRI Reagent (T9424, Sigma-Aldrich, Darmstadt, Germany) in accordance with the manufacturer's instructions. Two microliters of cDNA were subjected to semi-quantitative PCR using the subsequent primers: 5′-C CTT CTG GGT AGA CCT CTG GGA G-3′ and 5′-A AAC AGA GTA GCA GCT CAG ACT GC-3′. By staining 4% agarose gels with ethidium bromide and subjecting them to LAS 4000 (GE Healthcare, Chicago, IL, USA), fragments of 452 and 426 bps, which correspond to un-spliced and spliced XBP1 mRNA, were found.

2.7. Calcium Signaling Assay

Intracellular calcium concentrations were measured using a membrane-permeant acetoxymethyl ester form of Fura 2, the Fura 2-AM, a fluorescent indicator dye. Neuroblastoma cells (3×10^4 cells/plate) were seeded in 6-well tissue culture plates and treated as previously described.

At the final stage of the treatment, the cells were rinsed with phosphate-buffered saline (PBS), reconstituted, and incubated for 45 min in 1 mL of Hank's balanced salt solution (HBSS) that contained 5 μM Fura 2-AM.

After removing excess Fura 2-AM, SH-SY5Y cells were transferred to a cuvette for spectrofluorometer measurement (Per-kin-Elmer LS-55, Milano (MI), Italy). The cells were then rinsed with PBS buffer. The appropriate quantities of TG (1 nM) and Ionomycin (1 μM) were added to the cuvette in calcium-free HBSS/0.5 mM EGTA buffer to initiate treatment. At 515 nm, emission fluorescence was seen, with the excitation wavelength being varied between 340 and 380 nm. As previously reported [24], the fluorescence intensity ratio of 340/380 nm (F340/F380) was strongly correlated with intracellular free calcium. The TG or Ionomycin-induced increases in the fluorescence ratio (F340/F380 nm) were measured and reported as a delta (Δ) increase in the fluorescence ratio (F340/F380 nm).

2.8. Intracellular and Mitochondrial ROS Detection

Cytosolic ROS generation was evaluated in neuroblastoma cells (8×10^4 cells/well) plated into 6-well plates and treated as depicted above. After the treatment, the cells were collected, washed twice with PBS, and then incubated in PBS containing 2′,7′-dichlorofluorescin diacetate (H_2DCF-DA; 10 μM) probe, at 37 °C for 30 min in the dark. Cell fluorescence was then measured using fluorescence-activated cell sorting (FACSscan; Becton–Dickinson) and analyzed with Cell Quest software.

Changes in mitochondrial O_2^- production were evaluated by fluorescent mitochondrial superoxide indicators (MitoSOX Red). Briefly, cells (8×10^4 cells/well) were incubated with MitoSOX Red (2.5 μM) for 15 min in the dark at 37 °C, followed by washout. Fluorogenic dye, MitoSOX Red, is used to detect superoxide very specifically in living cell mitochondria. Once in mitochondria, it is oxidized by superoxide and produces red fluorescence, which is measured by flow cytometry (FACScan; BD Biosciences, San Jose, CA, USA) and analyzed by Cell Quest software version 4.1.

2.9. Caspase 4 Measurement

Caspase 4 cleavage was analyzed by fluorescence-activated cell sorting (FACSscan; Becton–Dickinson). SH-SY5Y cells were cultured in a 24-well plate (8×10^4 cells/well) and, after 24 h of adhesion, were treated as previously described. Subsequently, the cells were collected and treated for 20 min with a fixing solution (2% FBS, 4% formaldehyde, and sodium azide 0.1% in PBS), permeabilized with a solution consisting of 4% formaldehyde, Triton X-0.1%, 2% FBS, 0.1% sodium azide, and PBS, and the samples were left for 30 min. Following this, anti-caspase 4 antibody was added, and a secondary antibody of goat Texas-Red was utilized. After washing, the cells were fixed and detected by flow cytofluorometry and analyzed by Cell Quest software. The data were represented as the percentage of positive cells.

2.10. Hypodiploid DNA Detection

The cells were plated (8×10^4 cells/well) in a 24-well plate and allowed to grow for 24 h and treated as described above. After two PBS washes, the fixed cells were resuspended in 500 μL of 0.1% sodium citrate buffer, 0.1% Triton X-100, and 50 μg/mL of propidium iodide (PI). The cells were then incubated for 30 min at 4 °C in the dark to analyze the DNA content. By applying Cell Quest software, flow cytofluorometry was used to analyze PI-stained cells. The study of cellular debris was stopped by raising the scatter threshold, and the logarithmic scale was used to record the amount of DNA in the nucleus. The percentage of the hypodiploid region is used to represent the results.

2.11. Analytical Statistics

The commercially available software GraphPad Prism8 (GraphPad Software Inc., San Diego, CA, USA) was used for data assessments and statistical analysis. The data are shown as the mean ± standard error of at least three distinct experiments that were carried out in technical triplicate. Statistical information was gathered using the non-parametric Mann–Whitney U technique between the experimental points. If the p values fell between <0.01 and 0.05, the differences were regarded as significant.

3. Results

3.1. Role of Vx-809 in UPR Pathway

TG mimics the ER stress condition by blocking the sarco/endoplasmic reticulum Ca^{2+}-ATPase (SERCA), disrupts Ca^{2+} homeostasis, and causes cell death [25]. Considering the above considerations, by using the MTT assay on neuroblastoma cells to evaluate the potential toxic effect and in our experimental model, using 300 nM TG, we observed cell viability higher than 50%.

ER homeostasis plays a vital role in cell physiological functions. Several factors can destroy ER homeostasis, triggering a stress condition which activates an UPR pathway. Vx-809 involvement on misfolding protein was evaluated by a Western blotting assay on cell lysates, analyzing some UPR pathway proteins after inducing ER stress in human neuroblastoma (SH-SY5Y) cells.

One of the most essential protective mechanisms induced by the UPR is the upregulation of the GRP78/BiP expression [26].

Western blotting analysis on SH-SY5Y extracts revealed that TG treatment significantly increased ($p < 0.001$) Grp78/BiP levels at all pretreatment times, confirming an ER stress condition.

Addition of Vx-809 reduced TG-induced Grp78/BiP overexpression, significantly ($p < 0.05$) at 30 min and 4 h ($p < 0.005$) pretreatment, as shown in Figure 2A. Moreover, RT-PCR experiments showed the corrective Vx-809 action on splicing of XBP1 (Figure 2B), mediated by IRE1 activation.

ER stress is a known inducer of ATF4 protein expression [27]. Accordingly, we tested the Vx-809 effect on ATF4 induction in response to chemically mediated ER stress. As expected, ATF4 protein was significantly induced ($p < 0.001$) at all time points in our experimental model, following TG treatment. Corrector Vx-809 treatment significantly reduced ($p < 0.005$) TG-induced ATF4 levels, confirming its effect on ATF4 activation in neuroblastoma cells (Figure 2C).

In mammalian cells ATF6 is an n-type membrane protein located in the ER. Several studies have shown that increased ATF6 expression regulates ER stress, reducing cellular damage and ultimately exerts a neuroprotective effect. Previous research has demonstrated that ATF6 deficiency enhances organ damage, as proven by the more severe functional damage and poorer prognosis exhibited in ATF6 knockout mice following cerebral ischemia. More current works have demonstrated that improving brain function is facilitated by activating the ATF6 signaling pathway in the brain [28–30]. The results obtained on neuroblastoma cells, by Western blotting analysis, showed that total ATF6 expression increased in cells pretreated at 1 h and 4 h with TG compared with control cells, confirming the induction of reticular stress and the onset of UPR. Vx-809 administration significantly reduced ($p < 0.05$) TG-induced total ATF6 levels, in particular at 4 h TG-pretreatment times (Figure 2D), restoring a physiological condition.

The PERK pathway is a crucial mediator in neurodegeneration observed in several protein misfolded diseases, suggesting that the general disruption of protein translation is the mechanism underlying neuronal dysfunction and degeneration. In a PD case, markers of PERK activation were found in PD postmortem tissues, where nigral dopaminergic neurons showing αSyn inclusion were also positive for phosphorylated PERK [31]. Therefore, using the SH-SY5Y cell line, we performed a Western blotting analysis of the phosphorylated form of PERK (p-PERK). First and foremost, immunoblots were used to identify

PERK phosphorylation. Figure 2E illustrates this process and shows the p-PERK band-shift that results from the increased molecular weight caused by autophosphorylation [9]. As predicted, p-PERK form was only seen in Vx-809 cells treated with TG, an ER stressor, and not in cells that were left untreated or treated. Moreover, p-PERK band-shift was decreased by Vx-809 therapy even after just one hour of TG pre-treatment.

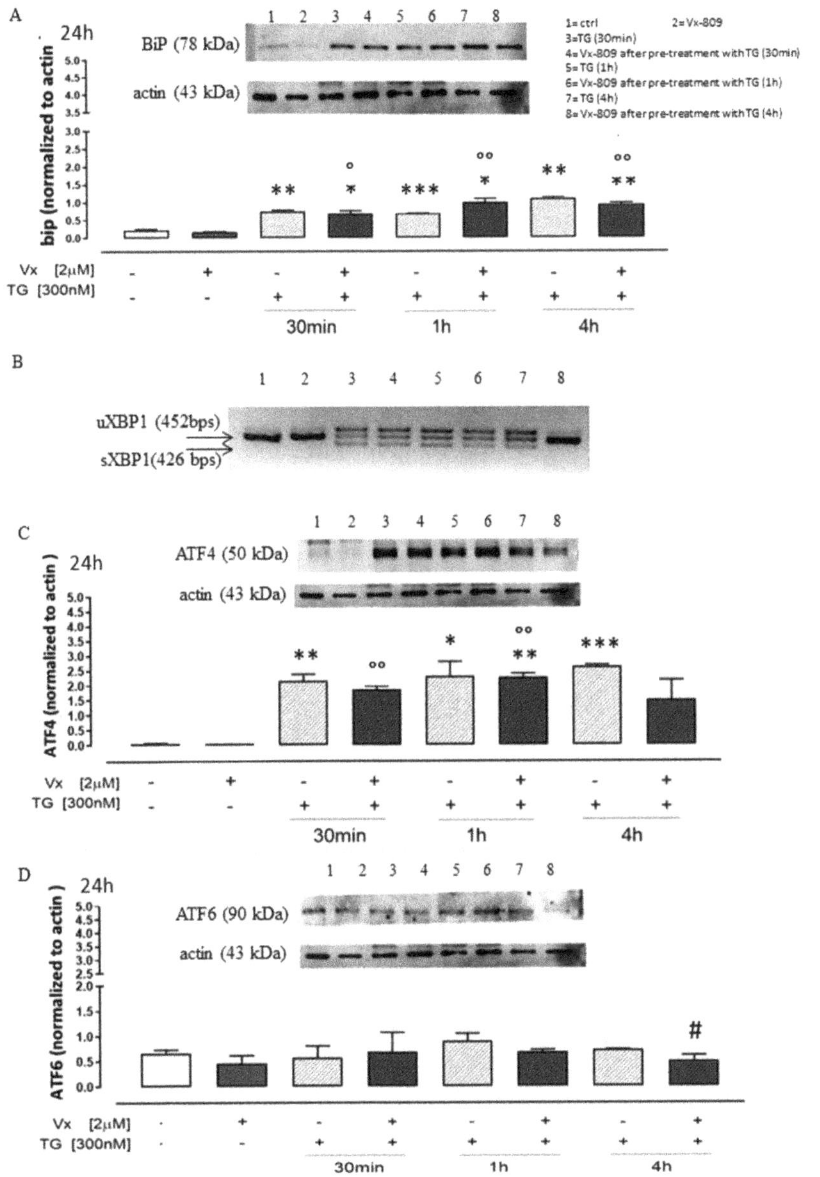

Figure 2. *Cont.*

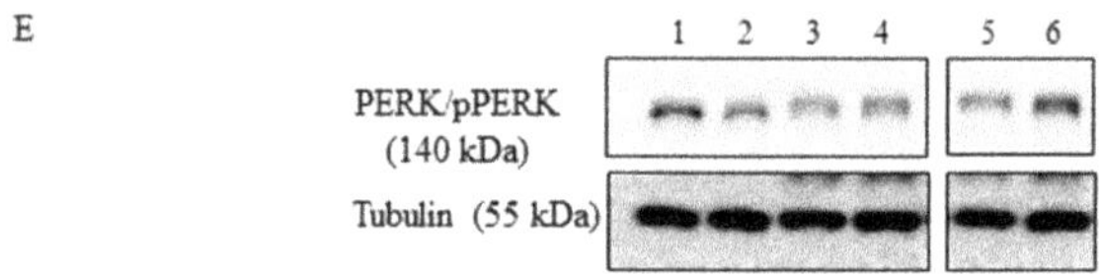

Figure 2. Vx-809 affects UPR activation. Cells were pretreated with 300 nM TG for 30 min or 2 or 4 h, to induce ER stress condition. Next, Vx-809 (2 μM) was added for 24 h. BiP (Panel (**A**)), ATF4 (Panel (**C**)), ATF6 (Panel (**D**)) and PERK/pPERK (Panel (**E**)) expressions in neuroblastoma cells were revealed by Western blotting analysis. Expression of actin or tubulin was employed as a loading control. Panel (**B**) illustrates the gel migration of the 452 bps unsplit fragment of XBP1 mRNA (XBP1 u) and the 426 bp split fragment (XBP1 s), achieved by RT-PCR. These results are presented as the average ± standard error of at least three separate, triplicate-performed studies. Data were processed according to the Mann–Whitney U-test. * $p < 0.05$, ** $p < 0.005$, and *** $p < 0.001$ vs. untreated cells; ° $p < 0.05$ and °° $p < 0.005$ vs. Vx-809-treated cells; # $p < 0.05$ vs. TG-treated cells.

3.2. "Corrector" Vx-809 Interferes on Calcium Signaling

Misfolded proteins causing AD, PD, and prion diseases cause increases in Ca^{2+} influx and ER Ca^{2+} dyshomeostasis, resulting in excitotoxicity and ER stress in affected neurons [32]. Since impaired calcium homeostasis has been implicated in various neurological disorders, we analyzed Vx-809 treatment effects on intracellular calcium concentrations by FURA 2-AM in a calcium-free incubation medium. TG (1 nM) was used to study reticular calcium content. As shown in Figure 3A, the delta increase in reticular calcium levels in Vx-809-treated cells previously pretreated with TG at 30 min and 1 h was significantly higher ($p < 0.05$) than that in TG-treated cells, indicating higher levels of calcium stored in the ER, improving calcium homeostasis.

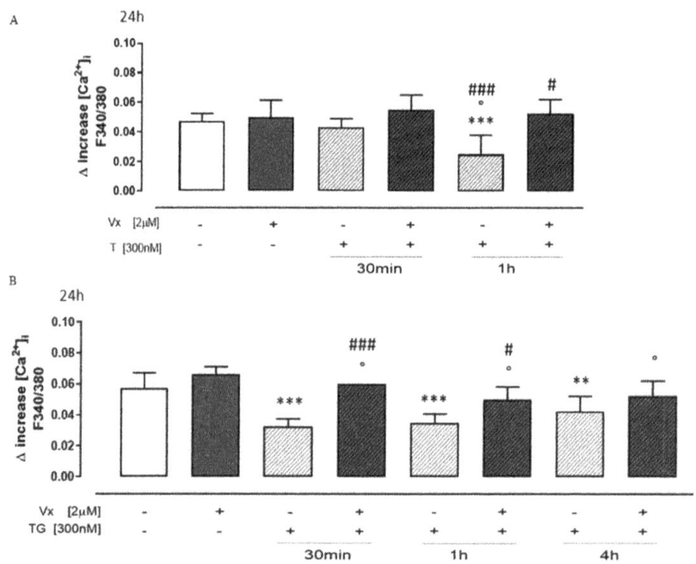

Figure 3. Vx-809 hampers calcium signaling. Cells were pretreated with 300 nM TG for 30 min or 1 or 4 h, to induce ER stress. Following this, Vx-809 (2 μM) was added for 24 h. After ER stress, the Vx-809 effect was determined on the reticular calcium pool in cells in calcium-free media in the presence of 1 nM TG (panel (**A**)), and intracellular calcium concentration was quantified using 1 μM

of ionomycin (panel (**B**)). The results show the mean ± S.E.M. of the delta (δ) increase in the fluorescence of the FURA 2 ratio (340/380 nm) from a minimum of three separate experiments, each carried out in duplicate. The findings are presented as the average ± standard error of duplicate data from a minimum of three separate and identical tests. The Mann–Whitney U test analysis was performed on the data. ** $p < 0.005$ and *** $p < 0.001$ vs. untreated cells; ° $p < 0.05$ vs. Vx-809-treated cells; # $p < 0.05$ and ### $p < 0.001$ vs. TG-treated cells.

Ionomycin (1 μM), a potent and selective Ca^{2+} ionophore, was used to study cytosolic calcium concentration. Our results show that, in Vx-809-treated cells previously pretreated with TG, the delta increase in intracellular calcium levels was higher than that in TG-treated cells, hypothesizing an improvement in intracellular calcium storage (Figure 3B) induced by treatment with a corrector.

3.3. Vx-809 Counteract Thapsigargin-Induced Oxidative Stress

Several NDs may be the result of a biochemical alteration, due to oxidative stress, in bimolecular components. Moreover, the neuronal membranes exhibit a high level of polyunsaturated fatty acids, which are highly susceptible to ROS [33].

To study the effects of Vx-809 on TG-induced cytosolic and mitochondrial ROS production, cytofluorimetric analyses were performed by fluorescent probe DCHF-DA and MitoSOX red, respectively. Our experiments show that Vx-809 treatment significantly decreased ($p < 0.001$) cytosolic (Figure 4A) and mitochondrial (Figure 4B) ROS production in TG-treated cells, at all experimental time points.

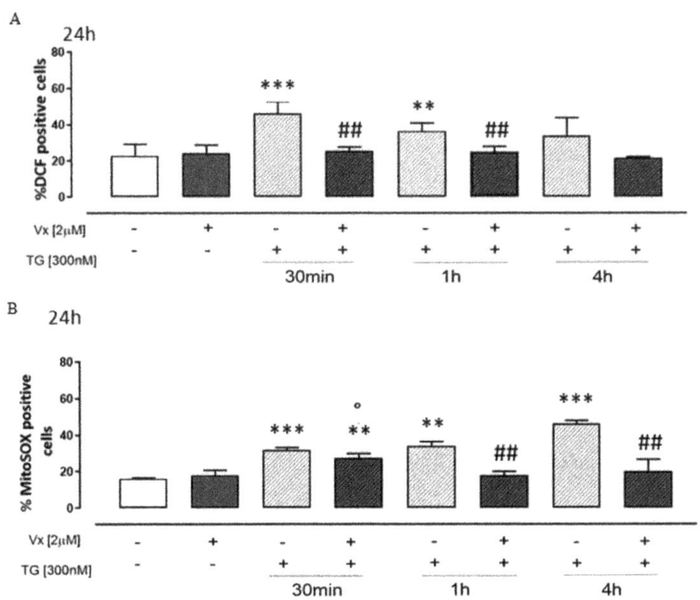

Figure 4. *Cont.*

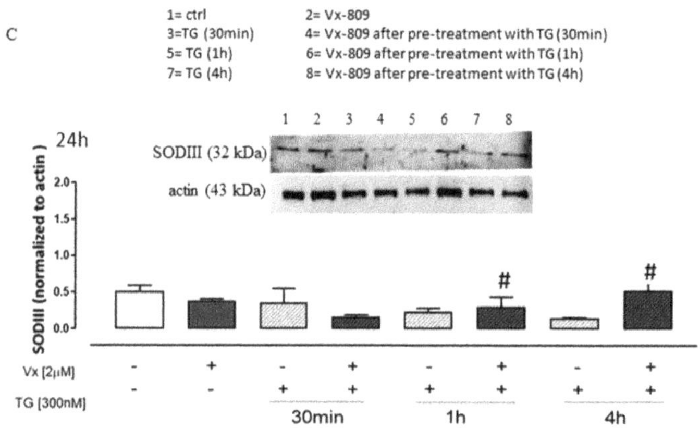

Figure 4. Vx-809 mitigates the oxidative damage caused by Thapsigargin. To cause ER stress, cells were pretreated with 300 nM TG for 30 min, 1 h, or 4 h. The corrector Vx-809 (2 μM) was then administered for a whole day. The probe 2′,7′-dichlorofluorescein diacetate (H_2DCF-DA) was used to measure the amount of ROS produced in SH-SY5Y cells (Panel (**A**)). The percentage of DCF-positive cells in at least three independent experiments, each conducted in duplicate, was used to express the mean ± SEM of ROS generation. Using the MitoSOX Red probe, flow cytometry analysis was used to measure the amount of superoxide produced by the mitochondria in cells (Panel (**B**)). The expression of mitochondrial superoxide generation was calculated as the mean ± standard error of the proportion of cells positive for MitoSOX in three separate tests, each carried out in duplicate. SODIII expressions (Panel (**C**)) on neuroblastoma cells were detected by a Western blotting assay. Actin protein expression was used as loading control. The Mann–Whitney U test was used to evaluate the data. ** $p < 0.005$ and *** $p < 0.001$ vs. untreated cells; ° $p < 0.05$ vs. Vx-809-treated cells; # $p < 0.05$ and ## $p < 0.005$ vs. TG-treated cells.

SODIII is the main body's antioxidant, capable of inhibiting active oxygen damage to the organism and repairing damage caused by free radicals. Moreover, SODIII is the main antioxidant enzyme that removes superoxide anions in cells, protecting one from brain injury [34]. Western blotting analysis showed a significant increase ($p < 0.05$) in SOD III expression at 1 and 4 h from treatment in Vx-809-treated cells after induction of reticular stress compared with TG-treated cells, as depicted in Figure 4C, probably to counteract the stress induced by the increase in ROS.

3.4. *Vx-809 Interferes with the Apoptotic Pathway*

Current studies have shown that the disruption of calcium homeostasis in ER initiates early signals of apoptosis [35,36]. Apoptosis appears to play a key role in the progression of several neurologic disorders, as demonstrated by studies in animal models and cell lines [37,38]. Thus, we evaluated the percentage of hypodiploid nuclei and caspase 4 activation.

In our experimental model, we show that Vx-809 administration induced a significant decrease ($p < 0.001$) in the percentage of hypodiploid nuclei in TG-pretreated SH-SY5Y cells (Figure 5A).

Caspase-4 is cleaved by calpain during ER stress, and suppression of caspase 4 activity partially inhibits cell death in humans. Therefore, caspase 4 plays a critical role in ER stress [39].

Flow cytometry analysis revealed a significant reduction in caspase 4 levels ($p < 0.001$) in treated neuroblastoma cells (Figure 5B) in ER stress conditions, suggesting that Vx-809 restores reticular homeostasis.

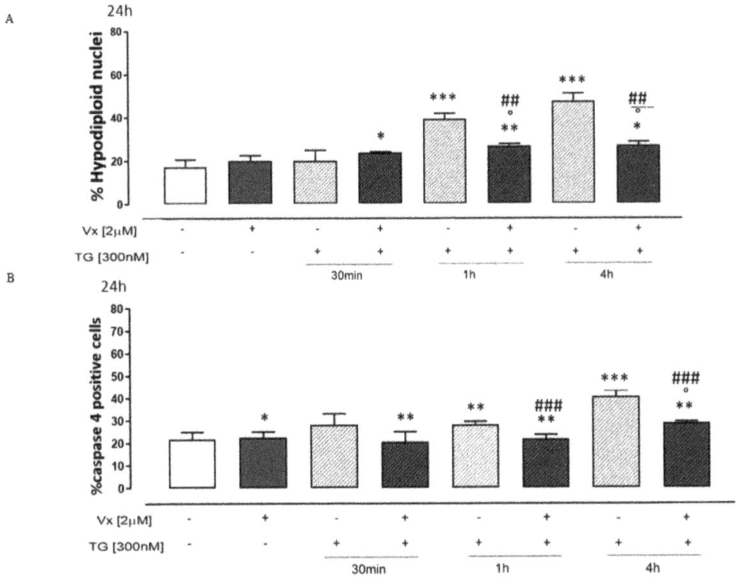

Figure 5. Vx-809 alters the process of apoptosis. Neuroblastoma cells were pretreated with 300 nM TG for 30 min, 2 h, or 4 h, to induce ER stress. Subsequently, 2 μM of the Vx-809 was administered for 24 h. After, the cells were stained by propidium iodide, and the fluorescence of individual nuclei was evaluated by flow cytometry (Panel (**A**)). The data are presented as the mean ± standard error of the percentage of hypodiploid nuclei from a minimum of three independent tests, each carried out in duplicate. The percentage of caspase 4 positive cells (Panel (**B**)) from at least three separate experiments, each carried out in duplicate, was given as mean ± S.E.M. The Mann–Whitney U test was utilized for data analysis. * $p < 0.05$, ** $p < 0.05$ and *** $p < 0.001$ vs. non-treated cells; ° $p < 0.05$ vs. Vx-809-treated cells; ## $p < 0.005$ and ### $p < 0.001$ vs. TG-treated cells.

4. Discussion

Neurodegenerative diseases such as AD, PD, Huntington's disease (HD), amyotrophic lateral sclerosis (ALS), and prion diseases (PrDs) have been found to share common cellular and molecular mechanisms including protein aggregation and formation of inclusion bodies. The initiation of misfolding in a particular cell may be a stochastic event, with constant risk throughout the individual's life [40]. Moreover, neurons lack the ability to remove or dilute toxic molecules by mitotic division since they are terminal, highly differentiated cells; therefore, they are very sensitive to misfolded proteins to an increasing extent with aging [41].

The broad tubular–reticular system in mammalian cells, referred to as the ER, serves as a gatekeeper for the synthesis and folding of transmembrane and secreted proteins and is essential for preserving the balance of calcium, cholesterol, and lipid synthesis. ER stress can be caused by physiological, pathological, and environmental factors that interfere with the folding of ER proteins [42].

A variety of factors that obstruct the ER's oxidative protein folding processes can cause ER stress and the buildup of intralumenal misfolded proteins [43]. When these proteins build up in the ER lumen, the UPR reaction is triggered, which can either lead to the restoration of protein homeostasis or, in the event of irreversible stress, cause cell death. A growing body of research indicates that AD-related hyperphosphorylated tau protein or Aβ peptides gradually accumulate or aggregate and cause irreversible ER stress, which in turn results in synaptic dysfunction and neurodegeneration [44]. As a matter of fact, protein misfolding-related neurodegenerative disorders are linked to the pathogenicity of chronic ER stress [43]. CFTR modulators, like Lumacaftor (Vx-809), are small molecules that bind to defective CFTR proteins and partially restore their function. Vx-809 was the first drug used in the treatment of clinical cystic fibrosis [45].

In this study, we evaluated an off-label Vx-809 use, hypothesizing that probably it does not interact directly with the mutant CFTR protein, responsible for cystic fibrosis, but with a yet unknown mechanism that acts indirectly on misfolded proteins, thus preventing the triggering of mechanisms involved in ER stress.

TG, is an experimental tool, commonly used as ER stressor, that by disturbing intracellular calcium homeostasis causes an accumulation of unfolded or misfolded proteins in the ER [9,46].

To demonstrate the neuroprotective mechanism of corrector Vx-809 on TG-induced ER stress in SH-SY5Y cells, we performed a Western blotting analysis showing that the corrector determines a significant reduction in GRP78/BiP, ATF4, ATF6, and pPERK expression, the main proteins involved in the UPR pathway, probably acting on restoring a stress-induced reticular physiological condition. Of note, our data demonstrate that the IRE1/XBP1 pathway of the UPR is blocked in Vx-809-treated cells, previously pretreated with TG. Thus, the transcription factor sXBP1 is not expressed in these cells.

Calcium is an intracellular messenger chemical found in neurons that is involved in many different activities, such as protein synthesis and energy metabolism [47,48]. The primary intracellular calcium reserve is found in the ER, which has luminal Ca^{2+} concentrations of 100–800 μM as opposed to the cytosol's 100 nM Ca^{2+}. Intraluminal chaperones, such as calnexin, calreticulin, and BiP, act as buffers by binding directly to calcium. Luminal calcium is essential for protein folding and maturation, as it binds to folding chaperones of ER and is necessary for their activity [47]. Alterations in ER calcium homeostasis are common pathological events observed in PrD models [43,48] and probably in other neuropathologies. Perturbation in calcium homeostasis directly correlated to the occurrence of ER stress and increased susceptibility to protein folding stress. Our results demonstrate, in our experimental model, that the proper restoration of protein folding, obtained by Vx-809 treatment, results in improved calcium homeostasis, by restoring the balance of reticular and cytosolic calcium, thereby reducing the free Ca^{2+} levels in neuronal cells.

The brain needs a lot of energy to function because it is one of the body's most active organs. However, as a substrate for the production of reactive oxygen species (ROS), which are essential in physiological communication systems associated with synaptic plasticity, cell–cell connections, development of memory, cell proliferation, and apoptotic processes, oxygen molecules can seriously harm the brain under a number of circumstances (e.g., ischemia reperfusion and misfolding proteins).

Misfolded/unfolded protein aggregation causes excessive oxidative stress, endogenous reticulum stress, and mitochondrial dysfunction in neurons. However, more ER stress increases ROS production, which intensifies oxidative stress [49]. The scientific literature is replete with evidence reflecting the role of ROS in the initiation and progression of several pathologies from cardiovascular diseases to neurodegenerative diseases [4,33,50]. In this study, we have shown that Vx-809 administration, in a reticular stress model, causes a decrease in intracellular and mitochondrial ROS levels and an increase in the antioxidant enzyme SODIII, mainly at 1 and 4 h from treatment, improving the cellular redox state.

UPR failure leads to the accumulation of protein aggregates that likely cause the activation of proapoptotic caspases and induce increased apoptosis of neurons [51]. ER stress-related apoptosis could be caused by increased ROS amounts and by caspase-4 cleavage, an ER-resident caspase known to be involved in ER stress-induced apoptosis [20,24]. Here, we have established that Vx-809 treatment affects protein folding, slowing down the apoptotic process. Furthermore, cytofluorimetric analysis demonstrated a decrease in caspase 4 levels in our experimental model, given by the reduction in ER stress.

In conclusion, we can state that the Vx-809 corrector decreases UPR activation, due to ER stress conditions in neuroblastoma cells. These findings are very promising, because neurodegenerative diseases, such as AD, PD, and ALS, have an etiopathogenesis based on the accumulation of protein aggregates causing chronic reticular stress, leading neuronal cells to apoptosis or loss of function. Vx-809 activity could, therefore, reverse this trend by repairing cellular damage and restoring homeostasis within neurons, making this drug, de facto, a valuable tool in the treatment of neurodegenerative diseases.

Author Contributions: Conceptualization, S.F., M.P. (Maria Pascale), and M.P. (Michela Pecoraro); methodology, M.P. (Michela Pecoraro) and A.S.; formal analysis, M.P. (Michela Pecoraro) and A.S.; investigation, S.F. and M.P. (Michela Pecoraro); data curation, M.P. (Michela Pecoraro); writing—original draft preparation, S.F. and M.P. (Michela Pecoraro); writing—review and editing, S.F., M.P. (Maria Pascale), and M.P. (Michela Pecoraro); supervision, S.F. and M.P. (Maria Pascale); and funding acquisition, S.F. and M.P. (Maria Pascale). All authors have read and agreed to the published version of the manuscript.

Funding: This research received no external funding.

Institutional Review Board Statement: Not applicable.

Informed Consent Statement: Not applicable.

Data Availability Statement: The authors confirm that the data supporting the findings of this study are available within this article.

Acknowledgments: We thank Bruno Maresca for the final revision of the manuscript.

Conflicts of Interest: The authors declare no conflicts of interest.

Abbreviations

AD	Alzheimer's disease
ER	Endoplasmic reticulum
UPR	Unfolded protein response
IRE1α	Inositol-requiring enzyme 1 α
PERK	Protein kinase RNA-like ER kinase
ATF6	Activating transcription Factor 6
GRP78/BiP	Glucose-regulated protein 78/binding immunoglobulin protein
eIF2α	Eukaryotic translation initiation factor 2A
ATF4	Activating transcription factor 4
CHOP	C/EBP homologous protein
ERAD	ER-associated degradation
Vx-809	Lumacaftor
CF	Cystic fibrosis
NBD1	Nucleotide-binding domain 1
TMD1	Transmembrane domain 1
TG	Thapsygargin
NDs	Neurodegenerative diseases
ROS	Reactive oxygen species
PD	Parkinson's disease
PrD	Prion disease
Xbp1	X-box binding protein 1
Xbp1s	Spliced Xbp1
CFTR	Cystic fibrosis transmembrane conductance regulator
SODIII	Superoxide dismutase III
DMEM	Dulbecco's modified Eagle's Medium
FBS	Fetal bovine serum
PBS	Phosphate-buffered saline
MTT	3-[4,5-dimetiltiazol]-2,5-diphenyl-2H-tetrazolium bromide
Sp	Staurosporine
ECL	Enhanced chemiluminescence

HBSS	Hank's balanced salt solution
H_2DCF-DA	2′,7′-dichlorofluorescin diacetate
MitoSOX	Mitochondrial superoxide
PI	Propidium iodide
SERCA	Sarco/endoplasmic reticulum Ca^{2+}-ATPase
ALS	Amyotrophic lateral sclerosis
IDP	Intrinsically disordered proteins

References

1. Oakes, S.A.; Papa, F.R. The role of endoplasmic reticulum stress in human pathology. *Annu. Rev. Pathol.* **2015**, *10*, 173–194. [CrossRef] [PubMed]
2. Rebecca, B.; Berlow, H.; Dyson, J.; Peter, E. Wright, Expanding the Paradigm: Intrinsically Disordered Proteins and Allosteric Regulation. *J. Mol. Biol.* **2018**, *430*, 2309–2320.
3. Soto, C.; Pritzkow, S. Protein misfolding, aggregation, and conformational strains in neurodegenerative diseases. *Nat. Neurosci.* **2018**, *21*, 1332–1340. [CrossRef]
4. Ghemrawi, R.; Khair, M. Endoplasmic Reticulum Stress and Unfolded Protein Response in Neurodegenerative Diseases. *Int. J. Mol. Sci.* **2020**, *21*, 6127. [CrossRef]
5. Ashraf, G.; Greig, N.; Khan, T.; Hassan, I.; Tabrez, S.; Shakil, S.; Sheikh, I.; Zaidi, S.; Akram, M.; Jabir, N.; et al. Protein Misfolding and Aggregation in Alzheimer's Disease and Type 2 Diabetes Mellitus. *CNS Neurol. Disord. Drug Targets* **2014**, *13*, 1280–1293. [CrossRef]
6. Hetz, C.; Saxena, S. ER stress and the unfolded protein response in neurodegeneration. *Nat. Rev. Neurol.* **2017**, *13*, 477–491. [CrossRef]
7. Frakes, A.E.; Dillin, A. The UPR^{ER}: Sensor and Coordinator of Organismal Homeostasis. *Mol. Cell* **2017**, *66*, 761–771. [CrossRef]
8. Li, Y.; Gao, S.; Meng, Y. Integrated analysis of endoplasmic reticulum stress regulators' expression identifies distinct subtypes of autism spectrum disorder. *Front. Psychiatry* **2023**, *17*, 1136154. [CrossRef]
9. Pecoraro, M.; Serra, A.; Pascale, M.; Franceschelli, S. Vx-809, a CFTR Corrector, Acts through a General Mechanism of Protein Folding and on the Inflammatory Process. *Int. J. Mol. Sci.* **2023**, *24*, 4252. [CrossRef]
10. Freeman, O.J.; Mallucci, G.R. The UPR and synaptic dysfunction in neurodegeneration. *Brain Res.* **2016**, *1648*, 530–537. [CrossRef]
11. Wang, M.; Kaufman, R.J. Protein misfolding in the endoplasmic reticulum as a conduit to human disease. *Nature* **2016**, *529*, 326–335. [CrossRef]
12. Hetz, C.; Zhang, K.; Kaufman, R.J. Mechanisms, regulation and functions of the unfolded protein response. *Nat. Rev. Mol. Cell Biol.* **2020**, *21*, 421–438. [CrossRef]
13. Lozada Ortiz, J.; Betancor, M.; Pérez Lázaro, S.; Bolea, R.; Badiola, J.J.; Otero, A. Endoplasmic reticulum stress and ubiquitin-proteasome system impairment in natural scrapie. *Front. Mol. Neurosci.* **2023**, *16*, 1175364. [CrossRef] [PubMed]
14. Kabir, F.; Atkinson, R.; Cook, A.L.; Phipps, A.J.; King, A.E. The role of altered protein acetylation in neurodegenerative disease. *Front. Aging Neurosci.* **2023**, *14*, 1025473. [CrossRef] [PubMed]
15. Moreno, J.A.; Halliday, M.; Molloy, C.; Radford, H.; Verity, N.; Axten, J.M.; Ortori, C.A.; Willis, A.E.; Fischer, P.M.; Barrett, D.A.; et al. Oral treatment targeting the unfolded protein response prevents neurodegeneration and clinical disease in prion-infected mice. *Sci. Transl. Med.* **2013**, *5*, 206ra138. [CrossRef]
16. Angelova, P.R.; Ludtmann, M.H.R.; Horrocks, M.H.; Negoda, A.; Cremades, N.; Klenerman, D.; Dobson, C.M.; Wood, N.W.; Pavlov, E.V.; Gandhi, S.; et al. Ca^{2+} is a key factor in α-synuclein-induced neurotoxicity. *J. Cell Sci.* **2016**, *129*, 1792–1801. [CrossRef] [PubMed]
17. Magrinelli, F.; Mehta, S.; Di Lazzaro, G.; Latorre, A.; Edwards, M.J.; Balint, B.; Basu, P.; Kobylecki, C.; Groppa, S.; Hegde, A.; et al. Dissecting the Phenotype and Genotype of PLA2G6-Related Parkinsonism. *Mov. Disord.* **2022**, *37*, 148–161. [CrossRef]
18. Goldsteins, G.; Hakosalo, V.; Jaronen, M.; Keuters, M.H.; Lehtonen, Š.; Koistinaho, J. CNS Redox Homeostasis and Dysfunction in Neurodegenerative Diseases. *Antioxidants* **2022**, *11*, 405. [CrossRef]
19. Wainwright, C.E.; Elborn, J.S.; Ramsey, B.W.; Marigowda, G.; Huang, X.; Cipolli, M.; Colombo, C.; Davies, J.C.; De Boeck, K.; Flume, P.A.; et al. Lumacaftor-Ivacaftor in Patients with Cystic Fibrosis Homozygous for Phe508del CFTR. *N. Engl. J. Med.* **2015**, *373*, 220–231. [CrossRef]
20. Pecoraro, M.; Franceschelli, S.; Pascale, M. Lumacaftor and Matrine: Possible Therapeutic Combination to Counteract the Inflammatory Process in Cystic Fibrosis. *Biomolecules* **2021**, *11*, 422. [CrossRef]
21. Laselva, O.; Molinski, S.; Casavola, V.; Bear, C.E. Correctors of the Major Cystic Fibrosis Mutant Interact through Membrane-Spanning Domains. *Mol. Pharmacol.* **2018**, *93*, 612–618. [CrossRef] [PubMed]
22. Bardin, E.; Pastor, A.; Semeraro, M.; Golec, A.; Hayes, K.; Chevalier, B.; Berhal, F.; Prestat, G.; Hinzpeter, A.; Gravier-Pelletier, C.; et al. Modulators of CFTR. Updates on clinical development and future directions. *Eur. J. Med. Chem.* **2021**, *213*, 113195. [CrossRef] [PubMed]

23. Pecoraro, M.; Pinto, A.; Popolo, A. Inhibition of Connexin 43 translocation on mitochondria accelerates $CoCl_2$-induced apoptotic response in a chemical model of hypoxia. *Toxicol. In Vitro* **2018**, *47*, 120–128. [CrossRef] [PubMed]
24. Pecoraro, M.; Marzocco, S.; Belvedere, R.; Petrella, A.; Franceschelli, S.; Popolo, A. Simvastatin Reduces Doxorubicin-Induced Cardiotoxicity: Effects beyond Its Antioxidant Activity. *Int. J. Mol. Sci.* **2023**, *24*, 7573. [CrossRef]
25. Sehgal, P.; Szalai, P.; Olesen, C.; Praetorius, H.A.; Nissen, P.; Christensen, S.B.; Engedal, N.; Møller, J.V. Inhibition of the sarco/endoplasmic reticulum (ER) Ca^{2+}-ATPase by thapsigargin analogs induces cell death via ER Ca^{2+} depletion and the unfolded protein response. *J. Biol. Chem.* **2017**, *292*, 19656–19673. [CrossRef] [PubMed]
26. Sun, J.; Mai, K.; Ai, Q. Effects of GRP78 on Endoplasmic Reticulum Stress and Inflammatory Response in Macrophages of Large Yellow Croaker (*Larimichthys crocea*). *Int. J. Mol. Sci.* **2023**, *24*, 5855. [CrossRef]
27. Yang, J.; Kim, K.S.; Iyirhiaro, G.O.; Marcogliese, P.C.; Callaghan, S.M.; Qu, D.; Kim, W.J.; Slack, R.S.; Park, D.S. DJ-1 modulates the unfolded protein response and cell death via upregulation of ATF4 following ER stress. *Cell Death Dis.* **2019**, *10*, 135. [CrossRef]
28. Yu, Z.; Sheng, H.; Liu, S.; Zhao, S.L.; Glembotski, C.C.; Warneret, D.S.; Paschen, W.; Yang, W. Activation of the ATF6 branch of the unfolded protein response in neurons improves stroke outcome. *J. Cereb. Blood Flow Metab.* **2017**, *37*, 1069–1079. [CrossRef]
29. Shen, Y.T.; Li, R.; Yu, S.; Zhao, Q.; Wang, Z.R.; Sheng, H.X.; Yang, W.V. Activation of the ATF6 (Activating Transcription Factor 6) signaling pathway in neurons improves outcome after cardiac arrest in mice. *J. Am. Heart Assoc.* **2021**, *10*, e020216. [CrossRef]
30. Wang, L.; Liu, Y.; Zhang, X.; Ye, Y.; Xiong, X.; Zhang, S.; Gu, L.; Jian, Z.; Wang, H. Endoplasmic Reticulum Stress and the Unfolded Protein Response in Cerebral Ischemia/Reperfusion Injury. *Front. Cell. Neurosci.* **2022**, *16*, 864426. [CrossRef]
31. Mercado, G.; Castillo, V.; Soto, P.; Sidhu, A. ER stress and Parkinson's disease: Pathological inputs that converge into the secretory pathway. *Brain Res.* **2016**, *1648*, 626–632. [CrossRef] [PubMed]
32. Kim, S.; Kim, D.K.; Jeong, S.; Lee, J. The Common Cellular Events in the Neurodegenerative Diseases and the Associated Role of Endoplasmic Reticulum Stress. *Int. J. Mol. Sci.* **2022**, *23*, 5894. [CrossRef]
33. Singh, A.; Kukreti, R.; Saso, L.; Kukreti, S. Oxidative Stress: A Key Modulator in Neurodegenerative Diseases. *Molecules* **2019**, *24*, 1583. [CrossRef] [PubMed]
34. Sun, S.; Gao, N.; Hu, X.; Luo, H.; Peng, J.; Xia, Y. SOD3 overexpression alleviates cerebral ischemia-reperfusion injury in rats. *Mol. Genet. Genom. Med.* **2019**, *7*, e00831. [CrossRef] [PubMed]
35. Marchi, S.; Patergnani, S.; Missiroli, S.; Morciano, G.; Rimessi, A.; Wieckowski, M.R.; Giorgi, C.; Pinton, P. Mitochondrial and Endoplasmic Reticulum Calcium Homeostasis and Cell Death. *Cell Calcium* **2018**, *69*, 62–72. [CrossRef]
36. Cui, X.; Zhang, Y.; Lu, Y.; Xiang, M. ROS and Endoplasmic Reticulum Stress in Pulmonary Disease. *Front. Pharmacol.* **2022**, *13*, 879204. [CrossRef]
37. Wu, Y.; Chen, M.; Jiang, J. Mitochondrial dysfunction in neurodegenerative diseases and drug targets via apoptotic signaling. *Mitochondrion* **2019**, *49*, 35–45. [CrossRef]
38. Radi, E.; Formichi, P.; Battisti, C.; Federico, A. Apoptosis and oxidative stress in neurodegenerative diseases. *J. Alzheimers Dis.* **2014**, *42* (Suppl. S3), S125–S152. [CrossRef]
39. Chukai, Y.; Ito, G.; Konno, M.; Sakata, Y.; Ozaki, T. Mitochondrial calpain-5 truncates caspase-4 during endoplasmic reticulum stress. *Biochem. Biophys. Res. Commun.* **2022**, *608*, 156–162. [CrossRef]
40. Youssef, M.M.M.; Park, J. LONRF2 is a gatekeeper against protein aggregation in aging neurons. *Nat. Aging* **2023**, *3*, 913–914. [CrossRef] [PubMed]
41. Candelise, N.; Scaricamazza, S.; Salvatori, I.; Ferri, A.; Valle, C.; Manganelli, V.; Garofalo, T.; Sorice, M.; Misasi, R. Protein Aggregation Landscape in Neurodegenerative Diseases: Clinical Relevance and Future Applications. *Int. J. Mol. Sci.* **2021**, *22*, 6016. [CrossRef] [PubMed]
42. Coleman, O.I.; Haller, D. ER Stress and the UPR in Shaping Intestinal Tissue Homeostasis and Immunity. *Front. Immunol.* **2019**, *10*, 2825. [CrossRef] [PubMed]
43. Torres, M.; Castillo, K.; Armisén, R.; Stutzin, A.; Soto, C.; Hetz, C. Prion protein misfolding affects calcium homeostasis and sensitizes cells to endoplasmic reticulum stress. *PLoS ONE* **2010**, *5*, e15658. [CrossRef] [PubMed]
44. Ajoolabady, A.; Lindholm, D.; Ren, J.; Pratico, D. ER stress and UPR in Alzheimer's disease: Mechanisms, pathogenesis, treatments. *Cell Death Dis.* **2022**, *13*, 706. [CrossRef]
45. Regard, L.; Martin, C.; Burnet, E.; Da Silva, J.; Burgel, P.R. CFTR Modulators in People with Cystic Fibrosis: Real-World Evidence in France. *Cells* **2022**, *11*, 1769. [CrossRef]
46. Peng, S.Y.; Tang, J.Y.; Lan, T.H.; Shiau, J.P.; Chen, K.L.; Jeng, J.H.; Yen, C.Y.; Chang, H.W. Oxidative-Stress-Mediated ER Stress Is Involved in Regulating Manoalide-Induced Antiproliferation in Oral Cancer Cells. *Int. J. Mol. Sci.* **2023**, *24*, 3987. [CrossRef]
47. Lemmer, I.L.; Willemsen, N.; Hilal, N.; Bartelt, A. A guide to understanding endoplasmic reticulum stress in metabolic disorders. *Mol. Metab.* **2021**, *47*, 101169. [CrossRef]
48. Torres, M.; Encina, G.; Soto, C.; Hetz, C. Abnormal calcium homeostasis and protein folding stress at the ER: A common factor in familial and infectious prion disorders. *Commun. Integr. Biol.* **2011**, *4*, 258–261. [CrossRef]
49. Esmaeili, Y.; Yarjanli, Z.; Pakniya, F.; Bidram, E.; Łos, M.J.; Eshraghi, M.; Klionsky, D.J.; Ghavami, S.; Zarrabi, A. Targeting autophagy, oxidative stress, and ER stress for neurodegenerative disease treatment. *J. Control Release* **2022**, *345*, 147–175. [CrossRef]

50. Karvandi, M.S.; Sheikhzadeh Hesari, F.; Aref, A.R.; Mahdavi, M. The neuroprotective effects of targeting key factors of neuronal cell death in neurodegenerative diseases: The role of ER stress, oxidative stress, and neuroinflammation. *Front. Cell. Neurosci.* **2023**, *17*, 1105247. [CrossRef]
51. Ochneva, A.; Zorkina, Y.; Abramova, O.; Pavlova, O.; Ushakova, V.; Morozova, A.; Zubkov, E.; Pavlov, K.; Gurina, O.; Chekhonin, V. Protein Misfolding and Aggregation in the Brain: Common Pathogenetic Pathways in Neurodegenerative and Mental Disorders. *Int. J. Mol. Sci.* **2022**, *23*, 14498. [CrossRef] [PubMed]

current issues in molecular biology

Article

BDNF/Cyclin D1 Signaling System and Cognitive Performance After Perampanel and Lacosamide Treatment Singly or in Combination in an Experimental Model of Temporal Lobe Epilepsy

Michaela Shishmanova-Doseva [1,2,*] and Darina Barbutska [3,*]

1 Department of Pharmacology, Toxicology and Pharmacotherapy, Pharmacy Faculty, Medical University Plovdiv, 4002 Plovdiv, Bulgaria
2 Research Institute, Medical University Plovdiv, 4002 Plovdiv, Bulgaria
3 Department of Anatomy, Histology and Embryology, Medical Faculty, Medical University Plovdiv, 4002 Plovdiv, Bulgaria
* Correspondence: mihaela.shishmanova@mu-plovdiv.bg (M.S.-D.); darina.barbutska@mu-plovdiv.bg (D.B.)

Abstract: Epilepsy is a common brain function disorder. The present study aims to evaluate the long-term effect of perampanel (PRM) and lacosamide (LCM), administered singly in a high-dose or in a low-dose combination of both, on comorbid anxiety, cognitive impairment, BDNF, and Cyclin D1 hippocampal expression in an experimental model of temporal lobe epilepsy with lithium–pilocarpine. PRM (3 mg/kg, p.o.)/LCM (30 mg/kg, p.o.) or PRM+LCM (0.5 mg/kg + 3 mg/kg, p.o.) treatments were administered three hours after the lithium–pilocarpine-induced status epilepticus and continued for up to ten weeks in adult Wistar rats. Our study demonstrated that perampanel and lacosamide administered singly in high doses improved epilepsy-associated cognitive impairment through ameliorating anxiety and facilitating passive learning and memory, with spatial and recognition memory measured in the elevated plus maze, step-through, Y-maze, and object recognition tests, respectively. In addition, the combination of both drugs in low doses demonstrated similar anxiolytic and cognitive-improving effects compared to the singly administered drugs. Moreover, the three experimental groups enhanced the hippocampal expression of the neurotrophic factor BDNF and mitigated the increased levels of the apoptotic factor Cyclin D1. These beneficial effects could be essential mechanisms through which administered anticonvulsants preserve neuronal survival and homeostasis in the CNS and especially in the hippocampus.

Keywords: perampanel; lacosamide; lithium–pilocarpine; BDNF; cyclin D1; hippocampus; apoptosis

1. Introduction

Epilepsy is one of the most common brain function disorders, and most focal epilepsy crises arise in the temporal lobe of the brain [1,2]. Although the pathogenesis of epilepsy is still not fully elucidated, different molecular targets, such as neurotransmitters, ion channels, or synaptic proteins [3], can be influenced by existing anti-seizure medications (ASMs). It is well known that glutamate is the primary excitatory neurotransmitter in the central nervous system (CNS), and hyperactivation of its postsynaptic α-amino-3-hydroxy-5-methylisoxazole-4-propionic acid (AMPA) receptors plays a crucial role in the generation, synchronization, and spread of epileptic activity [4,5]. Perampanel (PRM) is a novel third-generation ASM. It is the first drug that belongs to the class of non-competitive, selective AMPA receptor antagonists [6]. PRM has been approved as an adjunctive treatment for focal epileptic seizures with or without secondary generalization in patients with epilepsy aged $\geq$ 4 years and for primary generalized tonic–clonic seizures in patients with idiopathic generalized epilepsy aged $\geq$7 years (EU only) or $\geq$12 years (USA only). In the USA, the drug can be prescribed as a monotherapy for the treatment of focal epileptic seizures [7].

Although most ASMs act on voltage-gated sodium channels, lacosamide (LCM) is a third-generation drug with a unique mechanism of action on these channels. It selectively enhances their slow inactivation by regulating their long-term availability [8]. Voltage-gated sodium channels are responsible for the generation of action potentials during normal brain function and high-frequency firing, which is a feature of epileptic discharges [9]. LCM has been approved for the treatment of focal seizures with or without secondary generalization as a monotherapy or an adjunctive drug for patients $\geq$16 years of age [10].

Different comorbidities, including cognitive deficits, depression, anxiety, migraine, and a tendency for falls and fractures, can be observed among epileptic patients [11]. Numerous ASMs have been shown to be clinically effective [3]. Despite the latter fact, more than 30% of patients remain refractory to seizure treatment, which requires the prescribing of two or more ASMs [12]. Combinations of different anticonvulsants can produce additive, synergistic, or antagonistic effects on seizure control, alongside some adverse effects [13]. From a pharmacological perspective, polytherapy includes two or more ASMs with different mechanisms of action that influence various targets for seizure control. Considering the large number of anticonvulsants available, the consequences of different drug combinations have, in general, not been well elucidated.

At this stage, there are not enough studies related to the influence of epileptic seizures on neuronal survival in the hippocampus. There is also a lack of research on the possibility that anticonvulsant drugs affect the expression of neurotrophic factors in the hippocampus, a brain structure extremely critical for memorizing and consolidating information from short- to long-term memory. Brain-derived neurotrophic factor (BDNF) is an endogenous protein that is a key regulator of brain development and neuronal formation. It promotes neurogenesis and synaptic activity, protects neurons from programmed cell death, and maintains cellular homeostasis [14–16]. In contrast, BDNF is a mediator of neuron-microglial interactions [17,18]. Many researchers consider BDNF to be the most important signaling molecule between neurons and glia, especially in conditions of injury and cellular stress [19]. According to several studies, microglia express BDNF, and in turn, the derived BDNF affects synaptic plasticity, influencing different neuronal structures and functions [20,21]. The released neurotrophic factor can affect neuronal survival and compensate for neuronal loss [20,21]. Whether and how these interactions are unidirectional and what their subtle mechanisms are is a question that has not been sufficiently investigated.

In recent years, there has been evidence of a cascade of processes occurring in cells as a result of active external factors (cellular stress, damage, and intake of certain drugs), such as the process of apoptosis. The latter is a complex process regulated by multiple pro- and anti-apoptotic genes; long-term damage to the balance between the two groups causes apoptotic changes in the brain cells [22]. The hippocampus is extremely sensitive to all external influences that cause oxidative stress in cells [23]. In this respect, the participation of programmed cell death in the mechanisms of epilepsy, as well as the causes leading to cognitive deficits, are also considered. The Cyclin D1 protein participates as a regulator of some manifestations of the apoptotic process. Moreover, increased expression of this protein has been revealed in hippocampal neurons and proliferating glia after epileptic seizures [24,25]. Therefore, Cyclin D1 has been a subject of research in two lines of investigation: participation in the cell cycle and provoking apoptotic changes in major damage to the cell's DNA [26]. The data suggests that Cyclin D1 is a convenient marker for detecting probable neuronal damage in the presence of apoptotic cell changes. Cyclin D1 is visualized histochemically in damaged neurons of the hippocampus and in some glial elements [27]. The probable control of neuronal functions and neurogenesis by astrocytes through the expression of Cyclin D1 has also been described [28].

Animal models of epilepsy have proven to be invaluable in the evaluation of ASMs on comorbidities and the possible mechanisms through which drugs affect these comorbidities [9]. The lithium–pilocarpine model is a reliable animal model for investigating epileptogenesis after status epilepticus (SE) and pathogenesis of temporal lobe epilepsy

(TLE), which is demonstrated by spontaneous motor seizures (SMS) and comorbid cognitive and psychological disorders during the chronic phase [2]. In this respect, we evaluated the long-term effect of PRM and LCM, administered singly in a high-dose or in a low-dose combination of both on comorbid anxiety, cognitive impairment, BDNF, and Cyclin D1 hippocampal expression in an experimental model of TLE.

2. Materials and Methods

2.1. Reagents and Drugs

Pilocarpine hydrochloride (Pilo, powder, P6503), lithium chloride (LiCl, powder, L9650), and scopolamine methyl bromide (Scop, powder, S8502) were purchased from Sigma Aldrich, St. Louis, MO, USA. Lacosamide (Vimpat®, USB Pharma, Brussels, Belgium), Perampanel (Fycompa®, Eisai Ltd., Frankfurt am Main, Germany), and Diazepam (Sopharma, Sofia, Bulgaria) were obtained from the pharmaceutical companies. The following reagents were used in the study: Bouen's Fluid Sigma, HT10132 (Aldrich Chemie GmbH, Taufkirchen, Germany); Gill's Hematoxylin Solution, No. 2, sc-24973A (Santa Cruz Biotechnology, Inc., Dallas, TX, USA); ImmunoCruz goat ABC Staining, sc-2023 (Santa Cruz Biotechnology, Inc., Dallas, TX, USA); pro BDNF (5H8), sc-65514; Cyclin D1 (A-12), sc-8396 (Santa Cruz Biotechnology, Inc., Dallas, TX, USA); and VectaMount® Express Mounting Medium, H-5700-60 (Vector Laboratories, Newark, CA, USA).

2.2. Animals

Forty-six mature male Wistar rats at 3 months of age weighing between 180 and 200 g were used in this study. They were obtained from the Animal Center of the Medical University, Plovdiv. The rats were housed in plastic cages (4–5 per cage) [29–31]. They were maintained at a constant temperature (22 ± 1 °C) and relative humidity (55–60%) under a 12 h/12 h light/dark cycle. The ventilation system was set between 15 and 20 air changes per hour. Food and drinking water were provided ad libitum. This study was performed in strict accordance with the guidelines of European Community Council Directives 86/609/EEC and 0.2010/63/EC. The experiments were approved by the Bulgarian Food Safety Agency No. 206/01.10.2018 and the Ethical Committee on Human and Animal Experimentation of Medical University—Plovdiv No. 1/28.02.2019.

2.3. Generation of Chronic Epilepsy Rats

The timeline of the experiment is shown in Figure 1. Thirty-eight rats were injected with LiCl 127 mg/kg intraperitoneally (i.p.) 24 h before the Pilo treatment. The rats were given 30 mg/kg i.p. Pilo, 30 min after the injection of scopolamine methyl bromide 1 mg/kg i.p. The latter was administered to reduce the peripheral cholinergic effects resulting in respiratory problems, which are one of the main reasons for the animal's death in this model. After the last injection, the animals were placed in separate cages, and their behavioral seizure severity was evaluated based on the Racine scale [32]: Stage 1—mouth and facial movements; Stage 2—head nodding; Stage 3—forelimb clonus; Stage 4—seizures characterized by rearing and continued forelimb clonus; Stage 5—seizures characterized by rearing, forelimb clonus, and falling. The criterion for reaching status epilepticus was a state when the animal reached stage 4 or 5 based on the Racine scale, followed by continuous motor activity (>9 motor seizures/h). After two hours of ongoing seizures, 10 mg/kg Diazepam was injected i.p. to relieve convulsions and prevent mortality. The dosage was repeated as needed. Six animals died during the SE. The remaining 32 rats were then randomly allocated to the four experimental groups (8 per group, from the second to the fifth one), and an additional 8 rats, in which no SE was induced, were allocated to the control group as follows:

- 1st group—C-veh (control animals treated only with saline 1 mL/kg p.os.);
- 2nd group—Li-Pilo-veh (this group was with the model of post-SE-induced TLE triggered by the i.p. administration of LiCl 127 mg/kg and Pilocarpine 30 mg/kg i.p. and was treated with saline 1 mL/kg p.os.);

- 3rd group—Li-Pilo-PRM (this group was with the model of post-SE-induced TLE triggered by the i.p. administration of LiCl 127 mg/kg and Pilocarpine 30 mg/kg i.p. and was treated with perampanel 3 mg/kg p.os.);
- 4th group—Li-Pilo-LCM (this group was with the model of post-SE-induced TLE triggered by the i.p. administration of LiCl 127 mg/kg and Pilocarpine 30 mg/kg i.p. and was treated with lacosamide 30 mg/kg p.os.);
- 5th group—Li-Pilo-PRM-LCM (this group was with the model of post-SE-induced TLE triggered by the i.p. administration of LiCl 127 mg/kg and Pilocarpine 30 mg/kg i.p. and was treated with perampanel 0.5 mg/kg p.os + lacosamide 3 mg/kg p.os).

Three hours after the Li-Pilo injections, the rats were injected subcutaneously (s.c.) with NaCl 0.9% and glucose 5% in equal volumes (up to 3% of body weight) to restore volume loss. This procedure was repeated over the next 5 days to increase the survival chances of the animals. Treatment with veh/PRM or LCM, administered orally by gavage, started three hours after the onset of SE and continued for up to 10 weeks. We used the pharmaceutically prepared solution for infusion of lacosamide (Vimpat® 200 mg/20 mL). Doses of 3 mg/kg (0.03 mL per 100 g) and 30 mg/kg (0.3 mL per 100 g) were administered per os from this solution. Perampanel (Fycompa 2 mg tab.) was dissolved in a three-component solvent (distilled water, DMSO, and propylene glycol) in a concentration of 1 mg/10 mL. Doses of 0.5 mg/kg (0.5 mL per 100 g) and 3 mg/kg (3 mL per 100 g) were administered per os [33]. Eight weeks after the Li-Pilo injection, all rats were subjected to a series of tests and were daily treated with the drugs.

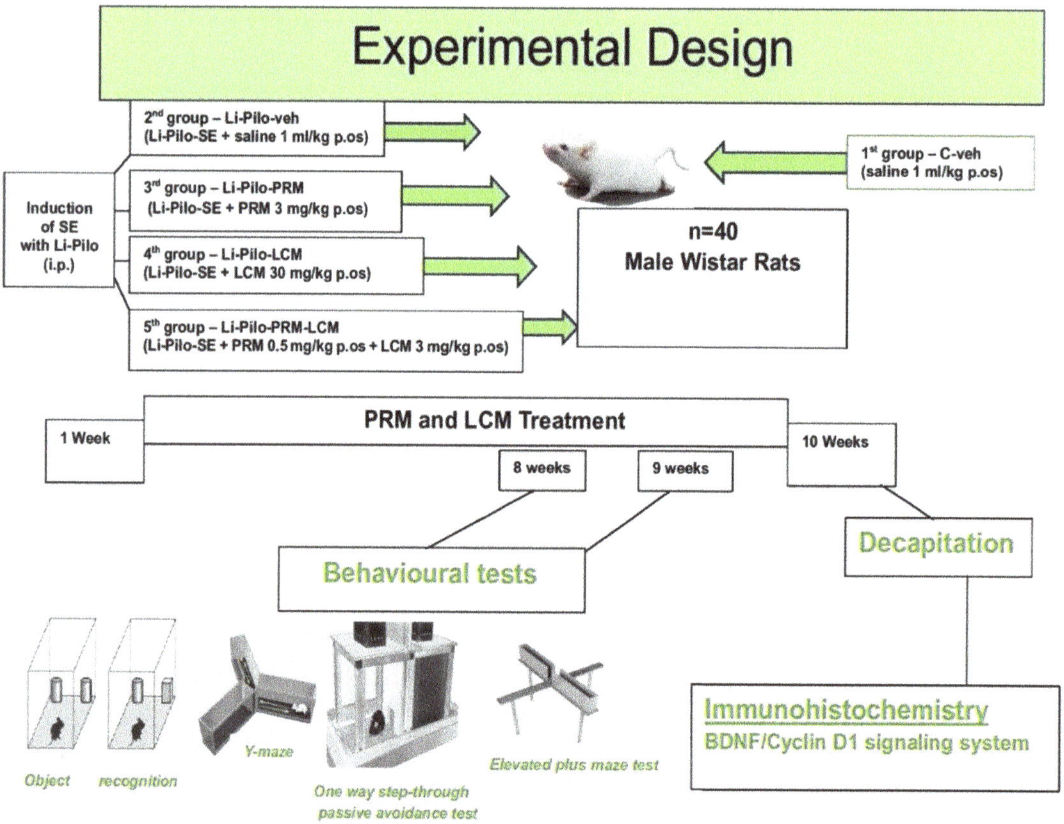

Figure 1. Timeline of the experiment.

2.4. Behavioral Tests

2.4.1. Object Recognition Test

The object recognition test (ORT) consisted of a training session (T1) and a test session (T2) conducted on two consecutive days. The object recognition test was performed in an open Plexiglas box (60 × 60 × 40 cm) with objects made of plastic, as previously described [34,35]. Briefly, during T1, each rat was allowed to explore two identical objects (A1 and A2) for 5 min. In the test session (T2), the rats were exposed to a familiar object (A1) and a novel object (B) for 5 min. The exploration time (s) for each object in the test session was recorded, and the discrimination index (DI) was defined as the difference in exploration time between the novel (TB) and familiar objects (TA) divided by the total time spent exploring the two objects in the discrimination phase: (TB − TA)/(TB + TA) = DI.

2.4.2. Y-Maze

The Y-maze is widely used to assess hippocampal-dependent spatial working memory by measuring the spontaneous alternations. This method utilizes the congenital tendency of rodents to explore novelty [36]. Black Plexiglas consisting of three equally spaced arms interconnected at 120° was used in the experiment. Each arm was designated as A, B, or C. At the beginning of the experiment, each animal was randomly placed at the end of one arm of the maze and allowed to explore the maze freely for a total trial duration of 7 min. Successful entry into an arm was considered when the animal entered the arm on all four paws. The number and sequence of arm entries were recorded manually. Spontaneous alternation occurs when the animal consecutively enters at least three of various combinations of arms; for example, ABC, CBA, CAB, BCA, etc. Spontaneous alternation (SA) % was calculated using the following formula: SA % = (number of alternations)/(total number of entries − 2) × 100.

2.4.3. One-Way Step-Through Passive Avoidance Test with Negative Reinforcement

The step-through apparatus (UgoBasile, Gemonio, Italy) consisted of two equal-sized dark and light compartments separated by a sliding automatic door. The experiment was conducted on two consecutive days: the 1st day was the learning session, which was performed with a schedule of 2 trainings with a 60 min interval between them, and the 2nd day was the retention test. During the learning session, the rats were placed in the light compartment. Immediately after the rat entered the dark chamber with all four feet inside, the door was closed and a short-lasting electrical foot shock (9 s, 0.4 mA, 50 Hz) was delivered. After 20 s, the animals were removed from the dark chamber and returned to their cages. Time (s) spent in the light compartment was recorded. Twenty-four hours after the last learning session, the memory retention test was performed. The experimental protocol was the same as above, except that no electrical shock was delivered to the rats. The test was concluded when the animal entered the dark compartment or remained in the light chamber for 178 s (cut-off time) [37].

2.4.4. Elevated Plus Maze Test

The apparatus consisted of two open arms (50 × 10 cm^2), two enclosed arms (50 × 10 × 50 cm^3), and a central platform (10 × 10 cm^2), elevated 50 cm above the floor. Rats were placed on the central square of the maze facing an open arm and allowed to freely explore the maze for 5 min. The calculated measures were: (1) the number of entries in open arms; (2) the number of entries in enclosed arms; (3) the time (s) spent in the open arms; and (4) the anxiety index (AI) = 1 − [(open arms time/total time) + (number of entries in open arms/total number of entries)/2]. Results close to 1 show anxious behavior [34,35].

After the last test, animals were decapitated under deep anesthesia with 0.2 mg/kg, i.p. of fentanyl and 0.3 mg/kg, i.p, of midazolam. Brains were removed immediately and collected for further investigations. Parts of the brains of experimental animals containing the hippocampus were fixed using Bouen's fluid for 24 h. After washing with xylol, the brain fragments stayed in liquid paraffin in a thermostat (at 56°) for 24 h, after which they were incorporated into paraffin. The paraffin blocks were cut into an automatic paraffin microtome (Leica 2055, Leica Biosystems, Deer Park, IL, USA). Paraffin histological sections (6 μm thick) were installed on silane-coated slides and were used for immunohistochemical analysis.

2.5. Immunohistochemistry

We used fragments of the hippocampus of the experimental animals, processed by protocol, included in paraffin, and prepared for immunohistochemical analysis. The cuts were mounted on silane-coated slides. The slides were dewaxed alternately with xylene and a descending alcohol battery. Then, we suppressed peroxidase with a solution of methanol and hydrogen peroxide for 30 min. The slides were kept in PBS (phosphate-buffered saline) for 15 min and in normal swine serum dissolved in PBS for 30 min. The expression of BDNF and Cyclin D1 was monitored using the ABC method with the ImmunoCruz™ rabbit ABC Staining System kit (Santa Cruz Biotechnology, Inc., USA), with DAB as chromogen and monoclonal primary anti-BDNF and anti-Cyclin D1 antibody (1:100; Santa Cruz Biotechnology, Inc., USA) [38,39]. Sections in which the primary antibody was substituted with PBS were used as negative controls. The duration of incubation was 24 h at 4° C in a humid (70%) chamber. After completion of the reaction, we rinsed with PBS, contrasted the nuclei with hematoxylin, dehydrated in alcohols of upward concentration, and covered with Vecta mount (Vector Laboratories, Newark, CA, USA).

The immunohistochemical manifestations of the investigated signal system are subjected to quantitative analysis of the intensity of reactions using specialized software, the Leica DM 3000 image system with Flexacam C3 (Leica Biosystems, Deer Park, IL, USA).

2.6. Quantitative Analysis of the Intensity of Immunohistochemical Reactions

The immunohistochemical analysis was performed on both brain hemispheres of all animals from the groups (n = 40), using specialized, highly sensitive software, the Olympus DP-Soft image system (version 4.1 for Windows), equipped with a Camedia-5050Z digital camera (Olympus, Japan). The intensity values of the reactions were in the range of 0–256, with 0 presenting white and 256 black. The specific staining of the fields was in the form of dark brown to black granules in the positive cells. The analysis was carried out on sections of the hippocampus of Wistar rats from all groups already described (n = 40). Series of simultaneous reactions involving material from all experimental groups were analyzed in order to determine the comparability of the results. The curve of the intensity of immune responses in the positive cells was calculated on different microscopic fields of sections (20 sections per animal, magnification ×400) of all hippocampal hemispheres of at least 100 cells. The mean value of the intensity of antigen expression for each animal in the groups was calculated, and BDNF/Cyclin D1 expression was recorded in relative units (RU).

2.7. Statistical Analysis

Experimental results were presented as mean ± SEM. The results were analyzed using parametric tests because of normally distributed data, as assessed by the Kolmogorov–Smirnov test. The different parameters of all behavioral tests—discrimination index, spontaneous alternations, step-through latency time, number of entries in open arms, time spent in open arms, and anxiety index, including BDNF and Cyclin D1 hippocampal expression—were assessed by one-way ANOVA. When the F-ratio was significant, the between-group differences were assessed by Tukey's post hoc test in case of justification. When the variances were significantly different, depending on the homogeneity of the dispersions (found by using the Levene's test), the Games–Howell post hoc test was applied. Statistical significance was set at $p < 0.05$. The analysis was conducted by using the IBM SPSS® (version 19.0.) statistical package.

3. Results

3.1. Object Recognition Test

The post hoc test demonstrated that the Li-Pilo-veh group had impaired object recognition memory compared to the C–veh group (−0.31 ± 0.09 vs. 0.57 ± 0.08, $p < 0.001$), while the long-term LCM treatment during the chronic phase of the TLE model managed to increase the discrimination index compared to the group with epilepsy (0.43 ± 0.09 vs. −0.31 ± 0.09, $p = 0.001$) (Figure 2). The Li-Pilo-PRM group singly did not increase the discrimination index, while the group treated with both drugs, PRM and LCM, managed to reduce the negative influence of epilepsy compared to the pilocarpine-treated animals (0.6 ± 0.09 vs. −0.31 ± 0.09, $p = 0.001$) and to the rats treated only with PRM (0.6 ± 0.09 vs. −0.01 ± 0.2, $p = 0.009$). No statistical significance was observed when the C-veh group was compared to the Li-Pilo-LCM and Li-Pilo-PRM-LCM animals as well as between the Li-Pilo-LCM and Li-Pilo-PRM-LCM rats.

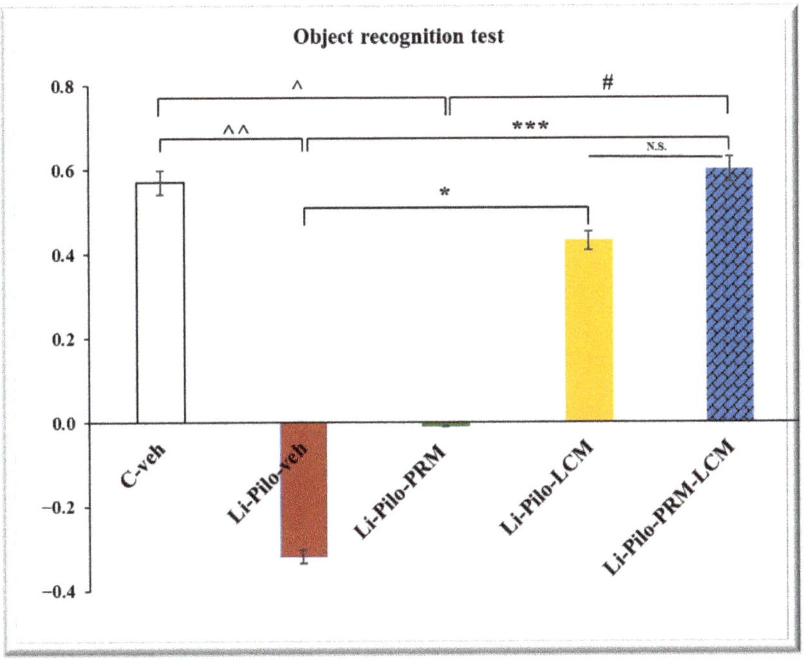

Figure 2. Effect of long-term treatment with perampanel (PRM) and lacosamide (LCM), singly or in combination, on the discrimination index in the object recognition test in animals with a model of temporal lobe epilepsy. ^^ $p < 0.01$ Li-Pilo-veh group vs. C-veh group; ^ $p < 0.05$ Li-Pilo-PRM vs. C-veh group, * $p < 0.05$ Li-Pilo-LCM vs. Li-Pilo-veh group; *** $p < 0.001$ Li-Pilo-PRM-LCM vs. Li-Pilo-veh group; # $p < 0.05$ Li-Pilo-PRM-LCM vs. Li-Pilo-PRM group; no significance (N.S.), $p > 0.05$ Li-Pilo-LCM vs. Li-Pilo-PRM-LCM group.

3.2. Y-Maze Test

In the Y-maze task, the Li-Pilo-veh group showed a significant decrease in the percentage of spontaneous alternations (SA) compared to the C-veh animals (31.17 ± 7.13 vs. 65.10 ± 4.66, $p = 0.001$) (Figure 3). Both groups, Li-Pilo-PRM and Li-Pilo-LCM, significantly increased spontaneous alternations compared to the animals with a model of epilepsy (69.29 ± 4.67 vs. 31.17 ± 7.13, $p < 0.001$ and 67.89 ± 6.63 vs. 31.17 ± 7.13, $p < 0.001$, respectively). The same positive effect on SA was observed in the group treated with both drugs (Li-Pilo-PRM-LCM) compared to the Li-Pilo-veh animals (58.34 ± 3.27 vs. 31.17 ± 7.13, $p = 0.012$). No statistical significance was observed when comparing the C-veh group and the three groups treated singly with PRM and LCM or in a combination of both drugs, $p > 0.05$. In addition, no difference was detected between the Li-Pilo-PRM and Li-Pilo-LCM groups when compared to the animals treated with both drugs (Li-Pilo-PRM-LCM), $p > 0.05$.

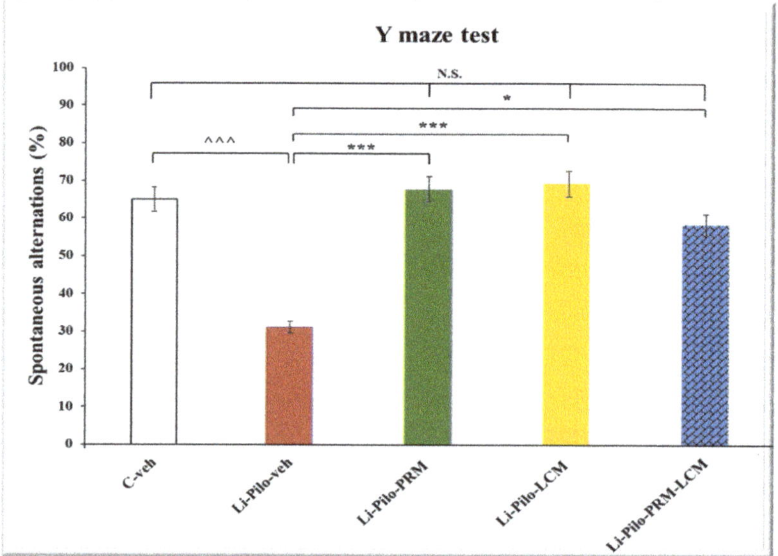

Figure 3. Effect of long-term treatment with perampanel (PRM) and lacosamide (LCM), singly or in combination, on the spontaneous alternations (%) in the Y-maze test in animals with a model of temporal lobe epilepsy. ^^^ $p < 0.001$ Li-Pilo-veh vs. C-veh group; *** $p < 0.001$ Li-Pilo-PRM vs. Li-Pilo-veh group; *** $p < 0.001$ Li-Pilo-LCM vs. Li-Pilo-veh group; * $p < 0.05$ Li-Pilo-PRM-LCM vs. Li-Pilo-veh group; no significance (N.S.), $p > 0.05$ C-veh group vs. Li-Pilo-PRM group; $p > 0.05$ C-veh group vs. Li-Pilo-LCM group; $p > 0.05$ C-veh group vs. Li-Pilo-PRM-LCM group; N.S., $p > 0.05$ Li-Pilo-PRM vs. Li-Pilo-PRM-LCM group; N.S., $p > 0.05$ Li-Pilo-LCM group vs. Li-Pilo-PRM-LCM group.

3.3. One-Way Step-Through Passive Avoidance Test with Negative Reinforcement

The post hoc test revealed that the Li-Pilo animals showed a decreased reaction time during the learning session (24.51 ± 5.83 vs. 77.13 ± 4.84, $p = 0.007$) and the memory retention test compared to the C-veh group (30.60 ± 6.61 vs. 137.58 ± 21.80, $p = 0.001$) (Figure 4A,B). The comparison between the Li-Pilo-veh rats and the group with a model of epilepsy treated with PRM showed that the animals treated with the anticonvulsant significantly increased their step-through latency time during both sessions on day 1 (86.98 ± 10.99 vs. 24.51 ± 5.83, $p = 0.001$) and day 2 (111.21 ± 25.41 vs. 30.60 ± 6.61, $p = 0.023$). The Li-Pilo-LCM group also showed an increase in the time for entering the dark compartment during the learning session (67.01 ± 15.49 vs. 24.51 ± 5.83, $p = 0.041$) and the memory retention test compared to the animals with a model of TLE (158.20 ± 19.80 vs. 30.60 ± 6.61, $p < 0.001$). Moreover, during the two experimental days, the group that was treated with both drugs showed a significant increase in the latency time compared to the Li-Pilo-veh animals (93.27 ± 9.95 vs. 24.51 ± 5.83, $p < 0.001$ for day 1 and 158.25 ± 6.28 vs. 30.60 ± 6.61, $p < 0.001$ for day 2). No statistical significance was observed when comparing the C-veh group and the three groups treated singly with PRM and LCM or a combination of both drugs, $p > 0.05$. Moreover, no difference was detected as well between the single-drug-treated groups when compared to the animals treated with both drugs (Li-Pilo-PRM-LCM), $p > 0.05$ during the learning session and memory retention test.

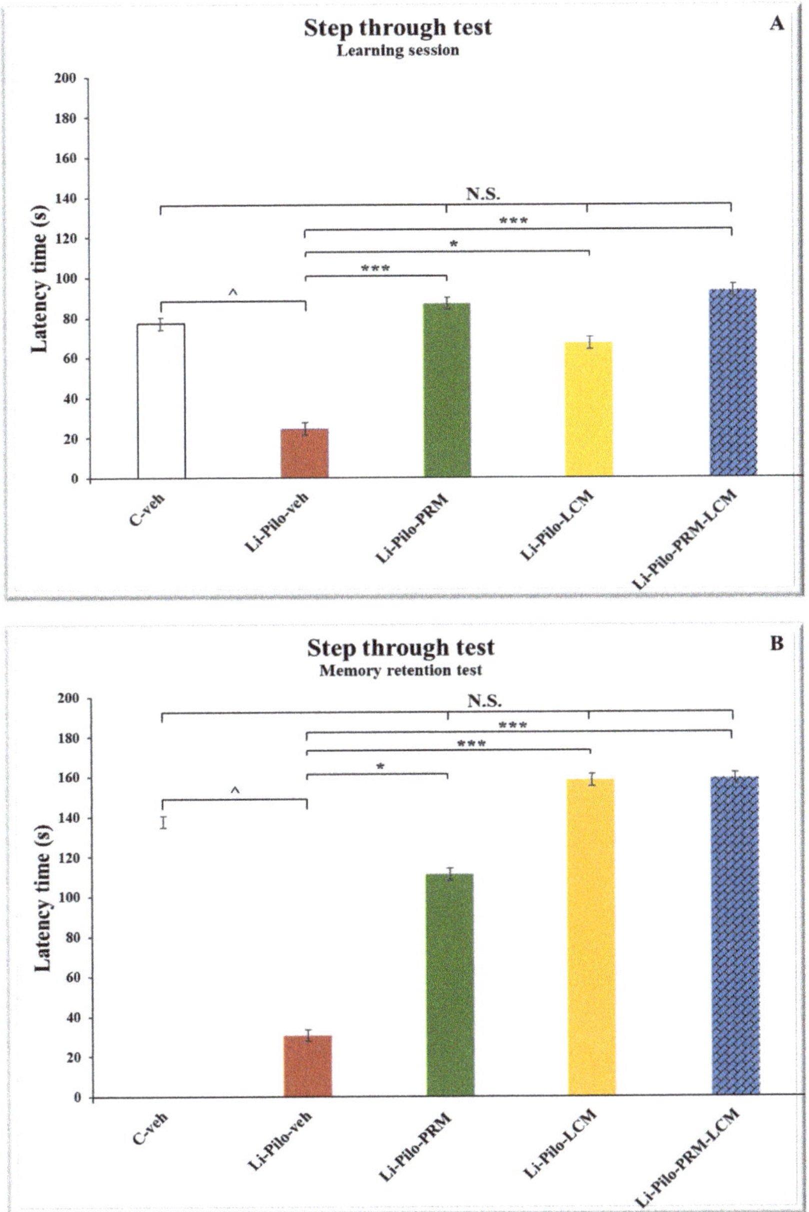

Figure 4. (**A**). Effect of long-term treatment with perampanel (PRM) and lacosamide (LCM), singly or in combination, on the latency time (s) during a learning session in the step-through passive avoidance test in animals with a model of temporal lobe epilepsy. ^ $p < 0.05$ Li-Pilo-veh vs. C-veh group; *** $p < 0.001$ Li-Pilo-PRM vs. Li-Pilo-veh group; * $p < 0.05$ Li-Pilo-LCM vs. Li-Pilo-veh group; *** $p < 0.001$ Li-Pilo-PRM vs. Li-Pilo-veh group; no significance (N.S.), $p > 0.05$ C-veh group vs. Li-Pilo-PRM group; $p > 0.05$ C-veh group vs. Li-Pilo-LCM group; $p > 0.05$ C-veh group vs. Li-Pilo-PRM-LCM group; N.S., $p > 0.05$ Li-Pilo-PRM vs. Li-Pilo-PRM-LCM group; N.S., $p > 0.05$ Li-Pilo-LCM group vs. Li-Pilo-PRM-LCM group. (**B**). Effect of long-term treatment with perampanel (PRM) and lacosamide

(LCM), singly or in combination, on the latency time (s) during a memory retention test in the step-through passive avoidance test in animals with a model of temporal lobe epilepsy. ^ $p < 0.05$ Li-Pilo-veh vs. C-veh group; * $p < 0.001$ Li-Pilo-PRM vs. Li-Pilo-veh group; *** $p < 0.001$ Li-Pilo-LCM vs. Li-Pilo-veh group; *** $p < 0.001$ Li-Pilo-PRM-LCM vs. Li-Pilo-veh group; no significance (N.S.), $p > 0.05$ C-veh group vs. Li-Pilo-PRM group; $p > 0.05$ C-veh group vs. Li-Pilo-LCM group; $p > 0.05$ C-veh group vs. Li-Pilo-PRM-LCM group; N.S., $p > 0.05$ Li-Pilo-PRM vs. Li-Pilo-PRM-LCM group; N.S., $p > 0.05$ Li-Pilo-LCM group vs. Li-Pilo-PRM-LCM group.

3.4. Elevated Plus Maze (EPM) Test

In the EPM test, both groups, Li-Pilo-PRM and Li-Pilo-LCM, had a higher number of entries in the open arms compared to the animals with a model of TLE ($p < 0.001$, respectively) (Figure 5). The group treated with both drugs, PRM and LCM, also showed an increased number of entries in comparison with the Li-Pilo animals ($p = 0.006$). The post hoc test demonstrated that only the Li-Pilo-LCM group had a significantly longer time in the aversive area compared to the Li-Pilo-veh group ($p = 0.009$) (Figure 6). The Li-Pilo-veh group showed a higher anxiety index compared to the C-veh animals ($p < 0.001$). The three groups treated with the drugs singly (Li-Pilo-PRM and Li-Pilo-LCM) or in combination of both (Li-Pilo-PRM-LCM) had lower anxiety index compared to the animals with a model of TLE ($p < 0.001$, $p < 0.001$, and $p = 0.001$, respectively) (Figure 7). The mean values and SEM found in the EPM test are presented in Supplementary Table S1.

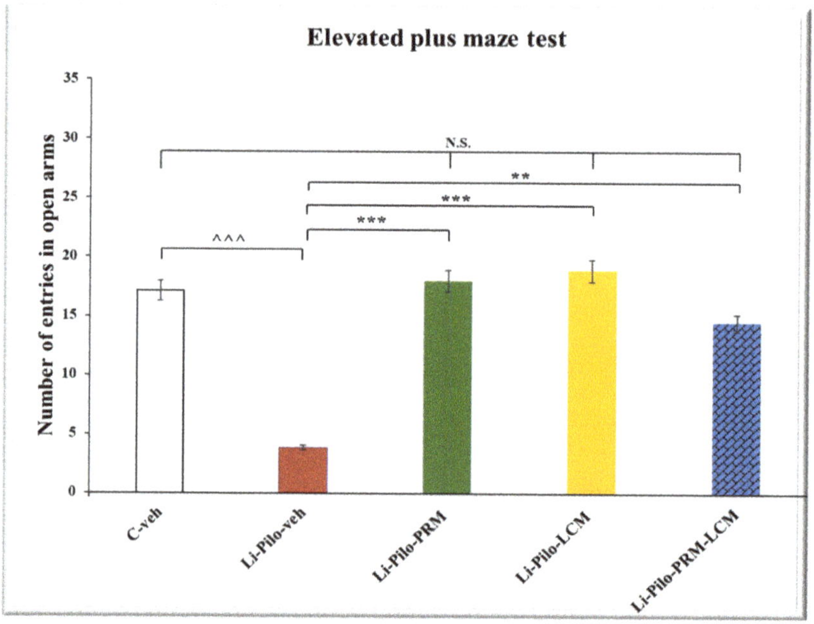

Figure 5. Effect of long-term treatment with perampanel (PRM) and lacosamide (LCM), singly or in combination, on the number of entries in open arms in the elevated plus maze test in animals with a model of temporal lobe epilepsy. ^^^ $p < 0.001$ Li-Pilo-veh vs. C-veh group; *** $p < 0.001$ Li-Pilo-PRM vs. Li-Pilo-veh group; *** $p < 0.001$ Li-Pilo-LCM vs. Li-Pilo-veh group; ** $p < 0.01$ Li-Pilo-PRM-LCM vs. Li-Pilo-veh group; no significance (N.S.), $p > 0.05$ C-veh group vs. Li-Pilo-PRM group; $p > 0.05$ C-veh group vs. Li-Pilo-LCM group; $p > 0.05$ C-veh group vs. Li-Pilo-PRM-LCM group; $p > 0.05$ Li-Pilo-PRM vs. Li-Pilo-PRM-LCM group; $p > 0.05$ Li-Pilo-LCM group vs. Li-Pilo-PRM-LCM group.

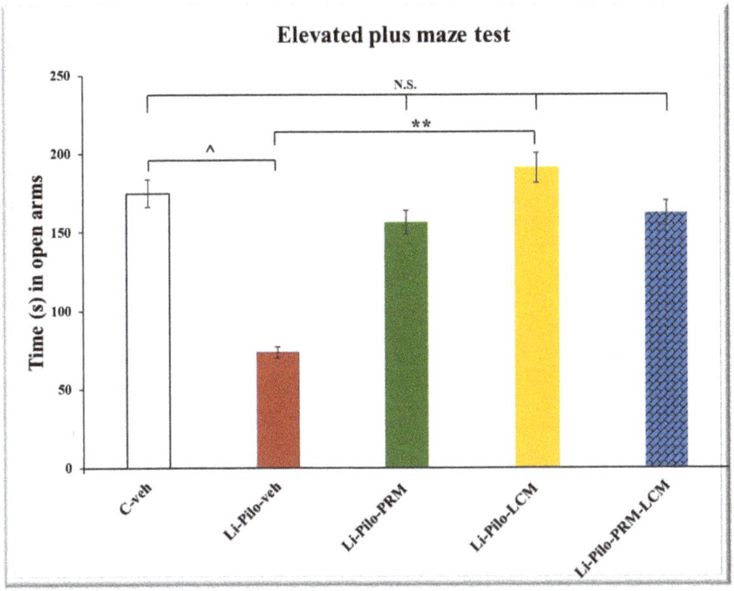

Figure 6. Effect of long-term treatment with perampanel (PRM) and lacosamide (LCM), singly or in combination, on the time (s) spent in open arms in the elevated plus maze test (300 s total time) in animals with a model of temporal lobe epilepsy. ^ $p < 0.05$ Li-Pilo-veh vs. C-veh group; ** $p < 0.01$ Li-Pilo-LCM vs. Li-Pilo-veh group; no significance (N.S.), $p > 0.05$ C-veh group vs. Li-Pilo-PRM group; $p > 0.05$ C-veh group vs. Li-Pilo-LCM group; $p > 0.05$ C-veh group vs. Li-Pilo-PRM-LCM group; $p > 0.05$ Li-Pilo-PRM vs. Li-Pilo-PRM-LCM group; $p > 0.05$ Li-Pilo-LCM group vs. Li-Pilo-PRM-LCM group.

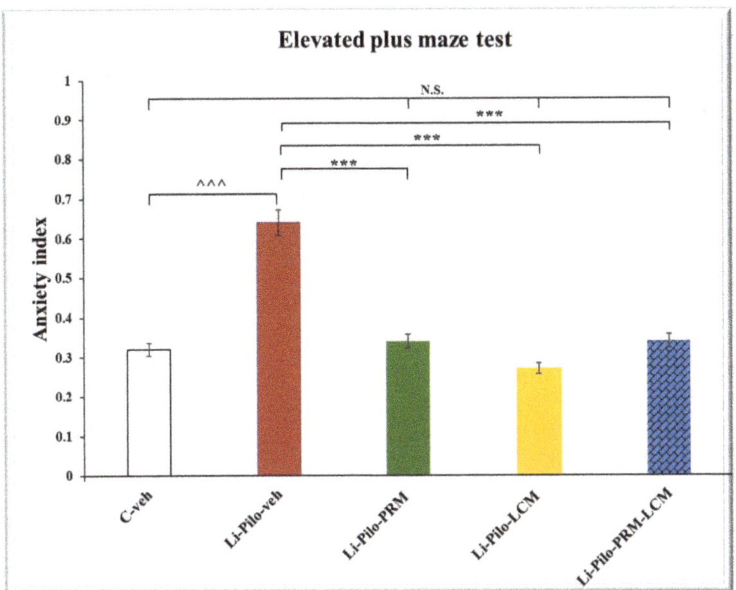

Figure 7. Effect of long-term treatment with perampanel (PRM) and lacosamide (LCM), singly or in combination, on the anxiety index in the elevated plus maze test in animals with a model of temporal

lobe epilepsy. ^^^ $p < 0.001$ Li-Pilo-veh vs. C-veh group; *** $p < 0.001$ Li-Pilo-PRM vs. Li-Pilo-veh group; *** $p < 0.001$ Li-Pilo-LCM vs. Li-Pilo-veh group; *** $p < 0.001$ Li-Pilo-PRM-LCM vs. Li-Pilo-veh group; no significance (N.S.), $p > 0.05$ C-veh group vs. Li-Pilo-PRM group; $p > 0.05$ C-veh group vs. Li-Pilo-LCM group; $p > 0.05$ C-veh group vs. Li-Pilo-PRM-LCM group; $p > 0.05$ Li-Pilo-PRM vs. Li-Pilo-PRM-LCM group; $p > 0.05$ Li-Pilo-LCM group vs. Li-Pilo-PRM-LCM group.

3.5. BDNF Immunohistochemical Expression

Immunohistochemical localization of BDNF in the dorsal hippocampus (Figure 8A–E) in cornu ammonis (CA1, CA2, and CA3) subfields, as well as in the granular cell layer in the dentate gyrus (GrDG).

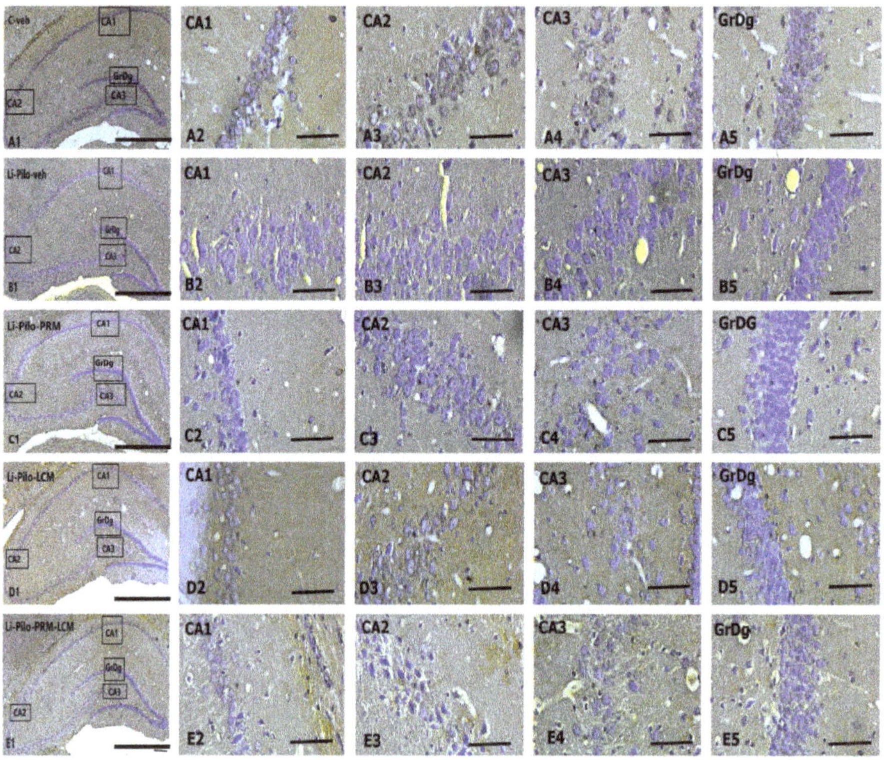

Figure 8. Immunohistochemical expression of BDNF in the dorsal hippocampus. C-veh group (**A1–A5**), Li-Pilo-veh group (**B1–B5**), Li-Pilo-PRM group (**C1–C5**), Li-Pilo-LCM group (**D1–D5**), Li-Pilo-PRM-LCM group (**E1–E5**). Higher magnifications of the rectangles in all five groups are given. Scale bars = 200 µm (**A1,B1,C1,D1,E1**); 50 µm (**A2–A5,B2–B5,C2–C5,D2–D5,E2–E5**).

Representative images showing BDNF immunostaining in the control C-veh group (A1–A5), Li-Pilo-veh group (B1–B5), Li-Pilo-PRM group (C1–C5), Li-Pilo-LCM group (D1–D5), and Li-Pilo-PRM-LCM group (E1–E5). Higher magnifications of the rectangles in all five groups are given. The immune response to BDNF in the C-veh group is moderate but strongly reduced in the Li-Pilo-veh group, especially in CA3 hippocampal fields (A4, B4). In the groups of experimental rats treated with antiepileptic drugs (Li-Pilo-PRM, Li-Pilo-LCM, and Li-Pilo-PRM-LCM group), we observed a significant improvement in BDNF levels, again, most detectable in the CA3 subfield (C4, D4, and E4) compared to the control group of rats undergoing epileptic seizures.

The post hoc test demonstrated that only the Li-Pilo animals showed a significant decrease in the BDNF expression in the CA1 (cornu ammonis 1) subfield of the hippocampus in comparison with the C-veh group ($p = 0.002$) (Figure 9A). The three experimental groups with a model of TLE, which are treated with PRM/LCM or both drugs, significantly increased the expression of the neurotrophic factor in the CA1 region compared to the Li-Pilo-veh animals ($p < 0.001$, respectively).

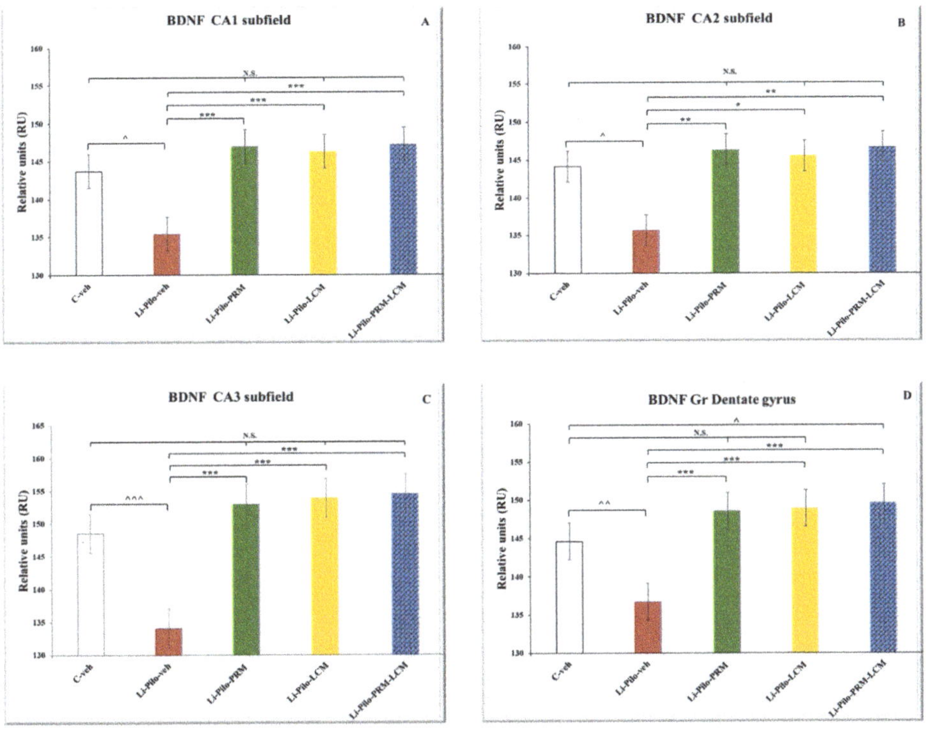

Figure 9. Effect of long-term treatment with perampanel (PRM) and lacosamide (LCM), singly or in combination, on the BDNF levels (RU) in animals with a model of temporal lobe epilepsy: (**A**) in the hippocampal CA1 subfield, ^ $p < 0.05$, Li-Pilo-veh vs. C-veh group; *** $p < 0.001$ Li-Pilo-PRM vs. Li-Pilo-veh group; *** $p < 0.001$ Li-Pilo-LCM vs. Li-Pilo-veh group; *** $p < 0.001$ Li-Pilo-PRM-LCM vs. Li-Pilo-veh group; no significance (N.S.), $p > 0.05$ C-veh group vs. Li-Pilo-PRM group; $p > 0.05$ C-veh group vs. Li-Pilo-LCM group; $p > 0.05$ C-veh group vs. Li-Pilo-PRM-LCM group; $p > 0.05$ Li-Pilo-PRM vs. Li-Pilo-PRM-LCM group; $p > 0.05$ Li-Pilo-LCM group vs. Li-Pilo-PRM-LCM group. (**B**) in the hippocampal CA2 subfield, ^ $p < 0.05$, Li-Pilo-veh vs. C-veh group; ** $p < 0.01$ Li-Pilo-PRM vs. Li-Pilo-veh group; * $p < 0.05$ Li-Pilo-LCM vs. Li-Pilo-veh group; ** $p < 0.01$ Li-Pilo-PRM-LCM vs. Li-Pilo-veh group; no significance (N.S.), $p > 0.05$ C-veh group vs. Li-Pilo-PRM group; $p > 0.05$ C-veh group vs. Li-Pilo-LCM group; $p > 0.05$ C-veh group vs. Li-Pilo-PRM-LCM group; $p > 0.05$ Li-Pilo-PRM vs. Li-Pilo-PRM-LCM group; $p > 0.05$ Li-Pilo-LCM group vs. Li-Pilo-PRM-LCM group; (**C**) in the hippocampal CA3 subfield, ^^^ $p < 0.001$, Li-Pilo-veh vs. C-veh group; *** $p < 0.001$ Li-Pilo-PRM vs. Li-Pilo-veh group; *** $p < 0.001$ Li-Pilo-LCM vs. Li-Pilo-veh group; *** $p < 0.001$ Li-Pilo-PRM-LCM vs. Li-Pilo-veh group; no significance (N.S.), $p > 0.05$ C-veh group vs. Li-Pilo-PRM group; $p > 0.05$ C-veh group vs. Li-Pilo-LCM group; $p > 0.05$ C-veh group vs. Li-Pilo-PRM-LCM group; $p > 0.05$ Li-Pilo-PRM vs. Li-Pilo-PRM-LCM group; $p > 0.05$ Li-Pilo-LCM group vs. Li-Pilo-PRM-LCM group and (**D**) in the granular cell layer in the dentate gyrus, ^^ $p < 0.01$, Li-Pilo-veh vs. C-veh group; *** $p < 0.001$ Li-Pilo-PRM vs. Li-Pilo-veh group; *** $p < 0.001$ Li-Pilo-LCM vs. Li-Pilo-veh group; *** $p < 0.001$ Li-Pilo-PRM-LCM vs. Li-Pilo-veh group; ^ $p < 0.05$ Li-Pilo-PRM-LCM vs. C-veh group; no significance (N.S.), $p > 0.05$ C-veh group vs. Li-Pilo-PRM group; $p > 0.05$ C-veh group vs. Li-Pilo-LCM group; $p > 0.05$ Li-Pilo-PRM vs. Li-Pilo-PRM-LCM group; $p > 0.05$ Li-Pilo-LCM group vs. Li-Pilo-PRM-LCM group.

In the CA2 subfield of the hippocampus, the Li-Pilo-veh group showed a significant decrease in the BDNF expression compared to the saline animals ($p = 0.04$) (Figure 9B). Chronic treatment with both groups, Li-Pilo-PRM and the one with the drug combination Li-Pilo-PRM-LCM, showed a significant increase in the neurotropic expression compared to the animals with a model of TLE ($p = 0.006$ and $p = 0.004$). The Li-Pilo-LCM group also showed higher expression of BDNF in the CA2 subfield in comparison with the animals with a model of TLE ($p = 0.012$).

The post hoc test revealed that the animals with epilepsy had a significantly lower BDNF expression in comparison with the C-veh group in the CA3 region of the hippocampus ($p < 0.001$) (Figure 9C). The three experimental groups treated with both drugs, PRM and LCM, singly or in combination, showed an increase in the expression of the neurotrophic factor compared to the Li-Pilo-veh rats in the same region ($p < 0.001$, respectively).

No statistical significance of the neurotrophic factor expression in the three subfields CA1, CA2, and CA3 was observed when comparing the C-veh group and the three groups treated singly with PRM and LCM or in combination with both drugs, $p > 0.05$. In addition, no difference was detected between the singly treated groups with PRM and LCM when compared to the animals treated with both drugs (Li-Pilo-PRM-LCM), $p > 0.05$.

The analyses of variance revealed that the Li-Pilo-veh group showed a significant decrease in the BDNF expression in the DG compared to the vehicle animals ($p < 0.01$), while only the Li-Pilo-PRM-LCM rats showed an increase in the expression of the neurotrophic factor compared to the C-veh group ($p = 0.022$) (Figure 9D). A tendency for a similar effect was also observed by the Li-Pilo-LCM animals ($p = 0.068$). All three groups treated with the ASMs—PRM and LCM singly or in combination with both—managed to increase the BDNF expression in the DG in comparison with the Li-Pilo animals ($p < 0.001$, respectively). No statistical significance of the neurotrophic factor expression in the DG was observed when comparing the C-veh group and the animals treated singly with PRM and LCM, $p > 0.05$. The mean values and S.E.M., found for BDNF expression, are presented in Supplementary Table S2.

3.6. Cyclin D1 Immunohistochemical Expression

Immunohistochemical localization of Cyclin D1 in the dorsal hippocampus (Figure 10A–E) in the cornu ammonis (CA1, CA2, and CA3) subfields, including in the dentate gyrus, and granular cell layer (GrDg).

Representative images showing Cyclin D1 immunoexpression in the control C-veh group (A1–A5), Li-Pilo-veh group (B1–B5), Li-Pilo-PRM group (C1–C5), Li-Pilo-LCM group (D1–D5), and Li-Pilo-PRM-LCM group (E1–E5). The insets show a higher magnification in the granular layer of the dentate gyrus and the three parts of the cornu ammonis hippocampal region. The immune response to Cyclin D1 is the most significant in the Li-Pilo-veh group, especially in the CA3 hippocampal fields (B4). In all experimental groups treated with antiepileptic drugs (Li-Pilo-PRM, Li-Pilo-LCM, and Li-Pilo-PRM-LCM groups), a significant decrease in Cyclin D1 levels was shown, again most detectable in the CA3 subfield (C4, D4, and E4).

The statistical analyses in the CA1 subfield of the hippocampus revealed that the animals with a model of TLE showed a significant increase in the Cyclin D1 expression ($p < 0.001$). The same effect was observed in the Li-Pilo-PRM and Li-Pilo-PRM-LCM animals when compared with the C-veh group ($p = 0.005$, $p < 0.001$, respectively) (Figure 11A). In contrast, all three groups with a model of epilepsy and treated with PRM/LCM singly or in combination showed a decrease in the cyclin expression compared to the Li-Pilo-veh animals ($p < 0.001$, respectively).

The post hoc test revealed that the animals with a model of epilepsy showed a significant overexpression of Cyclin D1 in the CA2 hippocampal region compared to the C-veh rats ($p < 0.001$) (Figure 11B). A decrease in cyclin expression was demonstrated by both groups with a model of TLE and treated with PRM and LCM in comparison with the

Li-Pilo-veh animals ($p = 0.033$ and $p = 0.012$, respectively). A tendency for such an effect was demonstrated by the group treated with both drugs ($p = 0.061$).

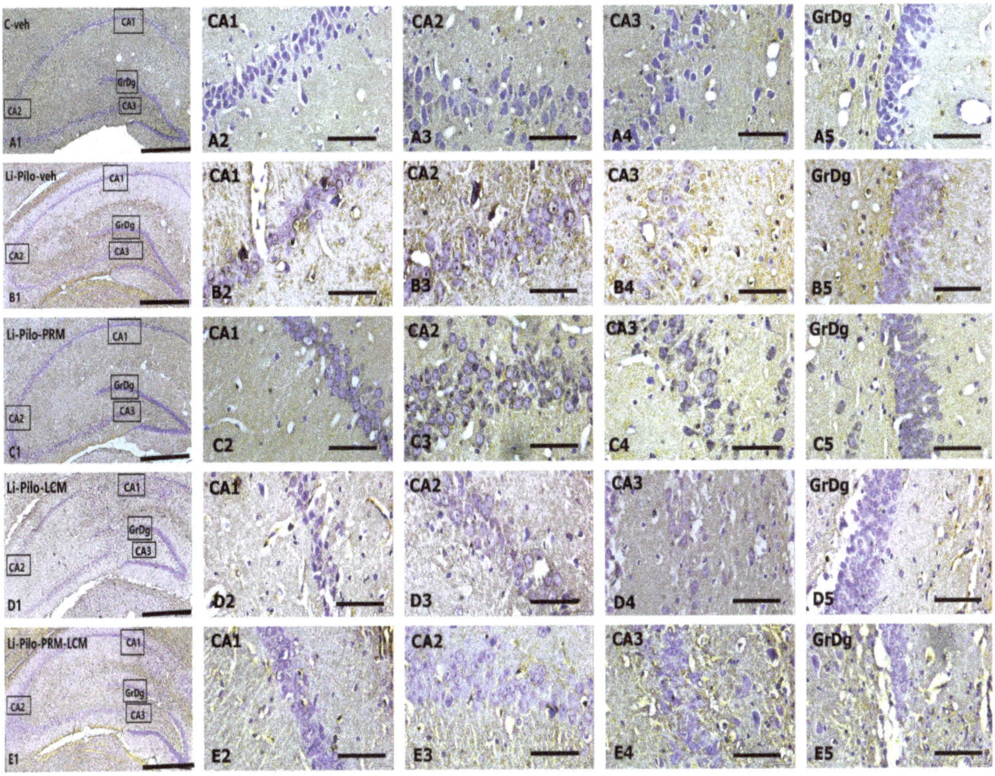

Figure 10. (**A–E**). Immunohistochemical expression of Cyclin D1 in the dorsal hippocampus. C-veh group (**A1–A5**), Li-Pilo-veh group (**B1–B5**), Li-Pilo-PRM group (**C1–C5**), Li-Pilo-LCM group (**D1–D5**), Li-Pilo-PRM-LCM group (**E1–E5**). Higher magnifications of the rectangles in all five groups are given. Scale bars = 200 μm (**A1,B1,C1,D1,E1**); 50 μm (**A2–A5,B2–B5,C2–C5,D2–D5,E2–E5**).

In the CA 3 hippocampal subfield, the Li-Pilo-veh animals had significantly higher Cyclin D1 protein expression ($p < 0.001$), while the opposite effect was observed in the three groups, Li-Pilo-PRM ($p = 0.002$), Li-Pilo-LCM ($p = 0.017$), and Li-Pilo-PRM-LCM ($p = 0.031$), compared to the C-veh rats (Figure 11C). Moreover, the same three experimental groups with a model of epilepsy and treated with drugs showed a decrease in the expression of the apoptotic factor compared to the Li-Pilo-veh animals ($p < 0.001$).

The analyses of variance demonstrated that the Li-Pilo-veh group showed a significant increase in the Cyclin D1 expression in the GrDG compared to the vehicle animals ($p < 0.001$). The same effect was observed in the three groups treated with the drugs singly or in combination ($p < 0.001$, Li-Pilo-PRM group compared to the C-veh group; $p = 0.002$, Li-Pilo-LCM group compared to the C-veh group, and $p < 0.001$, Li-Pilo-PRM-LCM group compared to the C-veh group) (Figure 11D). In contrast, the same three experimental groups, Li-Pilo-PRM, Li-Pilo-LCM, and Li-Pilo-PRM-LCM, showed significantly lower Cyclin D1 expression in this region in comparison with the Li-Pilo animals ($p < 0.001$, respectively).

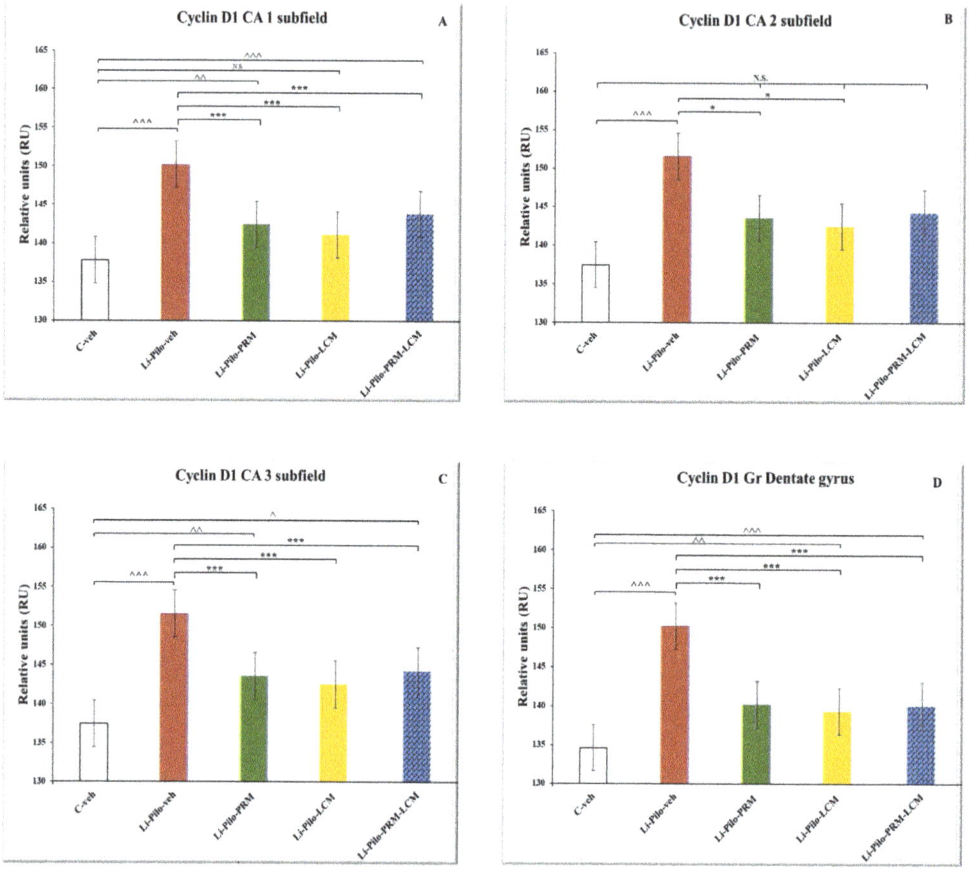

Figure 11. Effect of long-term treatment with perampanel (PRM) and lacosamide (LCM), singly or in combination, on the Cyclin D1 levels (RU) in (**A**) the hippocampal CA1 subfield, ^^^ $p < 0.001$ Li-Pilo-veh vs. C-veh group, ^^ $p < 0.01$ Li-Pilo-PRM vs. C-veh group, *** $p < 0.001$ Li-Pilo-PRM vs. Li-Pilo-veh group; *** $p < 0.001$ Li-Pilo-LCM vs. Li-Pilo-veh group; ^^^ $p < 0.001$ Li-Pilo-PRM-LCM vs. C-veh group, *** $p < 0.001$ Li-Pilo-PRM-LCM vs. Li-Pilo-veh group; no significance (N.S.), $p > 0.05$ C-veh group vs. Li-Pilo-LCM group, $p > 0.05$ Li-Pilo-PRM vs. Li-Pilo-PRM-LCM group; $p > 0.05$ Li-Pilo-LCM group vs. Li-Pilo-PRM-LCM group (**B**) CA2 subfield, ^^^ $p < 0.001$ Li-Pilo-veh vs. C-veh group, * $p < 0.05$ Li-Pilo-PRM vs. Li-Pilo-veh group; * $p < 0.05$ Li-Pilo-LCM vs. Li-Pilo-veh group; N.S., $p > 0.05$ C-veh group vs. Li-Pilo-PRM group; $p > 0.05$ C-veh group vs. Li-Pilo-LCM group; $p > 0.05$ C-veh group vs. Li-Pilo-PRM-LCM group; $p > 0.05$ Li-Pilo-PRM vs. Li-Pilo-PRM-LCM group; $p > 0.05$ Li-Pilo-LCM group vs. Li-Pilo-PRM-LCM group; $p > 0.05$ Li-Pilo-PRM-LCM vs. Li-Pilo-veh (**C**) CA3 subfield, ^^^ $p < 0.001$ Li-Pilo-veh vs. C-veh group; ^^^ $p < 0.01$ Li-Pilo-PRM vs. C-veh group; ^ $p < 0.05$, ^^ $p < 0.01$ Li-Pilo-LCM vs. C-veh group; ^ $p < 0.05$, ^^^ $p < 0.001$ Li-Pilo-PRM-LCM vs. C-veh group, *** $p < 0.001$ Li-Pilo-PRM vs. Li-Pilo-veh group; ^ $p < 0.05$, Li-Pilo-LCM vs. C-veh group; *** $p < 0.001$ Li-Pilo-LCM vs. Li-Pilo-veh group; ^ $p < 0.05$ Li-Pilo-PRM-LCM vs. C-veh group; *** $p < 0.001$ Li-Pilo-PRM-LCM vs. Li-Pilo-veh group and (**D**) in the granular cell layer in the dentate gyrus, ^^^ $p < 0.001$ Li-Pilo-veh vs. C-veh group; ^^^ $p < 0.001$ Li-Pilo-PRM vs. C-veh group; *** $p < 0.001$ Li-Pilo-PRM vs. Li-Pilo-veh group; ^^ $p < 0.01$ Li-Pilo-LCM vs. C-veh group; *** $p < 0.001$ Li-Pilo-LCM vs. Li-Pilo-veh group; ^^^ $p < 0.001$ Li-Pilo-PRM-LCM vs. C-veh group; *** $p < 0.001$ Li-Pilo-PRM-LCM vs. Li-Pilo-veh group.

In addition, no significant difference was detected between the singly treated groups with PRM and LCM when compared to the animals treated with both drugs (Li-Pilo-PRM-LCM), $p > 0.05$ on the Cyclin D1 hippocampal expression in all subfields and in the granular cell layer of the DG (Figure 11). The mean values and S.E.M., found for Cyclin D1 expression, are presented in Supplementary Table S3.

4. Discussion

The current study was conducted to investigate the tolerability and effectiveness of a single long-term administration and the combination of two third-generation ASMs with unique mechanisms of action of PRM and LCM. We found that the rats with the model of post-SE-induced TLE exerted various comorbidities such as impairment of different cognitive domains and exploratory behavior. In addition, the two anticonvulsants, PRM and LCM, administered singly in high doses, 3 mg/kg and 30 mg/kg, respectively, during the epileptogenesis and chronic state of the model of TLE, reversed the behavioral changes induced by SE. The combination of both drugs, administered in low doses of PRM (0.5 mg/kg) and LCM (3 mg/kg), demonstrated similar anxiolytic and cognitive-improving effects compared to the singly administered drugs in high doses. Moreover, in the animals with a model of epilepsy, an activated process of apoptosis accompanied by reduced levels of the neurotrophic factor was detected. In contrast, we observed a significant improvement in the neurotrophic factor BDNF levels and decreased expression of the apoptotic factor Cyclin D1 by the three groups treated with ASMs singly or in combination. All these data suggest a disease-modifying effect of both drugs, which could be closely related to their cognitive-enhancing effect.

Long-term neurophysiological deficits associated with epilepsy are strongly influenced by extrinsic factors, such as early-onset epilepsy, SE high frequency, poor seizure control, multiple polytherapy, etc. [40]. All these factors lead to progressive changes in brain connectivity, resulting in cognitive decline [40–42]. In line with other findings, in our study, the animals with a model of TLE showed impaired spatial working memory, deteriorated passive learning and memory, and decreased exploratory behavior. In contrast, long-term treatment with PRM singly at a dose of 3 mg/kg managed to weaken the negative effect of epilepsy and improve passive learning, facilitating the formation of spatial working memory and long-term memory traces. PRM enhanced exploratory behavior, although the drug failed to improve object recognition retrieval. Our data are in agreement with other experimental studies that have found that PRM preserves spatial and recognition memory as a result of the slowed-down appearance of spontaneous motor seizure activity and the reduced SE-induced hippocampal cell death [43]. In compliance with our results is the experimental model of ischemia where PRM (1.5 mg/kg) promotes memory consolidation and retrieval as a result of anti-inflammatory, antioxidant, and anti-apoptotic activities [44]. In the study of Martins et al. [45], the drug promotes spatial cognitive performance, and the observed result is due to the stimulation of GAP-43 expression, an essential protein for the neurotrophic effects of BDNF. Moreover, Aida et al. [46] demonstrated in an experimental model of traumatic brain injury that pre- and post-PRM treatment attenuates the increased hippocampal pro-apoptotic bax/bcl-xL ratio and reduces learning and memory deficits assessed by the Morris water maze test in male adult rats. Multiple lines of evidence suggest that different brain regions are associated with spatial and passive memory, namely the hippocampus, amygdala, and prefrontal cortex [47].

In the present study, we found that long-term LCM treatment (30 mg/kg) improved both spatial consolidation and retrieval and facilitated passive learning and formation of memory traces in an experimental lithium–pilocarpine model of TLE. These results are in agreement with our previous data in a similar model [34] and with other researchers who have found neuroprotective and cognitive-improving effects of the drug in different experimental models of hypoxic–ischemic brain injury [48], lipopolysaccharide-induced neuroinflammation [49], and traumatic spinal cord injury [50]. The authors associate most of these beneficial effects of LCM with antioxidant and anti-inflammatory activities, attenuated glial cell activation, and inhibited apoptosis in different brain regions, including the hippocampus, cortex, and cerebellum.

To the best of our knowledge, no study has investigated the long-term effect of the combination of low doses of PRM (0.5 mg/kg) and LCM (3 mg/kg) on cognitive performance and the underlying mechanisms of the observed effects during the chronic phase of an experimental model of TLE. We found that both drugs administered in low doses produced similar effects compared to the singly administered drugs in high doses, PRM (3 mg/kg) and LCM (30 mg/kg). Drug combination improved spatial working memory as well as passive learning and the formation of long-term memory. The two ASMs administered together managed to improve recognition memory while PRM failed to facilitate its consolidation and retrieval. These results complement other studies that have found a synergistic effect of PRM and zonisamide combination in a model of rat amygdala kindling of TLE [13]. The authors found a pronounced threshold increase when zonisamide administration is combined with different PRM doses. Moreover, better performance on the Rotarod test for assessing motor function was revealed for the drug combination. Additionally, it is important to note that zonisamide is an ASM and has a similar mechanism of action as LCM through influencing the slow inactivation of voltage-gated sodium channels [51]. The cognitive-enhancing effects of both drugs and their combination could be a real advantage when compared to many other anticonvulsants, especially the older ones, which usually lead to additional cognitive impairment in epileptic patients.

Anxiety is among the most common psychiatric comorbidity conditions that occur in patients with epilepsy [52]. Increased stress or anxiety can be a result of the disease process but, on the other hand, can also cause disease exacerbation. In the present study, we found that animals with a model of TLE had less time spent in the aversive area of the maze, and increased anxiety-like behavior was detected compared to the control rats. In contrast, both drugs administered singly or in combination led to a pronounced anxiolytic effect. Although data about the effect of PRM on levels of anxiety is quite scarce, a few recently published studies are in agreement with our results. The authors have demonstrated the anxiolytic activity of PRM in naïve rats [53], in mice subjected to maximal electroshock seizures [54], and in pentylenetetrazole-kindled mice [55]. The anxiolytic effect of LCM in the current study is in agreement with single-source data showing decreased levels of anxiety in patients with epilepsy [18,56–58].

Numerous molecular mechanisms could be underlying the pathogenesis of epilepsy and can be influenced by the administered drug therapy. As BDNF is an important neuronal modulator, regulating many critical aspects in the ontogenesis of neurons and the development of synapses [14], we investigated its hippocampal expression. Our results demonstrated impaired neuronal expression of the neurotrophic factor in the control group of animals undergoing seizures. These results are in accordance with other studies, showing that reduced hippocampal BDNF expression has been linked to impaired synaptic connections, inhibited process of neurogenesis, and cognitive impairment [16,59–62]. Identical manifestations of this neurotrophin are observed in activated microglia as well as in astrocytes. These results are in line with previous research, which considered BDNF as the most important signaling molecule between neurons and glia, especially in conditions of neuronal damage and cellular stress [19]. In our experiment, the two ASMs, PRM and LCM, administered singly or in a low-dose combination, led to a significant improvement of BDNF levels in all subfields of the hippocampus as well as in the GrDG. There is scarce data about the effect of different ASMs on the BDNF levels. Our results are in line with other studies revealing that combined drug interactions may affect, at least partially, the normalization of BDNF levels in the stressed hippocampus [61]. A recent clinical study revealed that serum BDNF levels are significantly increased in patients with epilepsy who have received PRM or valproate treatment [63]. In contrast, experimental studies reveal that some traditional ASMs like phenobarbital, topiramate, and lamotrigine can reduce mRNA levels of BDNF and lead to cognitive deficits [64]. The expression of the neurotrophic factor is increased during all processes of learning and memory in the hippocampus, which is related to improved cognitive function [16,65,66]. The neuroprotective microglia-neuron physical interactions lead to the preservation of homeostasis in the CNS and, especially, in the hippocampus [67].

Recent evidence reveals that epileptic seizures and the intake of certain medications cause neuronal damage, leading to apoptotic changes in hippocampal cells and arrest of the cell cycle. Therefore, the study of the expression of the apoptotic protein Cyclin D1 would determine the severity and direction of programmed cell death and could detect probable neuronal damage with the presence of apoptotic cell changes [27,28]. In addition, the correlation between neurotrophic and pro-apoptotic factors in the hippocampus has been established for its ontogenesis but has not yet been sufficiently studied. Moreover, there is a lack of information about the effect of different ASMs on Cyclin D1 expression.

According to Timsit et al. [27], Cyclin D1 is expressed histochemically in damaged neurons of the hippocampus. Our results on the activity of cyclin D1, which has the highest expression in the control group undergoing only epileptic seizures, are in line with the above-mentioned study. On the other hand, we observed a significant reduction in protein expression in all hippocampal subfields (CA1, CA2, and CA3, as well as in GrDG) in the three groups treated with both ASMs, PRM and LCM, singly or in combination. These results confirm the hypothesis that neuronal damage triggers the release of cell cycle proteins, resulting in increased cell death [22,24,25]. Furthermore, neurodegenerative manifestations are accompanied by microglial dystrophy, which, in turn, enhances neuronal dystrophy [68,69]. Significant expression of Cyclin D1 in astrocytic glia has also been reported [28,70], with neuron-astrocyte metabolic coupling given a crucial role in learning and long-term memory [28,71]. All mentioned studies determine the Cyclin D1 manifestation exclusively in cells that undergo apoptotic changes after ischemic damage or epileptic seizures. Therefore, many authors define Cyclin D1 as a kind of marker for the occurrence of programmed cell death [27,72,73]. The consequences of epileptic damage in the hippocampus are most significant in the vulnerable CA3 region, which is in line with our results [27,74,75]. The correlation between neurotrophic and apoptotic factors in the hippocampus is also different at different stages of injury. Cell signaling in the epileptic hippocampus is defective at the beginning of the damage, while the neurotrophic factors do not have a significant effect in the initial phases of the injury, but they are leading at a later stage, especially in the granular cells of the dentate gyrus [37]. This could be an important mechanism through which ASMs, which increase BDNF levels, improve cognitive functions in epileptic patients.

A limitation of the present study is the use of only male rats. The conduction of the experiment with female rats could be a subject of future research, as memory, anxiety levels, as well as the BDNF and Cyclin D1 expression, can be influenced by the natural fluctuations in the sex hormone levels during the ovarian cycle in female rats.

5. Conclusions

In conclusion, the present study demonstrates that chronic treatment with perampanel and lacosamide, singly in a high-dose or in a low-dose combination of both during epileptogenesis and chronic states of an experimental model of Li-Pilo TLE has pronounced cognitive-enhancing and anxiolytic effects. These beneficial outcomes could be associated with increased expression of the neurotrophic factor BDNF and decreased levels of the apoptotic factor Cyclin D1 in the neurons of the hippocampus. These additional mechanisms of both ASMs could be essential for preserving neuronal survival and homeostasis in the CNS and especially in the hippocampus, which could be an important advantage for their choice compared to many other anticonvulsants.

Supplementary Materials: The following supporting information can be downloaded at: https://www.mdpi.com/article/10.3390/cimb46120838/s1, Table S1: Summary of data of EPM test on mean values ± SEM; Table S2: Summary of data of BDNF expression in the hippocampus on mean values ± SEM; Table S3: Summary of data of Cyclin D1 expression in the hippocampus on mean values ± SEM.

Author Contributions: M.S.-D. and D.B. designed and performed the research study. M.S.-D. analyzed the data. Both authors contributed to writing the manuscript. All authors have read and agreed to the published version of the manuscript.

Funding: This research was funded by Medical University—Plovdiv, Bulgaria, grant number 6/2018 and the APC was funded by Medical University—Plovdiv, Bulgaria.

Institutional Review Board Statement: Animals were raised and obtained from the Animal Center of the Medical University, Plovdiv. This study was performed in strict accordance with the guidelines of European Community Council Directives 86/609/EEC. 0.2010/63/EC. The experiments were approved by the Bulgarian Food Safety Agency No. 206/01 October 2018 and the Ethical Committee on Human and Animal Experimentation of Medical University—Plovdiv No. 1/28 February 2019.

Data Availability Statement: All data reported in this paper will be shared by the lead contact upon request.

Acknowledgments: We thank Bogdana Adamu, who assisted with the preparation and proof-reading of the manuscript.

Conflicts of Interest: The authors declare no conflicts of interest.

References

1. Pascual, M.R. Temporal lobe epilepsy: Clinical semiology and neurophysiological studies. *Semin. Ultrasound CT MR* **2007**, *28*, 416–423. [CrossRef] [PubMed]
2. Kim, J.E.; Lee, D.S.; Park, H.; Kim, T.H.; Kang, T.C. AMPA Receptor Antagonists Facilitate NEDD4-2-Mediated GRIA1 Ubiquitination by Regulating PP2B-ERK1/2-SGK1 Pathway in Chronic Epilepsy Rats. *Biomedicines* **2021**, *9*, 1069. [CrossRef] [PubMed]
3. Wu, T.; Ido, K.; Ohgoh, M.; Hanada, T. Mode of seizure inhibition by sodium channel blockers, an SV2A ligand, and an AMPA receptor antagonist in a rat amygdala kindling model. *Epilepsy Res.* **2019**, *154*, 42–49. [CrossRef] [PubMed]
4. Michaelis, E.K. Molecular biology of glutamate receptors in the central nervous system and their role in excitotoxicity, oxidative stress and aging. *Prog. Neurobiol.* **1998**, *54*, 369–415. [CrossRef] [PubMed]
5. Kim, J.E.; Choi, H.C.; Song, H.K.; Kang, T.C. Perampanel Affects Up-Stream Regulatory Signaling Pathways of GluA1 Phosphorylation in Normal and Epileptic Rats. *Front. Cell. Neurosci.* **2019**, *13*, 80. [CrossRef]
6. Ahn, S.J.; Kim, T.J.; Cha, K.S.; Jun, J.S.; Byun, J.I.; Shin, Y.W.; Sunwoo, J.-S.; Lee, S.; Yu, K.-S.; Jang, I.-J. Effects of perampanel on cognition and quantitative electroencephalography in patients with epilepsy. *Epilepsy Behav.* **2021**, *115*, 107514. [CrossRef]
7. Witt, J.A.; Helmstaedter, C. The impact of perampanel on cognition: A systematic review of studies employing standardized tests in patients with epilepsy. *Seizure* **2022**, *94*, 107–111. [CrossRef]
8. Licko, T.; Seeger, N.; Zellinger, C.; Russmann, V.; Matagne, A.; Potschka, H. Lacosamide treatment following status epilepticus attenuates neuronal cell loss and alterations in hippocampal neurogenesis in a rat electrical status epilepticus model. *Epilepsia* **2013**, *54*, 1176–1185. [CrossRef]
9. Rogawski, M.A.; Tofighy, A.; White, H.S.; Matagne, A.; Wolff, C. Current understanding of the mechanism of action of the antiepileptic drug lacosamide. *Epilepsy Res.* **2015**, *110*, 189–205. [CrossRef]
10. Villanueva, V.; Giráldez, B.G.; Toledo, M.; De Haan, G.J.; Cumbo, E.; Gambardella, A.; De Backer, M.; Joeres, L.; Brunnert, M.; Dedeken, P.; et al. Lacosamide monotherapy in clinical practice: A retrospective chart review. *Acta Neurol. Scand.* **2018**, *138*, 186–194. [CrossRef]
11. Keezer, M.R.; Sisodiya, S.M.; Sander, J.W. Comorbidities of epilepsy: Current concepts and future perspectives. *Lancet Neurol.* **2016**, *15*, 106–115. [CrossRef] [PubMed]
12. Mahajan, S.S.; Prakash, A.; Sarma, P.; Niraj, N.; Bhattacharyya, A.; Medhi, B. Efficacy, tolerability and safety of perampanel in population with pharmacoresistant focal seizures: A systematic review and meta-analysis. *Epilepsy Res.* **2022**, *182*, 106895. [CrossRef] [PubMed]
13. Russmann, V.; Salvamoser, J.D.; Rettenbeck, M.L.; Komori, T.; Potschka, H. Synergism of perampanel and zonisamide in the rat amygdala kindling model of temporal lobe epilepsy. *Epilepsia* **2016**, *57*, 638–647. [CrossRef] [PubMed]
14. Kaplan, D.; Miller, F. Neurotrophin signal transduction in the nervous system. *Curr. Opin. Neurobiol.* **2000**, *10*, 381–391. [CrossRef]
15. Mowla, S.J.; Farhadi, H.F.; Pareek, S.; Atwal, J.K. Biosynthesis and post-translational processing of the precursor to brain-derived neurotrophic factor. *J. Biol. Chem.* **2001**, *276*, 12660–12666. [CrossRef]
16. Bhattarai, P.; Cosacak, M.I.; Mashkaryan, V.; Demir, S.; Popova, S.D.; Govindarajan, N.; Brandt, K.; Zhang, Y.; Chang, W.; Ampatzis, K.; et al. Neuron-glia interaction through Serotonin-BDNF-NGFR axis enables regenerative neurogenesis in Alzheimer's model of adult zebrafish brain. *PLoS Biol.* **2020**, *18*, e3000585. [CrossRef]
17. Wang, L.; Chang, X.; She, L.; Xu, D.; Huang, W.; Poo, M.M. Autocrine action of BDNF on dendrite development of adult-born hippocampal neurons. *J. Neurosci.* **2015**, *35*, 8384–8393. [CrossRef]
18. Onodera, J.; Nagata, H.; Nakashima, A.; Ikegaya, Y.; Koyama, R. Neuronal brain-derived neurotrophic factor manipulates microglial dynamics. *Glia* **2021**, *69*, 890–904. [CrossRef]

19. Charlton, T.; Prowse, N.; McFee, A.; Heiratifar, N.; Fortin, T.; Paquette, C.; Hayley, S. Brain-derived neurotrophic factor (BDNF) has direct anti-inflammatory effects on microglia. *Front. Cell. Neurosci.* **2023**, *17*, 1188672. [CrossRef]
20. Parkhurst, C.N.; Yang, G.; Ninan, I.; Savas, J.N.; Yates, J.R., 3rd; Lafaille, J.J.; Hempstead, B.L.; Littman, D.R.; Gan, W.-B. Microglia promote learning-dependent synapse formation through brain-derived neurotrophic factor. *Cell* **2013**, *155*, 1596–1609. [CrossRef]
21. Ferrini, F.; De Koninck, Y. Microglia control neuronal network excitability via BDNF signalling. *Neural Plast.* **2013**, *2013*, 429815. [CrossRef]
22. Bozec, A.; Chuzel, F.; Chater, S.; C Paulin, C.; Bars, R.; Benahmed, M.; Mauduit, C. The mitochondrial-dependent pathway is chronically affected in testicular germ cell death in adult rats exposed in utero to anti-androgens. *J. Endocrinol.* **2004**, *183*, 79–90. [CrossRef] [PubMed]
23. de Oliveira, L.; Spiazzi, C.M.; Bortolin, T.; Canever, L.; Petronilho, F.; Mina, F.G.; Dal-Pizzol, F.; Quevedo, J.; Zugno, A.I. Different sub-anaesthetic doses of ketamine increase oxidative stress in the brain of rats. *Prog. Neuropsychopharmacol. Biol. Psychiatry* **2009**, *33*, 1003–1008. [CrossRef] [PubMed]
24. Herrup, K.; Yang, Y. Cell cycle regulation in the postmitotic neuron: Oxymoron or new biology? *Nat. Rev. Neurosci.* **2007**, *8*, 368–378. [CrossRef] [PubMed]
25. Koeller, H.; Elizabeth-Ross, M.; Glickstein, S. Cyclin D1 in Excitatory Neurons of the Adult Brain Enhances Kainate-induced Neurotoxicity. *Neurobiol. Dis.* **2008**, *31*, 230–241. [CrossRef] [PubMed]
26. Beumer, T.L.; Roepers-Gajadien, H.L.; Gademan, I.S.; Kal, H.B.; de Rooij, D.G. Involvement of the D-type cyclins in germ cell proliferation and differentiation in the mouse. *Biol. Reprod.* **2000**, *63*, 1893–1898. [CrossRef]
27. Timsit, S.; Rivera, S.; Ouaghi, P.; Guischard, F.; Tremblay, E.; Ben-Ari, Y.; Khrestchatisky, M. Increased cyclin D1 in vulnerable neurons in the hippocampus after ischaemia and epilepsy: A modulator of in vivo programmed cell death? *Eur. J. Neurosci.* **1999**, *11*, 263–278. [CrossRef]
28. Ciapa, B.; Granon, S. Expression of Cyclin-D1 in Astrocytes Varies During Aging. *Front. Aging Neurosci.* **2018**, *10*, 104. [CrossRef]
29. Smolensky, I.V.; Zubareva, O.E.; Kalemenev, S.V.; Lavrentyeva, V.V.; Dyomina, A.V.; Karepanov, A.A.; Zaitsev, A.V. Impairments in cognitive functions and emotional and social behaviors in a rat lithium-pilocarpine model of temporal lobe epilepsy. *Behav. Brain Res.* **2019**, *372*, 112044. [CrossRef]
30. Sharma, H.; Reeta, K.H.; Sharma, U.; Suri, V.; Singh, S. AMPA receptor modulation through sequential treatment with perampanel and aniracetam mitigates post-stroke damage in experimental model of ischemic stroke. *Naunyn. Schmiedebergs Arch. Pharmacol.* **2023**, *396*, 3529–3545. [CrossRef]
31. Guignet, M.; Campbell, A.; Vuong, J.; Whittington, D.; White, H.S. Perampanel's forgiveness factor in a variable medication adherence paradigm in a rat model of chronic epilepsy. *J. Transl. Med.* **2023**, *21*, 642. [CrossRef] [PubMed]
32. Racine, R.J. Modification of seizure activity by electrical stimulation. II. Motor seizure. *Electroencephalogr. Clin. Neurophysiol.* **1972**, *32*, 281–294. [CrossRef] [PubMed]
33. Mareš, P.; Kubová, H. Perampanel exhibits anticonvulsant action against pentylentetrazol-induced seizures in immature rats. *Epilepsy Res.* **2021**, *169*, 106523. [CrossRef] [PubMed]
34. Shishmanova-Doseva, M.; Atanasova, D.; Uzunova, Y.; Yoanidu, L.; Peychev, L.; Marinov, P.; Tchekalarova, J. Effects of Lacosamide Treatment on Epileptogenesis, Neuronal Damage and Behavioral Comorbidities in a Rat Model of Temporal Lobe Epilepsy. *Int. J. Mol. Sci.* **2021**, *22*, 4667. [CrossRef]
35. Shishmanova-Doseva, M.; Atanasova, D.; Ioanidu, L.; Uzunova, Y.; Atanasova, M.; Peychev, L.; Tchekalarova, J. The anticonvulsant effect of chronic treatment with topiramate after pilocarpine-induced status epilepticus is accompanied by a suppression of comorbid behavioral impairments and robust neuroprotection in limbic regions in rats. *Epilepsy Behav.* **2022**, *134*, 108802. [CrossRef]
36. Miedel, C.J.; Patton, J.M.; Miedel, A.N.; Miedel, E.S.; Levenson, J.M. Assessment of Spontaneous Alternation, Novel Object Recognition and Limb Clasping in Transgenic Mouse Models of Amyloid-β and Tau Neuropathology. *J. Vis. Exp.* **2017**, *28*, 55523. [CrossRef] [PubMed] [PubMed Central]
37. Moosavi, M.; SoukhakLari, R.; Moezi, L.; Pirsalami, F. Scopolamine-induced passive avoidance memory retrieval deficit is accompanied with hippocampal MMP2, MMP-9 and MAPKs alteration. *Eur. J. Pharmacol.* **2018**, *819*, 248–253. [CrossRef]
38. Jadhav, R.; Kulkarni, Y.A. Effects of baicalein with memantine on aluminium chloride-induced neurotoxicity in Wistar rats. *Front. Pharmacol.* **2023**, *14*, 1034620. [CrossRef]
39. Mendiburu-Eliçabe, M.; García-Sancha, N.; Corchado-Cobos, R.; Martínez-López, A.; Chang, H.; Mao, J.H.; Blanco-Gómez, A.; García-Casas, A.; Castellanos-Martín, A.; Salvador, N.; et al. NCAPH drives breast cancer progression and identifies a gene signature that predicts luminal a tumour recurrence. *Clin. Transl. Med.* **2024**, *14*, e1554. [CrossRef]
40. Operto, F.F.; Pastorino, G.M.G.; Viggiano, A.; Dell'Isola, G.B.; Dini, G.; Verrotti, A.; Coppola, G. Epilepsy and Cognitive Impairment in Childhood and Adolescence: A Mini-Review. *Curr. Neuropharmacol.* **2023**, *21*, 1646–1665. [CrossRef]
41. Holmes, G.L. Cognitive impairment in epilepsy: The role of network abnormalities. *Epileptic Disord.* **2015**, *17*, 101–116. [CrossRef] [PubMed]
42. Sandouka, S.; Singh, P.K.; Saadi, A.; Taiwo, R.O.; Sheeni, Y.; Zhang, T.; Deeb, L.; Guignet, M.; White, S.H. Repurposing dimethyl fumarate as an antiepileptogenic and disease-modifying treatment for drug-resistant epilepsy. *J. Transl. Med.* **2023**, *21*, 796. [CrossRef] [PubMed]
43. Mohammad, H.; Sekar, S.; Wei, Z.; Moien-Afshari, F.; Taghibiglou, C. Perampanel but Not Amantadine Prevents Behavioral Alterations and Epileptogenesis in Pilocarpine Rat Model of Status Epilepticus. *Mol. Neurobiol.* **2019**, *56*, 2508–2523. [CrossRef] [PubMed]

44. Nakajima, M.; Suda, S.; Sowa, K.; Sakamoto, Y.; Nito, C.; Nishiyama, Y.; Aoki, J.; Ueda, M.; Yokobori, S.; Yamada, M.; et al. AMPA Receptor Antagonist Perampanel Ameliorates Post-Stroke Functional and Cognitive Impairments. *Neuroscience* **2018**, *386*, 256–264. [CrossRef] [PubMed]
45. Martins, C.W.; de Melo Rodrigues, L.C.; Nitsche, M.A.; Nakamura-Palacios, E.M. AMPA receptors are involved in prefrontal direct current stimulation effects on long-term working memory and GAP-43 expression. *Behav. Brain Res.* **2019**, *362*, 208–212. [CrossRef]
46. Aida, V.; Niedzielko, T.L.; Szaflarski, J.P.; Floyd, C.L. Acute administration of perampanel, an AMPA receptor antagonist, reduces cognitive impairments after traumatic brain injury in rats. *Exp. Neurol.* **2020**, *327*, 113222. [CrossRef]
47. Gibson, B.M.; Mair, R. A pathway for spatial memory encoding. *Learn. Behav.* **2016**, *44*, 97–98. [CrossRef]
48. Kim, G.H.; Byeon, J.H.; Eun, B.L. Neuroprotective Effect of Lacosamide on Hypoxic-Ischemic Brain Injury in Neonatal Rats. *J. Clin. Neurol.* **2017**, *13*, 138–143. [CrossRef]
49. Savran, M.; Ozmen, O.; Erzurumlu, Y.; Savas, H.B.; Asci, S.; Kaynak, M. The Impact of Prophylactic Lacosamide on LPS-Induced Neuroinflammation in Aged Rats. *Inflammation* **2019**, *42*, 1913–1924. [CrossRef]
50. Demiroz, S.; Ur, K.; Ulucan, A.; Bengu, A.S.; Ur, F.D.; Gergin, O.O.; Erdem, S. Neuroprotective Effects of Lacosamide in Experimental Traumatic Spinal Cord Injury in Rats. *Turk. Neurosurg.* **2019**, *29*, 718–723. [CrossRef]
51. Hakami, T. Neuropharmacology of Antiseizure Drugs. *Neuropsychopharmacol. Rep.* **2021**, *41*, 336–351. [CrossRef] [PubMed]
52. Dhir, A.; Bruun, D.A.; Guignet, M.; Tsai, Y.H.; González, E.; Calsbeek, J.; Vu, J.; Saito, N.; Tancredi, D.J.; Harvey, D.J.; et al. Allopregnanolone and perampanel as adjuncts to midazolam for treating diisopropylfluorophosphate-induced status epilepticus in rats. *Ann. N. Y. Acad Sci.* **2020**, *1480*, 183–206. [CrossRef] [PubMed]
53. Bektas, N.; Arslan, R.; Alyu, F. The anxiolytic effect of perampanel and possible mechanisms mediating its anxiolytic effect in mice. *Life Sci.* **2020**, *261*, 118359. [CrossRef]
54. Meirinho, S.; Rodrigues, M.; Santos, A.O.; Falcão, A.; Alves, G. Nose-to-brain delivery of perampanel formulated in a self-microemulsifying drug delivery system improves anticonvulsant and anxiolytic activity in mice. *Int. J. Pharm.* **2023**, *642*, 123145. [CrossRef]
55. Perveen, N.; Alqahtani, F.; Ashraf, W.; Fawad Rasool, M.; Muhammad Muneeb Anjum, S.; Kaukab, I.; Ahmad, T.; Alqarni, S.A.; Imran, I. Perampanel increases seizure threshold in pentylenetetrazole-kindled mice and improves behavioral dysfunctions by modifying mRNA expression levels of BDNF/TrkB and inflammatory markers. *Saudi Pharm. J.* **2024**, *32*, 101930. [CrossRef]
56. Moseley, B.D.; Cole, D.; Iwuora, O.; Strawn, J.R.; Privitera, M. The effects of lacosamide on depression and anxiety in patients with epilepsy. *Epilepsy Res.* **2015**, *110*, 115–118. [CrossRef]
57. Rocamora, R.; Ley, M.; Molins, A.; Toledo, M.; Sansa, G.; Bertol, V.; Becerra, J.-L.; Carreño, M.; Mauri, J. Effect of lacosamide on depression and anxiety symptoms in patients with focal refractory epilepsy: A prospective multicenter study. *Epilepsy Behav.* **2018**, *79*, 87–92. [CrossRef]
58. Alfaro, A.; Asensio, M.; García-Escrivá, A.; Medrano, V.; Salom, J.M.; Tortosa, D.; Palao, S.; Lezcano, M.; Berenguer, L.; Navarro, M.; et al. LAM study: Effects of lacosamide on behaviour and quality of life in patients with epilepsy. [Article in English, Spanish]. *Neurologia* **2019**, *34*, 1–6. [CrossRef]
59. Pittenger, C.; Duman, R.S. Stress, depression, and neuroplasticity: A convergence of mechanisms. *Neuropsychopharmacology* **2008**, *33*, 88–109. [CrossRef]
60. Duman, R.S.; Aghajanian, G.K.; Sanacora, G.; Krystal, J.H. Synaptic plasticity and depression: New insights from stress and rapid-acting antidepressants. *Nat. Med.* **2016**, *22*, 238–249. [CrossRef]
61. Li, K.; Shen, S.; Ji, Y.T.; Li, X.Y.; Zhang, L.S.; Wang, X.D. Melatonin Augments the Effects of Fluoxetine on Depression-Like Behavior and Hippocampal BDNF-TrkB Signaling. *Neurosci. Bull.* **2018**, *34*, 303–311. [CrossRef] [PubMed]
62. Tchekalarova, J.; Atanasova, M.; Ivanova, N.; Boyadjiev, N.; Mitreva, R.; Georgieva, K. Endurance training exerts time-dependent modulation on depressive responses and circadian rhythms of corticosterone and BDNF in the rats with pinealectomy. *Brain Res. Bull.* **2020**, *162*, 40–48. [CrossRef] [PubMed]
63. McGonigal, A.; Becker, C.; Fath, J.; Hammam, K.; Baumstarck, K.; Fernandes, S.; Giusiano, B.; Dufau, S.; Rheims, S.; Maillard, L.; et al. BDNF as potential biomarker of epilepsy severity and psychiatric comorbidity: Pitfalls in the clinical population. *Epilepsy Res.* **2023**, *195*, 107200. [CrossRef] [PubMed]
64. Shi, X.Y.; Wang, J.W.; Cui, H.; Li, B.M.; Lei, G.F.; Sun, R.P. Effects of antiepileptic drugs on mRNA levels of BDNF and NT-3 and cell neogenesis in the developing rat brain. *Brain Dev.* **2010**, *32*, 229–235. [CrossRef]
65. Waterhouse, E.G.; An, J.J.; Orefice, L.L.; Baydyuk, M.; Liao, G.Y.; Zheng, K. BDNF promotes differentiation and maturation of adult-born neurons through GABAergic transmission. *J. Neurosci.* **2012**, *32*, 14318–14330. [CrossRef]
66. Quesseveur, G.; David, D.J.; Gaillard, M.C.; Pla, P.; Wu, M.V.; Nguyen, H.T. BDNF overexpression in mouse hippocampal astrocytes promotes local neurogenesis and elicits anxiolytic-like activities. *Transl. Psychiatry* **2013**, *3*, e253. [CrossRef]
67. Eyo, U.B.; Peng, J.; Murugan, M.; Mo, M.; Lalani, A.; Xie, P.; Xu, P.; Margolis, D.J.; Wu, L.J. Regulation of Physical Microglia-Neuron Interactions by Fractalkine Signaling after Status Epilepticus. *eNeuro* **2017**, *3*, ENEURO.0209-16.2016. [CrossRef]
68. Streit, W.J.; Sammons, N.W.; Kuhns, A.J.; Sparks, D.L. Dystrophic microglia in the aging human brain. *Glia* **2004**, *45*, 208–212. [CrossRef]
69. Streit, W.J.; Braak, H.; Xue, Q.; Bechmann, I. Dystrophic (senescent) rather than activated microglial cells are associated with tau pathology and likely precede neurodegeneration in Alzheimer's disease. *Acta Neuropathol.* **2009**, *118*, 475–485. [CrossRef]
70. Aroeira, R.I.; Sebastião, A.M.; Valente, C.A. BDNF, via truncated TrkB receptor, modulates GlyT1 and GlyT2 in astrocytes. *Glia* **2015**, *63*, 2181–2197. [CrossRef]

71. Tadi, M.; Allaman, I.; Lengacher, S.; Grenningloh, G.; Magistretti, P.J. Learning-induced gene expression in the hippocampus reveals a role of neuron-astrocyte metabolic coupling in long term memory. *PLoS ONE* **2015**, *10*, e0141568. [CrossRef] [PubMed]
72. Small, D.L.; Monette, R.; Fournier, M.C.; Zurakowski, B.; Fiander, H.; Morley, P. Characterization of cyclin D1 expression in a rat global model of cerebral ischemia. *Brain Res.* **2001**, *900*, 26–37. [CrossRef] [PubMed]
73. Pittaras, E.; Callebert, J.; Chennaoui, M.; Rabat, A.; Granon, S. Individual behavioral and neurochemical markers of unadapted decisionmaking processes in healthy inbred mice. *Brain Struct. Funct.* **2016**, *221*, 4615–4629. [CrossRef] [PubMed]
74. Kaya, S.S.; Mahmood, A.; Li, Y.; Yavuz, E.; Göksel, M.; Chopp, M. Apoptosis and expression of p53 response proteins and cyclin D1 after cortical impact in rat brain. *Brain Res.* **1999**, *818*, 23–33. [CrossRef]
75. Ferrer, I. Cell signaling in the epileptic hippocampus. *Rev. Neurol.* **2002**, *34*, 544–550.

current issues in
molecular biology

MDPI

Review

Unlocking the Potential: Semaglutide's Impact on Alzheimer's and Parkinson's Disease in Animal Models

Andreea Daniela Meca [1,†], Ianis Kevyn Stefan Boboc [1,†], Liliana Mititelu-Tartau [2,*] and Maria Bogdan [1,*]

1 Department of Pharmacology, Faculty of Pharmacy, University of Medicine and Pharmacy, 200349 Craiova, Romania; andreea_mdc@yahoo.com (A.D.M.); kevynboboc@gmail.com (I.K.S.B.)
2 Department of Pharmacology, Faculty of Medicine, 'Grigore T. Popa' University of Medicine and Pharmacy, 700115 Iasi, Romania
* Correspondence: liliana.tartau@umfiasi.ro (L.M.-T.); maria.bogdan@umfcv.ro (M.B.)
† These authors contributed equally to this work.

Abstract: Semaglutide (SEM), a glucagon-like peptide-1 receptor agonist, has garnered increasing interest for its potential therapeutic effects in neurodegenerative disorders such as Alzheimer's disease (AD) and Parkinson's disease (PD). This review provides a comprehensive description of SEM's mechanism of action and its effects in preclinical studies of these debilitating conditions. In animal models of AD, SEM has proved beneficial effects on multiple pathological hallmarks of the disease. SEM administration has been associated with reductions in amyloid-beta plaque deposition and mitigation of neuroinflammation. Moreover, SEM treatment has been shown to ameliorate behavioral deficits related to anxiety and social interaction. SEM-treated animals exhibit improvements in spatial learning and memory retention tasks, as evidenced by enhanced performance in maze navigation tests and novel object recognition assays. Similarly, in animal models of PD, SEM has demonstrated promising neuroprotective effects through various mechanisms. These include modulation of neuroinflammation, enhancement of mitochondrial function, and promotion of neurogenesis. Additionally, SEM has been shown to improve motor function and ameliorate dopaminergic neuronal loss, offering the potential for disease-modifying treatment strategies. Overall, the accumulating evidence from preclinical studies suggests that SEM holds promise as a novel therapeutic approach for AD and PD. Further research is warranted to elucidate the underlying mechanisms of SEM's neuroprotective effects and to translate these findings into clinical applications for the treatment of these devastating neurodegenerative disorders.

Keywords: semaglutide; neuroprotective; Alzheimer's disease; Parkinson's disease; animal models

1. Introduction

Alzheimer's disease (AD) is a neurodegenerative condition marked by cognitive decline, memory impairment, and eventual loss of executive function [1,2]. It accounts for 50% to 75% of diagnosed dementia cases [3]. AD is classified into two types: senile (sporadic), which is predominant in 95–98% of cases, and presenile (familial) [4,5]. It is hypothesized that the neurodegenerative processes associated with sporadic AD may begin as early as 20 years before the onset of clinical symptoms [6].

Parkinson's disease (PD) is a prevalent condition among the elderly, characterized by progressive neurodegeneration that significantly impacts patients' lives, particularly when left unmanaged [7,8]. Typically initiating around the ages of 60–65, though occasionally manifesting earlier, it ranks among the most prevalent movement disorders [9–12]. Primarily triggered by dopamine deficiency, PD chiefly involves the degeneration of neurons responsible for dopamine production within the substantia nigra [10–14].

Various analogs of glucagon-like peptide-1 (GLP-1) have been examined for their potential in AD and PD, including those that activate receptors for a single type of incretin [single incretin receptor agonists—exenatide, liraglutide, lixisenatide, and semaglutide

(SEM)] and those that activate receptors for both types of incretins (dual incretin receptor agonists—Peptide 19, DA4-JC, DA5-CH, DA3-CH) [12–16].

SEM, a long-acting peptide-modified human GLP-1 receptor agonist resistant to protease, has been shown to significantly reduce blood glucose and glycated hemoglobin (HbA1c) levels compared to short-acting agents [16–20]. It was approved for type 2 diabetes in the USA in 2017 and in Canada and Europe in 2018 for 1 mg SEM administered subcutaneously once weekly, exhibiting a safety profile similar to other antidiabetic agents and offering additional advantages [21,22]. In 2019 in the USA and 2020 in Europe, an oral dose of a maximum of 14 mg daily of SEM received approval as type 2 diabetes pharmacotherapy [10,21,22] so that doctors can choose the most suitable formulation for the patients' necessities (Figure 1) [10].

Semaglutide	Subcutaneous injection	Oral
Storage	- refrigerator at a temperature between 2°C to 8°C	- in original packaging to protect from light and moisture - no special temperature conditions required
Administration	- once per week	- once per day
Dosing	- no specific instructions	- should follow specific instructions daily
Benefits	- convenience for frequent travelling patients - stability of blood medication level - easy to use prefilled pen device - reduced risk of medication-related side effects - decreased frequency of medical visits	- patients with injection fears (fear of pain, concerns about correct administration, and side effects) - flexibility in dosing, allowing patients to take their medication without the need for refrigeration or special storage conditions
Adherence	- often better with once-weekly administration due to increased convenience and reduced frequency of dosing	- improved compared to injectables - dosing conditions must be acceptable
Costs	- assess cost-effectiveness relative to other treatments, factoring in formulary and reimbursement considerations	- assess cost-effectiveness relative to other treatments, factoring in formulary and reimbursement considerations

Figure 1. Characteristics of subcutaneous and oral formulations of SEM.

Nevertheless, in 2021, the FDA offered an additional approval for 2.4 mg of SEM, administered once a week subcutaneously, as an adjunct able to reduce caloric intake in individuals diagnosed with obesity (BMI higher than 30 kg/m^2 or higher than 27 kg/m^2 with at least one comorbidity related to weight) [10,21,22]. Due to its pharmacokinetic profile, SEM presents a slightly different toxicity profile when compared to other GLP-1 receptor agonists, such as less frequent injection site effects and hypoglycemic risk (that can further increase when associated with insulin or sulfonylureas), but also more frequent vomiting [9].

SEM boasts an extended half-life of 7 days in the bloodstream, allowing for once-weekly administration at any time of the day, with or without food. The initial injectable dose typically starts at 0.25 mg, while the regular dosage ranges from 0.5 to 1 mg [20]. Additionally, it is available in oral tablet form in strengths of 3, 7, or 14 mg, exhibiting similar efficacy to subcutaneous doses. SEM stands out as the sole GLP-1 receptor agonist offered in both injectable and oral pharmaceutical formulations [9,14,23]. With a 94% homology to native GLP-1, SEM results in only 1% presence of antibodies against SEM or GLP-1 post-treatment, thus minimizing the risk of allergic reactions [23,24]. Furthermore, it can be excreted via both urine and feces, eliminating the need for dose adjustment in cases of renal insufficiency [25,26]. An absorption enhancer (SNAC or sodium N-[8-(2-hydroxybenzoyl)]-aminocaprylate) for SEM has been noticed due to its ability to protect this GLP-1 agonist from proteolytic degradation within the stomach and also to facilitate active intestinal transport [9].

The objective of this review is to offer an extensive description of SEM's involvement in the pathophysiology of AD and PD, emphasizing the drug's mechanism of action and its relevance in animal models of these disorders.

2. SEM Mechanism of Action

GLP-1 receptor agonists, also referred to as incretin analogs, play a crucial role in maintaining glycemic control by stimulating natural mechanisms and responses to nutrient intake [25]. This process involves the release of the incretin hormone GLP-1 from intestinal L cells following meals [26–28]. GLP-1 receptor agonists bind to specific receptors distributed widely throughout the body, including pancreatic islets, renal, pulmonary, cardiovascular, gastrointestinal, immune, and brain cells [19]. GLP-1 and GIP (glucose-dependent insulinotropic polypeptide) receptors belong to the G protein-coupled B1 class receptors (the secretin family), which can trigger the production of cAMP (cyclic adenosine monophosphate) and undergo conformational changes upon activation [27]. The activation of GLP-1 and GIP hormones consequently leads to delayed gastric emptying and modulation of insulin secretion [24,25]. However, shortly after their release, GLP-1 and GIP are broken down by the enzyme dipeptidyl peptidase-4 (DPP-4), resulting in their short half-lives as endogenous molecules [27–29].

As versatile peptides, GLP-1 receptor agonists, such as SEM, play a role in enhancing insulin and amylin secretion by stimulating pancreatic β-cells while simultaneously inhibiting glucagon secretion from pancreatic α-cells in a glucose-dependent manner. They also decrease hepatic glucose production, increase feelings of satiety, and regulate appetite through central mechanisms [19,29,30]. Additionally, GLP-1 is involved in promoting pancreatic β-cell proliferation and preventing apoptosis [25]. SEM promotes insulin uptake in peripheral tissues, resulting in weight loss, reduced risk of hepatic steatosis, and increased lipolysis, making them beneficial for patients with type 2 diabetes and obesity [19,28]. Activation of GLP-1 receptors correlates with increased intracellular calcium levels and ERK1/2 phosphorylation to stimulate insulin production [25,28]. Furthermore, SEM can enhance glycolysis by upregulating GLUT2 transporters and glucokinase expression. SEM also regulates tissue sensitivity to insulin [26].

These benefits arise from the activation of peripheral and central intestinal and brain receptors, particularly those located in hypothalamic satiety centers, which are also involved in regulating perceptions of motivation and reward-related to food intake [19,23]. Acting as a multifunctional peptide, brain-derived GLP-1 is synthesized by pre-proglucagon neurons situated in the caudal area of the nucleus tractus solitarius (NTS) [30]. GLP-1 receptors are expressed in various regions of the brain, including the frontal cortex, hippocampus, substantia nigra, and cerebellum [24]. Moreover, GLP-1 has the capacity to modulate diverse brain functions such as water intake, energy homeostasis, thermogenesis, neural genesis, degeneration, and responses to stress [31]. The amelioration of cognitive impairment has led to the recommendation of GLP-1 receptor agonists for neurological deficits associated with type 2 diabetes and obesity [28]. Additionally, most GLP-1 receptor agonists can penetrate the blood-brain barrier (BBB) and initiate neuroprotective effects, as shown in a murine study for the i.v. injection of 1×10^6 counts per minute of radioactively labeled exenatide, lixisenatide, Peptide 17, Peptide 21, DA3-CH, DA4-JC [18,32].

GLP-1 receptor agonists are distinguished by their prolonged half-life compared to endogenous GLP-1, allowing them to remain bound to specific receptors for an extended period [31]. Their safety profile includes a low risk of hypoglycemia, facilitation of weight loss, beneficial cardiovascular and renal effects, reduced dosing frequency, and decreased injection burden, leading to improved treatment adherence among patients [19,20]. Additionally, one of the most significant advantages of GLP-1 receptor agonists is their ability to traverse the BBB to varying extents within the class [9,10]. Even when compared to other long-acting agents, such as exenatide with extended release and dulaglutide, subcutaneous SEM has demonstrated superior efficacy in improving glycemic control [28]. Furthermore, SEM exhibits pleiotropic effects by correcting insulin resistance, protecting against glucolipotoxicity, and inhibiting apoptosis [14,28]. This GLP-1 receptor agonist can also enhance lipid profiles by activating an intrinsic gut–liver signaling pathway, thereby reducing VLDL production [14]. Moreover, SEM has been shown to lower systolic blood pressure, protect renal function, improve insulin resistance, and induce anti-obesity effects [14,32]. However, recent research has focused on investigating the potential of SEM to provide neuroprotection and mitigate the progression of various neurodegenerative diseases. In this review, we examine the therapeutic potential of SEM and its underlying neuroprotective pathways in both AD and PD.

3. Therapeutic Potential of SEM in Neurodegenerative Diseases

Impaired cognitive function is associated with insulin resistance, as neuronal metabolism and synaptic efficacy suffer from the desensitization of insulin signaling pathways [33,34]. Insulin is crucial in activating various growth factors that further stimulate brain receptors, thereby regulating mitochondrial functionality, cellular energy utilization, cell survival, and synaptic processes [33,35]. Reduced or delayed neuronal repair due to impaired insulin signaling has been correlated with an increased risk of developing neurodegenerative pathologies [33,35]. Since neurons cannot produce or store glucose, they rely on the activation and sensitization of specific proteins acting as glucose transporters to prevent neurodegeneration [35]. GLP-1 receptor agonists, more specifically SEM, can compensate for deficiencies in insulin signaling by activating the same growth factor cascades as insulin [33,34]. Moreover, recent research has unveiled the neurotrophic and neuroprotective activities of GLP-1 [36,37].

Neuronal loss in AD has been associated with neurocyte apoptosis [36,38]. However, both insulin resistance and hyperinsulinemia can contribute to cognitive impairment in adults, highlighting impaired tissue sensitivity to insulin as a pathogenic mechanism in AD [29]. As demonstrated by Yu et al. in their experimental study using the water navigation task, liraglutide has shown efficacy in preventing neuronal apoptosis [38]. GLP-1 receptor activation can also mitigate tau phosphorylation and amyloid β deposition, critical factors in delaying the progression of AD [29,30]. GLP-1 receptor agonists (especially SEM) have been found to reduce neuronal apoptosis, neuroinflammation, synapse loss, and brain accumulation of advanced glycation end products, as concluded by a systematic review [25].

Moreover, the onset of PD has been linked to type 2 diabetes and desensitized insulin signaling [23,34,39]. In various mouse models of PD, GLP-1 mimetics have shown efficacy in reducing chronic neuronal inflammation, dopaminergic neuron loss, oxidative stress, and α-synuclein levels, ultimately leading to improved motor coordination [23,34]. Activation of GLP-1 brain receptors has been found to mitigate microglial neurotoxicity by inhibiting A1 astrocyte activity, thereby delaying neuronal death in neurodegenerative disorders [29]. Notably, liraglutide and lixisenatide demonstrated superior efficacy compared to other short-acting agents in maintaining tyrosine hydroxylase expression, a crucial enzyme in dopamine production [34]. In experimental mouse models, exenatide restored motor functionality, while SEM prevented the loss of dopaminergic neurons by down-regulating microgliosis and astrogliosis, thus reducing chronic inflammation [20,23,25]. Furthermore, SEM normalized the expression of autophagy-related proteins in the substantia nigra and striatum in mice, including P62, ATG7, Beclin, and LC3, leading to the alleviation of oxidative stress and promotion of neurovascular reconstruction [31,32,39]. When compared in equivalent doses in experimental PD models, SEM exhibited superior efficacy in restoring mitochondrial functionality and antioxidative balance by enhancing autophagy [23,39].

SEM has been shown to reduce oxidative stress, a critical factor in NMDA excitotoxicity. By lowering oxidative stress levels, SEM can help mitigate the damage caused by excessive Ca^{2+} influx and reactive oxygen species (ROS) generation [40]. This reduction in oxidative stress also helps preserve the integrity and function of cholinergic neurons, thereby supporting acetylcholine production [41,42].

SEM has been found to improve mitochondrial function, which could help protect neurons from excitotoxic damage. Enhancing mitochondrial efficiency is crucial for maintaining neuronal health and preventing the cascade of events leading to cell death in AD [23,43].

By modulating the release and uptake of glutamate, SEM could help prevent the overactivation of NMDA receptors, thereby reducing excitotoxicity. This regulation of glutamate dynamics is essential for protecting neurons from the harmful effects of excessive glutamate signaling [44–46].

Chronic neuroinflammation is a hallmark of AD and is exacerbated by NMDA excitotoxicity. SEM exhibits anti-inflammatory properties, reducing the release of pro-inflammatory cytokines and potentially lessening the neuronal damage associated with excitotoxicity [44,47,48].

Although SEM's primary mechanism is not the inhibition of acetylcholinesterase, there is some evidence to suggest that GLP-1 receptor agonists can reduce the activity of acetylcholinesterase, increasing the availability of acetylcholine in the brain, albeit this effect is less pronounced compared to traditional acetylcholinesterase inhibitors used in AD treatment. Furthermore, SEM can enhance the cholinergic system function by supporting the growth and maintenance of cholinergic synapses [41,45].

Figure 2 shows the pathogenic mechanisms of AD and PD and the effects (decrease/increase) produced by SEM therapy.

Various experimental studies have shown the neurotrophic effects of GLP-1 agonists, although the exact mechanism of neuroprotection is not yet fully understood [18,20]. SEM, especially, is considered a versatile multifaceted agent [49,50]; it can activate both the production and signaling of neuronal stem cells [49].

Incretin signaling has also proven beneficial with regard to the outgrowth of the essential synaptic components called neurites through a mechanism similar to that of the nerve growth factor (NGF) [20,51]. Nevertheless, chronic administration of GLP-1 agonists (for more than 4 weeks) in mice models of diabetes has led to early DCX-positive neurons in the dentate gyrus area [51]. Neuronal precursors and other immature nervous cells usually express DCX, a microtubule-associated protein, suggesting an active division process and multiplication [51]. After binding and activating GLP-1 receptors, cAMP levels increase rapidly and activate two pathways through PI3K (phosphoinositide 3-kinase) and protein kinase A, being involved in protein and mitochondrial biogenesis while inhibiting neuronal apoptosis [20,51]. Therefore, GLP-1 agonists have been associated with neurotrophic effects.

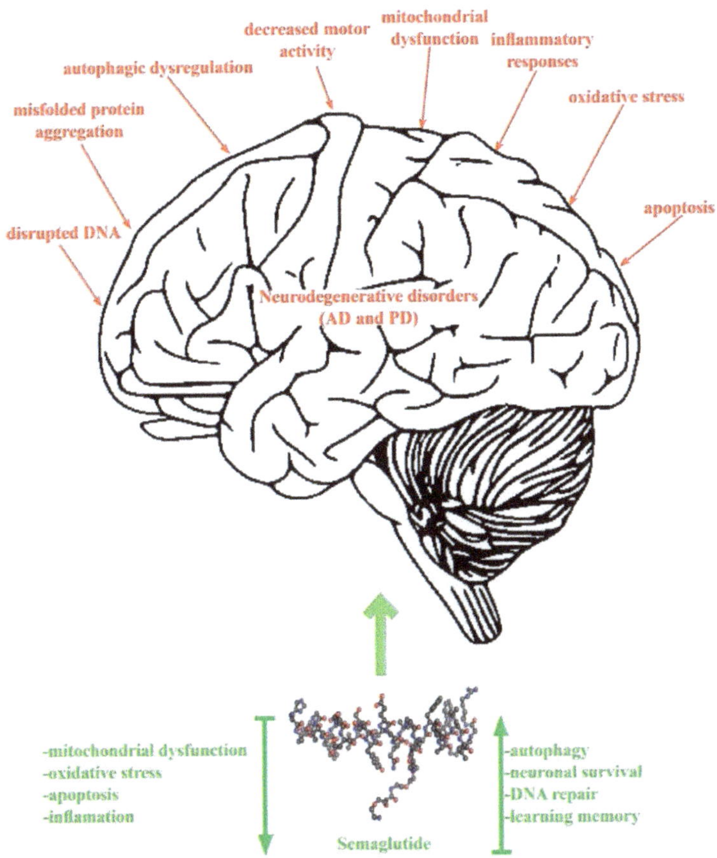

Figure 2. The pathogenesis of AD and PD and the effects of SEM.

The PI3K/Akt signaling pathway has been experimentally correlated with the neuroprotective properties of SEM due to enhanced mitochondrial functionality and reduction of neuro-apoptotic reactions [20]. Another GLP-1 agonist, exenatide, has initiated cellular stem proliferation through ciliary neurotrophic factor (CNTF), increased Ki-67 gene expression, and also induced microglial activation with reduction of astrogliosis [51], suggesting GLP-1 agonists utility in both AD and PD.

Even more, SEM PI3K/Akt pathway activation led to inhibition of a proinflammatory and neurodegenerative serine/threonine kinase (GSK3β or glycogen synthase kinase-3), noted in various nervous system diseases [52,53]. However, regulation of GSK3β by treatment GLP-1 agonists is complex and needs to be investigated in further experimental or clinical studies. Among its neuroprotective and neurotrophic effects, SEM has activated proteolytic and autophagic mechanisms that further led to the diminished accumulation of α-synuclein and therefore maintained an equilibrium among dopaminergic neurons in the substantia nigra in experimental-induced PD models [29,49]. This suggests a strong correlation between SEM treatment and improved mitochondrial functionality with reduced impairment of autophagic and lysosomal pathways, which needs to be monitored in clinical studies [20].

4. SEM Pharmacokinetics in Animal Models

SEM, an acylated GLP-1 analog, emerges as a distinctive contender among the insulin receptor agonists (IRAs) scrutinized by the Salameh team [18]. Unlike linear peptides such as exenatide and lixisenatide, SEM exhibits acylation, a characteristic it shares with liraglutide. Notably, the acylated dual agonist, Peptide 19, stands out for its significantly greater lipid solubility compared to its counterparts, including liraglutide and SEM. This heightened lipid solubility could potentially influence the pharmacokinetics and distribution of Peptide 19 in vivo. Moreover, SEM demonstrates remarkable stability, with less than 2% degradation in serum and less than 12% in the whole brain over the specified time frame of 60 min [18,54–57]. In another study [58], the stability of SEM was evaluated under four different storage conditions (i.e., 4 h at room temperature, 7 days at −70 °C, 24 h in the autosampler, and freeze/thaw cycles). It was found that SEM exhibited average stability ranging from 93.94% to 106.13% in plasma and 91.64% to 107.31% in brain tissue, with no significant deviations observed under all tested conditions [58]. Such robust stability positions SEM favorably when compared to other IRAs like DA3-CH, which experiences higher degradation rates, indicating that SEM remains stable for routine analysis. These structural and stability distinctions underscore SEM's potential advantages in bioavailability and durability, contributing to its unique profile within the landscape of insulin receptor agonists [18,58–60].

Following intravenous administration, SEM plasma concentrations exhibited a multi-exponential decline, with an average half-life (T1/2) of 9.26 ± 1.06 h and an average clearance and distribution volume estimated at 0.21 mL/min/kg (0.10 L/kg) [58]. In a study on CD-1 mice conducted by Salameh's team, the serum clearance of SEM labeled with mCi Na 125I was 2.5 h. Concerning subcutaneous administration, SEM plasma concentration increased gradually, reaching peak concentration between 3 and 12 h, and decreased with an average half-life of 7.22–8.99 h [18]. The absolute bioavailability of SEM in rats was reported to be 76.65–82.85%. However, in humans, the half-life after s.c. administration ranges between 165 and 183 h, with the highest bioavailability (89%) among all GLP-1 agonists [59–62].

Brain influx rates were analyzed to assess SEM's ability to cross the BBB. It was observed that there was no significant correlation between blood-to-serum (B/S) ratios and exposure time, indicating a lack of transport. Additionally, SEM, along with other tested IRAs, exhibited varying capabilities in accessing the brain parenchyma. Within a 15 min timeframe after i.v. injection, the majority of DA4-JC, DA3-CH, exenatide, Peptide 17, and lixisenatide successfully entered the brain parenchyma. Conversely, Peptide 21 and liraglutide were predominantly sequestered in brain endothelial cells during the same period, indicating an obstacle to complete passage across the capillary wall. Notably, SEM and Peptide 19 encountered challenges in reliable detection within the brain parenchyma [18,58,63].

Despite the assertion that SEM generally does not penetrate the BBB, there is intriguing evidence of localized distribution of SEM within the brain, particularly in the hypothalamus [63,64]. Concentrations of SEM in the hypothalamus were notably higher than those observed in other brain regions, exhibiting an average concentration and blood-brain partition coefficient (Kp) that were 2.26- and 1.82-fold higher, respectively, compared to the total brain following both intravenous and subcutaneous injections [58].

This localized distribution in the hypothalamus is significant as it aligns with the proposed effects of SEM in the brain, such as neuroprotection. These effects are believed to be associated with the interaction of SEM with GLP-1 receptors in the brain [64–68]. This paradoxical finding underscores the complexity of SEM's interaction with the brain and challenges the conventional understanding of its BBB permeability.

5. SEM Potential Mechanism of Action in AD

AD is a progressive neurodegenerative disorder characterized by a decline in cognitive function, memory impairment, and changes in behavior and personality. It is the most common cause of dementia among older adults. The pathological disturbances in AD are multifaceted and involve a combination of genetic, molecular, and cellular mechanisms. The primary pathological hallmarks of AD include amyloid-beta (Aβ) plaques, neurofibrillary tangles (NFTs), neuroinflammation, and synaptic and neuronal loss [69].

Aβ plaques are extracellular deposits of amyloid-beta peptides that accumulate in the brain. These peptides are derived from the amyloid precursor protein (APP), which is cleaved by the enzymes β-secretase and γ-secretase. The accumulation of Aβ is thought to result from an imbalance between production and clearance. The aggregation of Aβ peptides leads to the formation of soluble oligomers, which are neurotoxic, and eventually to the deposition of insoluble fibrils in plaques. The toxic oligomers disrupt synaptic function, impairing communication between neurons. They also induce oxidative stress and inflammatory responses, contributing to neuronal damage and cell death [70].

NFTs are intracellular aggregates of hyperphosphorylated tau protein. Tau is normally associated with microtubules, aiding in their stabilization and function in neuronal transport. In AD, tau becomes abnormally phosphorylated, leading to its detachment from microtubules and aggregation into paired helical filaments that form NFTs. The formation of NFTs disrupts the microtubule network, impairing axonal transport and leading to neuronal dysfunction and death. The spread of tau pathology follows a stereotypical pattern, starting in the entorhinal cortex and hippocampus before progressing to other brain regions [71].

Neuroinflammation is a significant component of AD's pathology. It involves activating microglia and astrocytes, the brain's resident immune cells, in response to Aβ plaques and NFTs. Activated microglia and astrocytes release pro-inflammatory cytokines and chemokines, contributing to a chronic inflammatory environment. This inflammation exacerbates neuronal injury and promotes further Aβ and tau pathology. Additionally, chronic neuroinflammation can disrupt the BBB, leading to further neuronal damage [72].

Synaptic loss and neuronal death are key features of AD, leading to the clinical symptoms of cognitive decline and memory impairment. The combined effects of Aβ toxicity, tau pathology, and neuroinflammation result in synaptic dysfunction and loss. Synapses are the primary sites of neural communication, and their loss directly correlates with cognitive deficits. Neuronal death occurs through various mechanisms, including apoptosis and necrosis, leading to brain atrophy [73].

Genetic factors play a significant role in AD, especially in early-onset cases. Mutations in genes such as APP, PSEN1, and PSEN2 are associated with familial forms of AD, leading to increased production of Aβ [74,75].

Cerebrovascular disease and impaired cerebral blood flow are increasingly recognized as contributing factors in AD. Vascular dysfunction can exacerbate Aβ deposition and tau pathology by impairing clearance mechanisms and promoting hypoxia and oxidative stress. This can further enhance neuroinflammation and neuronal damage [76].

Increased oxidative stress, resulting from an imbalance between the production of ROS and antioxidant defenses, is observed in AD. This leads to lipid peroxidation, protein oxidation, and DNA damage, contributing to neuronal injury. Impaired mitochondrial function is a hallmark of AD, leading to reduced energy production, increased ROS, and activation of apoptotic pathways [77,78].

5.1. Cell Viability

SEM has shown protective effects against the detrimental effects of Aβ25-35 on SH-SY5Y cells [35] and has also been found to activate the SIRT1/GLUT4 pathway [33,36,64–68,79,80].

5.2. Apoptosis Inhibition

SEM prevents Aβ25-35-induced apoptosis [39], as evidenced by elevated levels of the prosurvival BCl2 protein and reduced levels of the proapoptotic Bax protein. BCl2 is recognized for its anti-apoptotic function, whereas Bax promotes apoptosis [35]. This alteration in their equilibrium implies a protective effect against programmed cell death [33,35,36].

5.3. Enhanced Autophagy

Initially, Aβ25-35 inhibits autophagy, but this inhibition is reversed in the presence of SEM [24,32,35,39]. Autophagy is a cellular process involving the degradation and recycling of cellular components. The reversal is confirmed by alterations in the expression of key autophagy-related proteins: LC3II (a marker of autophagosome formation) increases; ATG7 (an essential autophagy-related protein) exhibits enhanced expression; P62 (a protein degraded during autophagy) decreases; Beclin1 (a regulator of autophagy initiation) shows increased expression [35,68,80].

5.4. SIRT1/GLUT4 Pathway

SEM enhances the expression of Sirtuin 1 (SIRT1), a protein involved in various cellular processes such as glucose metabolism, energy regulation, and cellular stress response, as well as the expression of GLUT4 (Glucose transporter 4), a pivotal protein facilitating glucose transport into cells. GLUT4 holds particular significance in glucose metabolism [33,36]. The interplay between SIRT1 and GLUT4, known as the SIRT1/GLUT4 pathway, appears to be crucial [33,36,68]. This pathway likely contributes to the regulation of glucose metabolism, potentially augmenting glucose uptake by cells, particularly in regions like the hippocampal CA3 region [33,36,68].

5.5. Improved Aβ and Tau Pathology

SEM appears to mitigate Aβ pathology in the hippocampal CA3 region, implying a potential therapeutic effect on the aggregation or build-up of Aβ, a hallmark of AD [33,36,81,82]. Tau pathology involves the accumulation of abnormal tau protein, resulting in neurofibrillary tangles within nerve cells [33,36]. Tau pathology is another prominent characteristic of AD. SEM also exhibits the ability to alleviate tau pathology in the same hippocampal CA3 region, suggesting a potential influence on the abnormal aggregation or alteration of tau proteins, thereby contributing to the amelioration of AD-related pathological changes [33,36,82–86].

5.6. Reduction of Neuroinflammation

Another potential mechanism proposed for SEM in the context of dementia, which may also be extrapolated to AD, involves neuroprotection through the reduction of neuroinflammation [84,85,87], particularly concerning microglial involvement in neurodegenerative diseases. SEM has been demonstrated to decrease markers of systemic inflammation in patients, and both liraglutide and SEM have exhibited anti-inflammatory effects by mitigating the development of atherosclerotic plaques in mouse models deficient in APOE and LDLr [84,85,87].

6. SEM Potential Mechanism of Action in PD

The pathological disturbances in PD are complex and involve a combination of genetic, molecular, and cellular mechanisms. The primary pathological hallmarks include the loss of dopaminergic neurons in the substantia nigra, the presence of Lewy bodies, neuroinflammation, oxidative stress, and mitochondrial dysfunction. The most prominent pathological feature of PD is the selective loss of dopaminergic neurons in the substantia nigra pars compacta. The degeneration of these neurons leads to a significant reduction in dopamine levels in the striatum, a critical brain region involved in regulating movement. The loss of dopamine disrupts the balance between the excitatory and inhibitory pathways in the basal ganglia, leading to the characteristic motor symptoms of PD [16].

Lewy bodies are intracytoplasmic inclusions composed primarily of α-synuclein, a presynaptic neuronal protein. The presence of Lewy bodies is a key histopathological hallmark of PD. α-Synuclein undergoes misfolding and aggregation, forming insoluble fibrils that are deposited as Lewy bodies within neurons. The aggregation of α-synuclein is believed to impair various cellular functions, including synaptic vesicle trafficking, mitochondrial function, and protein degradation pathways, contributing to neuronal death [88,89].

Neuroinflammation is a significant feature of PD, involving the activation of microglia and astrocytes, the brain's resident immune cells. Activated microglia and astrocytes release pro-inflammatory cytokines and chemokines, creating a chronic inflammatory environment. This inflammation contributes to neuronal injury and exacerbates the progression of the disease. Neuroinflammation may be triggered by the presence of α-synuclein aggregates and other cellular debris resulting from neuronal degeneration.

Oxidative stress plays a crucial role in the pathogenesis of PD. It results from an imbalance between the production of ROS and the brain's ability to detoxify these reactive intermediates. Dopaminergic neurons are especially vulnerable to oxidative stress due to dopamine metabolism, which generates ROS. Oxidative stress can damage cellular components, including lipids, proteins, and DNA, leading to neuronal dysfunction and death. The accumulation of oxidized dopamine and α-synuclein also contributes to the formation of Lewy bodies [90,91].

Mitochondrial dysfunction is a well-established feature of PD, affecting neurons' energy metabolism and viability. Mitochondria are responsible for ATP production through oxidative phosphorylation. In PD, there is evidence of impaired mitochondrial function, including deficiencies in complex I activity of the electron transport chain. This leads to reduced ATP production, increased ROS generation, and the activation of apoptotic pathways, contributing to neuronal death [92,93].

Genetic factors contribute significantly to the pathogenesis of PD, especially in familial cases. Mutations in these genes are associated with autosomal recessive forms of PD. They are involved in mitochondrial quality control, and their dysfunction leads to impaired mitochondrial function and increased susceptibility to oxidative stress [94]. Another pathological feature in PD is impairment of the ubiquitin-proteasome system and autophagy-lysosome pathway. These pathways are essential for the clearance of damaged proteins and organelles. Dysfunction in these systems leads to the accumulation of misfolded proteins and cellular debris, contributing to neuronal death [95,96].

6.1. Inhibition of Cell Death and Neurodegeneration

Following the 6-OHDA treatment, there was a notable decrease in cell viability. Nonetheless, the administration of either SEM or liraglutide reversed this decline in cell viability. Notably, no discernible differences were observed between the effects of SEM and liraglutide treatments [23].

Treatment with SEM improved neurodegeneration, especially in the ventral posterior medial and lateral nuclei of the thalamus (VPM/VPL) in Pla2g6−/− mice [97].

Untreated PD mice exhibited significant downregulation of BClxL and BCl2. However, SEM treatment increased levels of both BClxL and BCl2, restoring them to levels found in wild-type controls [97]. Zhang et al. (2018) demonstrated that MPTP induces apoptosis by inhibiting mitochondrial enzyme complex I, and SEM partly reverses this process by modulating BCl2 and Bax levels (Table 1) [32]. Additionally, SEM interferes with mechanisms leading to the accumulation and aggregation of α-synuclein (α-syn), reducing α-syn expression and potentially preventing the spread of toxic forms of α-syn between neurons, thus promoting neuronal survival [24,31,35,97–103].

Table 1. Characteristics of animal studies that analyze the impact of SEM in PD.

Article	Animals/Cells	Study Design (Randomization, Blind)	Pathology Model	Biochemical Tests	Behavior Tests	SEM (dose, Administration, Period of Time)	Other Drugs
Poupon-Bejuit 2022 [97]	Mice	Randomized, double-blind	Pla2g6−/− transgenic mice	- Hematoxylin/eosin staining - PAS staining. - Immunohistochemistry: CD68, NeuN, GFAP, Iba-1. - Western blot: RIP1, RIP3, β-actin. - PCR: GLP-1R gene, ATF-3, BCl2, BClxL Bax. - Stereology: pan-neuronal marker NeuN. - Blood analysis: total white blood cell count, neutrophils, lymphocytes, monocytes, eosinophils and basophils count, hematocrit, platelets, red blood cells, hemoglobin, and mean corpuscular volume.	Open field Rotarod Vertical pole	0.5, 0.25, 0.15 µg/g, i.p. injected once a week until the end of the experiment	No
Zhang 2018 [32]	Mice	Randomized	MPTP 20 mg/kg i.p. once daily for 7 days	- Immunohistochemistry: TH, GFAP, Iba-1, 4-HNE, BCl2, Bax. - Western blot: BCl2, Bax, β-actin, ATC7, LC2, Beclin1, SQSTM1, P62.	Open field Rotarod Footprint	25 nmol/kg, i.p., once daily for 7 days	Liraglutide 25 nmol/kg i.p. once daily for 7 days
Zhang 2019 [103]	Mice	In vivo, randomized	MPTP 20 mg/kg i.p. once daily for 30 days	- Immunohistochemistry: TH, GFAP, Iba-1, 4-HNE. - Western blot: BCl2, Bax, β-actin, α-Syn, ATC7, LC3, Beclin1, SQSTM1, GDNF.	Open field Rotarod Footprint gait Grip strength	25 nmol/kg, i.p., once daily for 30 days	Liraglutide 25 nmol/kg i.p. once daily for 30 days
Zhang 2022 [20]	Rats	Randomized, blind	6-OHDA	- ELISA: DA, TNF-α, IL-1β. - Western blot: TH, α-syn, IRS-1, IRS-1(phospho-S312), β-actin, GAPDH. - Immunofluorescence: TH.	Apomorphine Rotation	25 nmol/kg, i.p., once daily for 30 days postlesion	DA5-CH 25 nmol/kg, i.p., once daily for 30 days postlesion

Table 1. *Cont.*

Article	Animals/ Cells	Study Design (Randomization, Blind)	Pathology Model	Biochemical Tests	Behavior Tests	SEM (dose, Administration, Period of Time)	Other Drugs
Liu 2022 [23]	SH-SY5Y cells	In vitro	6-OHDA	- MTT method. - Western blot: LC3II, LC3I, Beclin1, P62, β-actin, ATG7. - Flow cytometry: measurement of ROS levels, membrane potential.	Not applicable	0, 1, 10, 100 nmol/L semaglutide	Liraglutide 0, 1, 10, 100 nmol/L

Abbreviations: Pla2g6−/−—Phospholipase A2, group VI knockout (a genetic modification where the Pla2g6 gene is knocked out), PAS—Periodic Acid-Schiff stain (a staining method used to detect glycogen and other carbohydrates), CD68—Cluster of differentiation 68 (a marker for macrophages and monocytes), NeuN—Neuronal Nuclei (a neuron-specific nuclear protein), GFAP—glial fibrillary acidic protein (a marker for astrocytes), Iba-1—Ionized calcium-binding adapter molecule 1 (a marker for microglia), RIP1—Receptor-interacting protein 1, RIP3—rRceptor-interacting protein 3, β-actin—Beta-actin (a cytoskeletal protein often used as a loading control in Western blots), PCR—Polymerase chain reaction, GLP-1R gene—Glucagon-like peptide-1 receptor gene, ATF-3—activating transcription Factor 3, BCl2—B-cell lymphoma 2 (anti-apoptotic protein), BClxL—B-cell lymphoma-extra large (anti-apoptotic protein), Bax—Bcl-2-associated X protein (pro-apoptotic protein), MPTP—1-Methyl-4-phenyl-1,2,3,6-tetrahydropyridine (a neurotoxin), TH—Tyrosine Hydroxylase (an enzyme involved in dopamine synthesis), 4-HNE—4-Hydroxynonenal (a marker of oxidative stress), ATC7—Autophagy-related gene 7 (part of the autophagy process), LC2—Light chain 2 (part of the autophagy process), Beclin1—Bcl-2-interacting myosin-like coiled-coil protein 1, SQSTM1—Sequestosome-1 (also known as P62, a protein involved in autophagy), P62—Sequestosome-1, α-Syn—Alpha-synuclein (a protein associated with neurodegenerative disorders), LC3—Microtubule-associated protein 1A/1B-light chain 3 (part of the autophagy process), GDNF—Glial cell-derived neurotrophic Factor, 6-OHDA—6-Hydroxydopamine (a neurotoxin), DA—Dopamine, TNF-α—Tumor necrosis factor-alpha, IL-1β—Interleukin-1 beta, IRS-1—Insulin receptor substrate 1, IRS-1(phospho-S312)—Phosphorylated form of IRS-1 at serine 312, GAPDH—Glyceraldehyde-3-phosphate dehydrogenase (a common housekeeping gene used as a loading control in experiments), DA5-CH—Dopamine-5,6-chlorohydroxydihydroxyphenylalanine, ATG7—Autophagy-related gene 7, LC3II—Microtubule-associated protein 1A/1B-light chain 3 (processed form), LC3I—Microtubule-associated protein 1A/1B-light chain 3 isoform I, ROS—Reactive oxygen species.

In the MPTP murine model of PD, which disrupts dopamine synthesis in the brain, both SEM and liraglutide restore dopamine synthesis. SEM proves more effective than liraglutide in normalizing TH expression [14,24,30,32], potentially by reducing the number of damaged dopaminergic neurons [30,32]. SEM's efficacy in this context might be attributed to its ability to protect dopaminergic neurons against stress and damage rather than directly enhancing dopamine synthesis. In another murine PD model involving 6-hydroxydopamine (6-OHDA), SEM shields against 6-OHDA-induced damage to dopaminergic neurons in the substantia nigra [20,30]. Another potential mechanism involves restoring glial cell line-derived neurotrophic factor levels (GDNF), crucial for the survival of midbrain dopamine neurons implicated in PD [20,24,30,32,99–101]. Interestingly, SEM does not significantly impact the recovery of dopamine synthesis in the substantia nigra; however, the administration of DA5-CH exhibits higher dopamine levels [30,32,99–101]. This suggests that while SEM plays a critical role in maintaining the viability and function of dopaminergic neurons, its effects on dopamine synthesis might be indirect, focusing more on neuronal survival and health rather than directly increasing dopamine production (Figure 3).

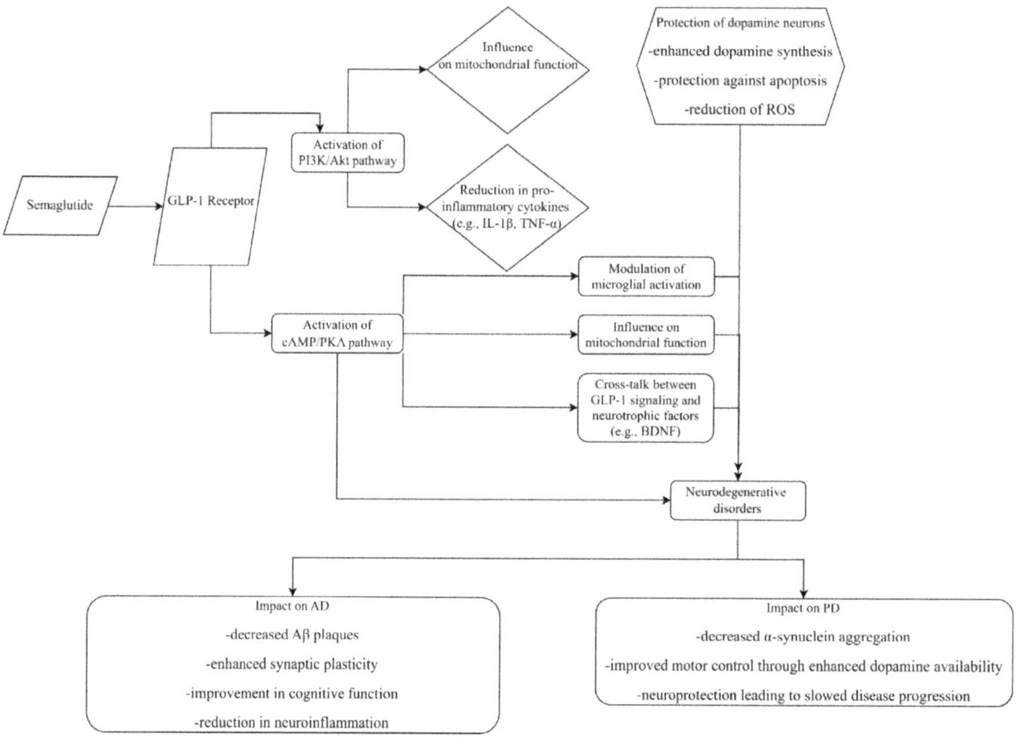

Figure 3. Mechanism of action of SEM and its impact on dopamine in AD and PD.

SEM activates GLP-1 receptors, triggering cAMP/PKA and PI3K/Akt pathways, reducing oxidative stress and pro-inflammatory cytokines. This protects dopaminergic neurons therefore enhancing dopamine synthesis and preventing apoptosis. In PD, it improves motor control and slows neurodegeneration. In AD, it reduces beta-amyloid plaques and enhances cognitive function.

6.2. GSK3β Levels

Treatment with SEM improved GSK3β levels in a murine model of PD, restoring them to levels comparable to those seen in wild-type animals. Additionally, phosphorylated GSK3β Y216 protein levels, which were elevated in untreated PD mice, returned to wild-type levels after SEM treatment (Table 1) [97].

6.3. CREB Gene Expression

Treatment with SEM elevated CREB mRNA levels in Pla2g6−/− mice, reinstating expression levels to those seen in wild-type controls [97].

6.4. Inflammation Response

Treatment with SEM markedly decreased CD68 immunoreactivity in all affected brain areas compared to controls [97].

Untreated mice displayed significantly heightened microglial activation compared to wild-type controls in various brain regions. SEM treatment notably decreased microglial activation, except in the cerebellum [97]. The study conducted by Zhang's team [20,30,32] also revealed a decrease in microgliosis in the substantia nigra, thereby improving the chronic inflammation response in the brain. PD animals exhibited significant astrogliosis in various brain regions; SEM treatment alleviated astrogliosis, particularly in the hippocampus, with no statistically significant difference observed in the thalamus and cerebellum [97], but also in the substantia nigra [20,30,32]. SEM demonstrates greater efficacy in reducing astrogliosis and microgliosis compared to liraglutide [30,32,103].

6.5. Oxidative Stress

Both SEM and liraglutide reduce oxidative stress, as measured by 4-hydroxynonenal biomarker levels. SEM displays greater effectiveness in diminishing oxidative stress by inhibiting the formation of ROS [20,30,32,102]. Both SEM and liraglutide protect against the detrimental effects of 6-OHDA by suppressing the elevation of ROS levels within cells. While exposure to 6-OHDA resulted in a notable increase in ROS levels, neither SEM nor liraglutide alone affected ROS levels compared to the control group. However, when combined with 6-OHDA, both SEM and liraglutide effectively lowered ROS levels, with SEM exhibiting superior efficacy in reducing ROS levels compared to liraglutide (Table 1) [23].

6.6. Autophagy Regulation

The activation of Beclin-1 [20,23,32] initiates autophagosome formation, initiating the process of autophagy. The protein ATG7 is essential for lysosome formation and contributes to the delayed neurodegeneration of dopamine (DA) neurons. P62, a critical cargo adaptor for selective autophagy, plays a central role in clearing misfolded proteins. SEM enhances the expression of Beclin-1, ATG7, and LC3 (leading to increased conversion of LC3B-I to LC3B-II) [20,30,32], as well as P62. This suggests that the drug mitigates autophagy of dopaminergic neurons, potentially promoting neuroprotection [32].

6.7. Effects on Mitochondrial Membrane Potential ($\Delta\Psi m$)

Both SEM and liraglutide counteract the damage inflicted by 6-OHDA on $\Delta\Psi$m and mitochondrial dysfunction. Administration of either SEM or liraglutide alone does not impact $\Delta\Psi$m levels [23]. However, when SEM or liraglutide is co-administered with 6-OHDA, there is a significant improvement in $\Delta\Psi$m levels, indicating the prevention of 6-OHDA-induced mitochondrial toxicity. Notably, SEM demonstrates greater efficacy than liraglutide in enhancing $\Delta\Psi$m levels [23].

7. SEM Effects on Motor Recovery

7.1. AD

7.1.1. Open Field Test

There were no statistically significant differences observed in the total motor distance and the percentage of time spent in the central area among the four groups. The drug interventions did not influence the motor ability and spatial exploration ability of the mice [33,36].

7.1.2. Novel Object Recognition Test

During the familiarization phase, no statistically significant differences were observed in the percentage of time spent exploring the first and second objects among the groups. However, in the testing phase, there was a significant difference in the novel object index (NOI) among the groups. The transgenic PD mice demonstrated a decreased NOI compared to WT mice ($p < 0.01$), and treatment with SEM increased NOI in PD mice ($p < 0.05$). Notably, this effect was reversed by the SIRT1 inhibitor EX527 [33,36].

7.1.3. Y-Maze Task

No significant variance was observed in the total number of arm entries across the various groups. However, a notable distinction was evident in the percentage of correct spontaneous alternations among the groups. Notably, transgenic PD mice displayed a decrease compared to WT mice ($p < 0.05$), and treatment with SEM partially mitigated this decline ($p < 0.05$). It is noteworthy the protective effect was reversed by EX527 [33,36].

7.2. PD

7.2.1. Rotarod Test

Pla2g6−/− mice untreated demonstrated significant progressive deficits from 10 to 14 weeks compared to age-matched wild-type controls [97]. However, Pla2g6−/− mice treated with 0.5 µg/g SEM did not display significant deficits in rotarod performance at any measured time point compared to wild-type controls [97]. MPTP impeded the mice's ability to remain on the rotating rod for 3 min [32,103]. Post-hoc analysis revealed no difference between the control and SEM or liraglutide groups but a notable distinction between the control and MPTP groups. Both liraglutide and SEM ameliorated bradykinesia and imbalance induced by MPTP, with SEM showing greater efficacy [32,103].

7.2.2. Vertical Pole Test

Commonly employed to evaluate locomotor function and hind limb strength, the vertical pole test revealed that untreated Pla2g6−/− mice exhibited notable progressive deficits beginning at 9 weeks. Administration of 0.5 µg/g SEM led to a marked enhancement in vertical pole test performance from weeks 9 to 13, although statistical significance was not sustained at 14 weeks [97].

7.2.3. Open Field Test

Untreated Pla2g6−/− mice exhibited mobility parameter abnormalities at 12 weeks compared to the wild-type controls. Pla2g6−/− mice treated with high-dose SEM (0.5 µg/g—more than three times higher than the equivalent dose given to adult diabetics via subcutaneous administration) showed similar results to age-matched wild-type controls for most parameters, with notable differences observed in freezing time at 12 weeks [97]. Conversely, MPTP injection decreased spontaneous locomotion and overall travel time in mice [30,32]. Post-hoc analyses revealed no distinction between the control and liraglutide or SEM groups but a significant contrast between the control and MPTP groups [32]. SEM demonstrated greater efficacy than liraglutide in restoring MPTP-induced impairments in locomotor and exploratory activity [32]. In another study by Zhang et al. [103], there was an overall disparity in distance traveled, with no discrepancy between the control group and groups treated with liraglutide or SEM. However, significant variances were noted between the control and MPTP groups, MPTP + liraglutide and MPTP + SEM [103]. Both liraglutide and SEM normalized MPTP-induced impairments in locomotor and exploratory activity [103]. No significant distinction was observed between the MPTP + SEM and MPTP + liraglutide groups [103], despite SEM demonstrating superior benefits over liraglutide in the previous study [32].

7.2.4. Footprint Test (Motor Coordination)

MPTP induced postural and gait abnormalities in mice, resulting in a significant overall difference between groups. Post-hoc analyses showed no distinction between the control and liraglutide or SEM groups but a notable difference between the control and MPTP groups. Both liraglutide and SEM ameliorated the abnormal posture and gait induced by MPTP, with SEM demonstrating greater effectiveness [32,103].

7.2.5. Grip Strength Test

SEM and liraglutide both enhanced muscle strength impaired by MPTP, with SEM showing greater efficacy compared to liraglutide [103].

7.2.6. Apomorphine-Induced Rotation

Variations in rotational behavior among the experimental conditions were evident, with significant differences observed across all groups [30]. The sham + saline group did not display contralateral rotations upon apomorphine challenge [30]. Both the 6-OHDA + saline group and the 6-OHDA + SEM group exhibited a notable increase in contralateral rotations following apomorphine injection compared to the sham + saline group ($p < 0.0001$) [30]. The 6-OHDA + SEM group showed a significant difference from the 6-OHDA + saline group ($p < 0.001$). Moreover, the 6-OHDA + DA5-CH group displayed significant differences from both the 6-OHDA + saline group ($p < 0.001$) and the 6-OHDA + SEM group ($p < 0.0004$) [30]. The study suggests that DA5-CH exhibits greater potency than SEM in safeguarding the brain against 6-OHDA toxicity [30].

8. Conclusions

In summary, the studies indicate a diverse potential for SEM in alleviating neurodegenerative mechanisms, offering valuable perspectives for its therapeutic use in associated conditions. The literature collectively presents compelling evidence regarding the neuroprotective capabilities of SEM in AD and PD. The drug mitigates AD pathology and associated symptoms, such as memory impairment, by fostering glycolysis through the GLP-1/SIRT1/GLUT4 pathway.

SEM proves effective in normalizing impaired motor function, preserving dopamine levels, reducing inflammation, oxidative stress, and apoptosis, and enhancing autophagy to safeguard against dopaminergic neuron loss in models of motor impairment.

Despite the promising preclinical results, further research is essential to fully elucidate the underlying mechanisms of SEM's neuroprotective effects. Understanding these mechanisms is imperative for optimizing SEM's therapeutic potential.

The ongoing clinical trials of SEM in AD and PD aim to provide crucial insights into SEM's therapeutic potential, mechanisms of action, and optimal dosing strategies. Successful outcomes from these trials could lead to new, effective treatment options for millions of individuals affected by AD and PD, ultimately improving their quality of life and offering hope for better disease management.

Author Contributions: Conceptualization and methodology, A.D.M., I.K.S.B. and M.B.; writing—original draft preparation, A.D.M. and I.K.S.B.; writing—review and editing, L.M.-T. and M.B.; supervision, L.M.-T. and M.B. All authors have read and agreed to the published version of the manuscript.

Funding: This research received no external funding.

Conflicts of Interest: The authors declare no conflicts of interest.

References

1. Su, M.; Nizamutdinov, D.; Liu, H.; Huang, J.H. Recent Mechanisms of Neurodegeneration and Photobiomodulation in the Context of Alzheimer's Disease. *Int. J. Mol. Sci.* **2023**, *24*, 9272. [CrossRef]
2. Bano, D.; Ehninger, D.; Bagetta, G. Decoding metabolic signatures in Alzheimer's disease: A mitochondrial perspective. *Cell Death Discov.* **2023**, *9*, 432. [CrossRef]
3. Tahami Monfared, A.A.; Byrnes, M.J.; White, L.A.; Zhang, Q. Alzheimer's Disease: Epidemiology and Clinical Progression. *Neurol. Ther.* **2022**, *11*, 553–569. [CrossRef]
4. Ferrer, I. Hypothesis review: Alzheimer's overture guidelines. *Brain Pathol.* **2023**, *33*, e13122. [CrossRef] [PubMed]
5. Theron, D.; Hopkins, L.N.; Sutherland, H.G.; Griffiths, L.R.; Fernandez, F. Can Genetic Markers Predict the Sporadic Form of Alzheimer's Disease? An Updated Review on Genetic Peripheral Markers. *Int. J. Mol. Sci.* **2023**, *24*, 13480. [CrossRef] [PubMed]
6. Wei, P. Ultra-Early Screening of Cognitive Decline Due to Alzheimer's Pathology. *Biomedicines* **2023**, *11*, 1423. [CrossRef]
7. Prajjwal, P.; Flores Sanga, H.S.; Acharya, K.; Tango, T.; John, J.; Rodriguez, R.S.C.; Dheyaa Marsool Marsool, M.; Sulaimanov, M.; Ahmed, A.; Hussin, O.A. Parkinson's disease updates: Addressing the pathophysiology, risk factors, genetics, diagnosis, along with the medical and surgical treatment. *Ann. Med. Surg.* **2023**, *85*, 4887–4902. [CrossRef]
8. Adam, H.; Gopinath, S.C.B.; Md Arshad, M.K.; Adam, T.; Parmin, N.A.; Husein, I.; Hashim, U. An update on pathogenesis and clinical scenario for Parkinson's disease: Diagnosis and treatment. *3 Biotech* **2023**, *13*, 142. [CrossRef]
9. Smits, M.M.; Van Raalte, D.H. Safety of Semaglutide. *Front. Endocrinol.* **2021**, *12*, 645563, Erratum in: *Front. Endocrinol.* **2021**, *12*, 786732. [CrossRef]
10. Meier, J.J. Efficacy of Semaglutide in a Subcutaneous and an Oral Formulation. *Front. Endocrinol.* **2021**, *12*, 645617. [CrossRef]
11. Nauck, M.A.; Quast, D.R.; Wefers, J.; Meier, J.J. GLP-1 receptor agonists in the treatment of type 2 diabetes—State-of-the-art. *Mol. Metab.* **2021**, *46*, 101102. [CrossRef] [PubMed]
12. Vilsbøll, T.; Bain, S.C.; Leiter, L.A.; Lingvay, I.; Matthews, D.; Simó, R.; Helmark, I.C.; Wijayasinghe, N.; Larsen, M. Semaglutide, Reduction in Glycated Haemoglobin and the Risk of Diabetic Retinopathy. *Diabetes Obes. Metab.* **2018**, *20*, 889–897. [CrossRef] [PubMed]
13. Gaborit, B.; Julla, J.B.; Besbes, S.; Proust, M.; Vincentelli, C.; Alos, B.; Ancel, P.; Alzaid, F.; Garcia, R.; Mailly, P.; et al. Glucagon-Like Peptide 1 Receptor Agonists, Diabetic Retinopathy and Angiogenesis: The AngioSafe Type 2 Diabetes Study. *J. Clin. Endocrinol. Metab.* **2020**, *105*, e1549-60. [CrossRef] [PubMed]
14. Chen, F.; Chen, S.; Si, A.; Luo, Y.; Hu, W.; Zhang, Y.; Ma, J. The long-term trend of Parkinson's disease incidence and mortality in China and a Bayesian projection from 2020 to 2030. *Front. Aging Neurosci.* **2022**, *14*, 973310. [CrossRef] [PubMed]
15. Ramesh, S.; Arachchige, A.S.P.M. Depletion of dopamine in Parkinson's disease and relevant therapeutic options: A review of the literature. *AIMS Neurosci.* **2023**, *10*, 200–231. [CrossRef] [PubMed]
16. Zhou, Z.D.; Yi, L.X.; Wang, D.Q.; Lim, T.M.; Tan, E.K. Role of dopamine in the pathophysiology of Parkinson's disease. *Transl. Neurodegener.* **2023**, *12*, 44. [CrossRef] [PubMed]
17. Cramb, K.M.L.; Beccano-Kelly, D.; Cragg, S.J.; Wade-Martins, R. Impaired dopamine release in Parkinson's disease. *Brain* **2023**, *146*, 3117–3132. [CrossRef] [PubMed]
18. Salameh, T.S.; Rhea, E.M.; Talbot, K.; Banks, W.A. Brain uptake pharmacokinetics of incretin receptor agonists showing promise as Alzheimer's and Parkinson's disease therapeutics. *Biochem Pharmacol.* **2020**, *180*, 114187, Erratum in: *Biochem Pharmacol.* **2023**, *210*, 115474. https://doi.org/10.1016/j.bcp.2023.115474. [CrossRef]
19. Cornell, S. A review of GLP-1 receptor agonists in type 2 diabetes: A focus on the mechanism of action of once-weekly agents. *J. Clin. Pharm. Ther.* **2020**, *45* (Suppl. S1), 17–27. [CrossRef]
20. Zhang, L.; Li, C.; Zhang, Z.; Zhang, Z.; Jin, Q.Q.; Li, L.; Hölscher, C. DA5-CH and Semaglutide Protect against Neurodegeneration and Reduce α-Synuclein Levels in the 6-OHDA Parkinson's Disease Rat Model. *Park. Dis.* **2022**, *2022*, 1428817. [CrossRef]
21. FDA Drug Approvals and Databases. Available online: https://www.fda.gov/drugs/drug-approvals-and-databases/drug-trial-snapshot-ozempic (accessed on 15 February 2024).
22. FDA Medicines. Available online: https://www.ema.europa.eu/en/medicines/human/EPAR/ozempic (accessed on 15 February 2024).
23. Liu, D.X.; Zhao, C.S.; Wei, X.N.; Ma, Y.P.; Wu, J.K. Semaglutide Protects against 6-OHDA Toxicity by Enhancing Autophagy and Inhibiting Oxidative Stress. *Park. Dis.* **2022**, *2022*, 6813017. [CrossRef] [PubMed]
24. Chen, S.D.; Chuang, Y.C.; Lin, T.K.; Yang, J.L. Alternative role of glucagon-like Peptide-1 receptor agonists in neurodegenerative diseases. *Eur. J. Pharmacol.* **2023**, *938*, 175439. [CrossRef] [PubMed]
25. Laurindo, L.F.; Barbalho, S.M.; Guiguer, E.L.; da Silva Soares de Souza, M.; de Souza, G.A.; Fidalgo, T.M.; Araújo, A.C.; de Souza Gonzaga, H.F.; de Bortoli Teixeira, D.; de Oliveira Silva Ullmann, T.; et al. GLP-1a: Going beyond Traditional Use. *Int. J. Mol. Sci.* **2022**, *23*, 739. [CrossRef] [PubMed]

26. Kabahizi, A.; Wallace, B.; Lieu, L.; Chau, D.; Dong, Y.; Hwang, E.S.; Williams, K.W. Glucagon-like peptide-1 (GLP-1) signalling in the brain: From neural circuits and metabolism to therapeutics. *Br. J. Pharmacol.* **2022**, *179*, 600–624. [CrossRef] [PubMed]
27. McLean, B.A.; Wong, C.K.; Campbell, J.E.; Hodson, D.J.; Trapp, S.; Drucker, D.J. Revisiting the Complexity of GLP-1 Action from Sites of Synthesis to Receptor Activation. *Endocr. Rev.* **2021**, *42*, 101–132. [CrossRef] [PubMed]
28. Mayendraraj, A.; Rosenkilde, M.M.; Gasbjerg, L.S. GLP-1 and GIP receptor signaling in beta cells—A review of receptor interactions and co-stimulation. *Peptides* **2022**, *151*, 170749. [CrossRef] [PubMed]
29. Kopp, K.O.; Glotfelty, E.J.; Li, Y.; Greig, N.H. Glucagon-like peptide-1 (GLP-1) receptor agonists and neuroinflammation: Implications for neurodegenerative disease treatment. *Pharmacol. Res.* **2022**, *186*, 106550. [CrossRef] [PubMed]
30. Zhang, L.; Zhang, W.; Tian, X. The pleiotropic of GLP-1/GLP-1R axis in central nervous system diseases. *Int. J. Neurosci.* **2023**, *133*, 473–491. [CrossRef] [PubMed]
31. Mahapatra, M.K.; Karuppasamy, M.; Sahoo, B.M. Therapeutic Potential of Semaglutide, a Newer GLP-1 Receptor Agonist, in Abating Obesity, Non-Alcoholic Steatohepatitis and Neurodegenerative diseases: A Narrative Review. *Pharm. Res.* **2022**, *39*, 1233–1248. [CrossRef]
32. Zhang, L.; Zhang, L.; Li, L.; Hölscher, C. Neuroprotective effects of the novel GLP-1 long acting analogue semaglutide in the MPTP Parkinson's disease mouse model. *Neuropeptides* **2018**, *71*, 70–80. [CrossRef]
33. Wang, Y.; Hu, H.; Liu, X.; Guo, X. Hypoglycemic medicines in the treatment of Alzheimer's disease: Pathophysiological links between AD and glucose metabolism. *Front. Pharmacol.* **2023**, *14*, 1138499. [CrossRef]
34. Mulvaney, C.A.; Duarte, G.S.; Handley, J.; Evans, D.J.; Menon, S.; Wyse, R.; Emsley, H.C. GLP-1 receptor agonists for Parkinson's disease. *Cochrane Database Syst. Rev.* **2020**, *7*, CD012990. [CrossRef]
35. Chang, Y.F.; Zhang, D.; Hu, W.M.; Liu, D.X.; Li, L. Semaglutide-mediated protection against Aβ correlated with enhancement of autophagy and inhibition of apotosis. *J. Clin. Neurosci.* **2020**, *81*, 234–239. [CrossRef] [PubMed]
36. Wang, Z.J.; Li, X.R.; Chai, S.F.; Li, W.R.; Li, S.; Hou, M.; Li, J.L.; Ye, Y.C.; Cai, H.Y.; Hölscher, C.; et al. Semaglutide ameliorates cognition and glucose metabolism dysfunction in the 3xTg mouse model of Alzheimer's disease via the GLP-1R/SIRT1/GLUT4 pathway. *Neuropharmacology* **2023**, *240*, 109716. [CrossRef]
37. Dai, C.; Tan, C.; Zhao, L.; Liang, Y.; Liu, G.; Liu, H.; Zhong, Y.; Liu, Z.; Mo, L.; Liu, X.; et al. Glucose metabolism impairment in Parkinson's disease. *Brain Res. Bull.* **2023**, *199*, 110672. [CrossRef] [PubMed]
38. Yu, C.J.; Ma, D.; Song, L.L.; Zhai, Z.N.; Tao, Y.; Zhang, Y.; Cai, L.Y.; Hou, Y.H.; Chen, H.Y.; Wang, L.; et al. The role of GLP-1/GIP receptor agonists in Alzheimer's disease. *Adv. Clin. Exp. Med.* **2020**, *29*, 661–668. [CrossRef] [PubMed]
39. Gouveri, E.; Popovic, D.S.; Papanas, N. Potential New Therapeutic Implications of Semaglutide: New Colours of the Rainbow? *Diabetes Ther.* **2024**, *15*, 13–18. [CrossRef] [PubMed]
40. Nowell, J.; Blunt, E.; Edison, P. Incretin and insulin signaling as novel therapeutic targets for Alzheimer's and Parkinson's disease. *Mol. Psychiatry* **2023**, *28*, 217–229. [CrossRef]
41. Reich, N.; Hölscher, C. The neuroprotective effects of glucagon-like peptide 1 in Alzheimer's and Parkinson's disease: An in-depth review. *Front Neurosci.* **2022**, *16*, 970925. [CrossRef]
42. Sadek, M.A.; Kandil, E.A.; El Sayed, N.S.; Sayed, H.M.; Rabie, M.A. Semaglutide, a novel glucagon-like peptide-1 agonist, amends experimental autoimmune encephalomyelitis-induced multiple sclerosis in mice: Involvement of the PI3K/Akt/GSK-3β pathway. *Int. Immunopharmacol.* **2023**, *115*, 109647. [CrossRef]
43. Plascencia-Villa, G.; Perry, G. Exploring Molecular Targets for Mitochondrial Therapies in Neurodegenerative Diseases. *Int. J. Mol. Sci.* **2023**, *24*, 12486. [CrossRef] [PubMed]
44. Tipa, R.O.; Balan, D.G.; Georgescu, M.T.; Ignat, L.A.; Vacaroiu, I.A.; Georgescu, D.E.; Raducu, L.; Mihai, D.A.; Chiperi, L.V.; Balcangiu-Stroescu, A.E. A Systematic Review of Semaglutide's Influence on Cognitive Function in Preclinical Animal Models and Cell-Line Studies. *Int. J. Mol. Sci.* **2024**, *25*, 4972. [CrossRef]
45. Chen, X.; Chen, S.; Li, Z.; Zhu, R.; Jia, Z.; Ban, J.; Zhen, R.; Chen, X.; Pan, X.; Ren, Q.; et al. Effect of semaglutide and empagliflozin on cognitive function and hippocampal phosphoproteomic in obese mice. *Front. Pharmacol.* **2023**, *14*, 975830. [CrossRef] [PubMed]
46. Rebosio, C.; Balbi, M.; Passalacqua, M.; Ricciarelli, R.; Fedele, E. Presynaptic GLP-1 receptors enhance the depolarization-evoked release of glutamate and GABA in the mouse cortex and hippocampus. *Biofactors* **2018**, *44*, 148–157. [CrossRef]
47. Park, J.S.; Kam, T.I.; Lee, S.; Park, H.; Oh, Y.; Kwon, S.H.; Song, J.J.; Kim, D.; Kim, H.; Jhaldiyal, A.; et al. Blocking microglial activation of reactive astrocytes is neuroprotective in models of Alzheimer's disease. *Acta Neuropathol. Commun.* **2021**, *9*, 78. [CrossRef] [PubMed]
48. Singh, B.; Day, C.M.; Abdella, S.; Garg, S. Alzheimer's disease current therapies, novel drug delivery systems and future directions for better disease management. *J. Control. Release* **2024**, *367*, 402–424. [CrossRef] [PubMed]
49. Lisco, G.; De Tullio, A.; Iovino, M.; Disoteo, O.; Guastamacchia, E.; Giagulli, V.A.; Triggiani, V. Dopamine in the Regulation of Glucose Homeostasis, Pathogenesis of Type 2 Diabetes, and Chronic Conditions of Impaired Dopamine Activity/Metabolism: Implication for Pathophysiological and Therapeutic Purposes. *Biomedicines* **2023**, *11*, 2993. [CrossRef]
50. Gentilella, R.; Pechtner, V.; Corcos, A.; Consoli, A. Glucagon-like peptide-1 receptor agonists in type 2 diabetes treatment: Are they all the same? *Diabetes Metab. Res. Rev.* **2019**, *35*, e3070. [CrossRef] [PubMed]
51. Kim, D.S.; Choi, H.I.; Wang, Y.; Luo, Y.; Hoffer, B.J.; Greig, N.H. A New Treatment Strategy for Parkinson's Disease through the Gut-Brain Axis: The Glucagon-Like Peptide-1 Receptor Pathway. *Cell Transplant.* **2017**, *26*, 1560–1571. [CrossRef]

52. Beurel, E.; Grieco, S.F.; Jope, R.S. Glycogen synthase kinase-3 (GSK3): Regulation, actions, and diseases. *Pharmacol. Ther.* **2015**, *148*, 114–131. [CrossRef]
53. Duda, P.; Wiśniewski, J.; Wójtowicz, T.; Wójcicka, O.; Jaśkiewicz, M.; Drulis-Fajdasz, D.; Rakus, D.; McCubrey, J.A.; Gizak, A. Targeting GSK3 signaling as a potential therapy of neurodegenerative diseases and aging. *Expert. Opin. Ther. Targets.* **2018**, *10*, 833–848. [CrossRef] [PubMed]
54. Kalinderi, K.; Papaliagkas, V.; Fidani, L. GLP-1 Receptor Agonists: A New Treatment in Parkinson's Disease. *Int. J. Mol. Sci.* **2024**, *25*, 3812. [CrossRef] [PubMed]
55. Diz-Chaves, Y.; Maastor, Z.; Spuch, C.; Lamas, J.A.; González-Matías, L.C.; Mallo, F. Glucagon-like peptide 1 receptor activation: Anti-inflammatory effects in the brain. *Neural Regen. Res.* **2024**, *19*, 1671–1677. [CrossRef] [PubMed]
56. Chao, A.M.; Tronieri, J.S.; Amaro, A.; Wadden, T.A. Semaglutide for the treatment of obesity. *Trends Cardiovasc. Med.* **2023**, *33*, 159–166. [CrossRef] [PubMed]
57. Bergmann, N.C.; Davies, M.J.; Lingvay, I.; Knop, F.K. Semaglutide for the treatment of overweight and obesity: A review. *Diabetes Obes. Metab.* **2023**, *25*, 18–35. [CrossRef] [PubMed]
58. Lee, T.S.; Park, E.J.; Choi, M.; Oh, H.S.; An, Y.; Kim, T.; Kim, T.H.; Shin, B.S.; Shin, S. Novel LC-MS/MS analysis of the GLP-1 analog semaglutide with its application to pharmacokinetics and brain distribution studies in rats. *J. Chromatogr. B Analyt Technol. Biomed. Life Sci.* **2023**, *1221*, 123688. [CrossRef] [PubMed]
59. Hall, S.; Isaacs, D.; Clements, J.N. Pharmacokinetics and Clinical Implications of Semaglutide: A New Glucagon-Like Peptide (GLP)-1 Receptor Agonist. *Clin. Pharmacokinet.* **2018**, *57*, 1529–1538. [CrossRef]
60. Secher, A.; Jelsing, J.; Baquero, A.F.; Hecksher-Sørensen, J.; Cowley, M.A.; Dalbøge, L.S.; Hansen, G.; Grove, K.L.; Pyke, C.; Raun, K.; et al. The arcuate nucleus mediates GLP-1 receptor agonist liraglutide-dependent weight loss. *J. Clin. Investig.* **2014**, *124*, 4473–4488. [CrossRef] [PubMed]
61. Jensen, C.B.; Pyke, C.; Rasch, M.G.; Dahl, A.B.; Knudsen, L.B.; Secher, A. Characterization of the Glucagonlike Peptide-1 Receptor in Male Mouse Brain Using a Novel Antibody and In Situ Hybridization. *Endocrinology* **2018**, *159*, 665–675. [CrossRef] [PubMed]
62. Kapitza, C.; Nosek, L.; Jensen, L.; Hartvig, H.; Jensen, C.B.; Flint, A. Semaglutide, a once-weekly human GLP-1 analog, does not reduce the bioavailability of the combined oral contraceptive, ethinylestradiol/levonorgestrel. *J. Clin. Pharmacol.* **2015**, *55*, 497–504. [CrossRef]
63. Smith, B.; Ownby, R.L. Disease-Modifying Treatments and Their Future in Alzheimer's Disease Management. *Cureus.* **2024**, *16*, e56105. [CrossRef] [PubMed]
64. Marbury, T.C.; Flint, A.; Jacobsen, J.B.; Derving Karsbøl, J.; Lasseter, K. Pharmacokinetics and Tolerability of a Single Dose of Semaglutide, a Human Glucagon-Like Peptide-1 Analog, in Subjects With and Without Renal Impairment. *Clin. Pharmacokinet.* **2017**, *56*, 1381–1390. [CrossRef] [PubMed]
65. Adem, M.A.; Decourt, B.; Sabbagh, M.N. Pharmacological Approaches Using Diabetic Drugs Repurposed for Alzheimer's Disease. *Biomedicines* **2024**, *12*, 99. [CrossRef]
66. Gabery, S.; Salinas, C.G.; Paulsen, S.J.; Ahnfelt-Rønne, J.; Alanentalo, T.; Baquero, A.F.; Buckley, S.T.; Farkas, E.; Fekete, C.; Frederiksen, K.S.; et al. Semaglutide lowers body weight in rodents via distributed neural pathways. *JCI Insight.* **2020**, *5*, e133429. [CrossRef] [PubMed]
67. Złotek, M.; Kurowska, A.; Herbet, M.; Piątkowska-Chmiel, I. GLP-1 Analogs, SGLT-2, and DPP-4 Inhibitors: A Triad of Hope for Alzheimer's Disease Therapy. *Biomedicines* **2023**, *11*, 3035. [CrossRef] [PubMed]
68. Cao, Y.; Yu, F.; Lyu, Y.; Lu, X. Promising candidates from drug clinical trials: Implications for clinical treatment of Alzheimer's disease in China. *Front. Neurol.* **2022**, *13*, 1034243. [CrossRef] [PubMed]
69. Vejandla, B.; Savani, S.; Appalaneni, R.; Veeravalli, R.S.; Gude, S.S. Alzheimer's Disease: The Past, Present, and Future of a Globally Progressive Disease. *Cureus* **2024**, *16*, e51705. [CrossRef] [PubMed]
70. Vogt, A.-C.S.; Jennings, G.T.; Mohsen, M.O.; Vogel, M.; Bachmann, M.F. Alzheimer's Disease: A Brief History of Immunotherapies Targeting Amyloid β. *Int. J. Mol. Sci.* **2023**, *24*, 3895. [CrossRef] [PubMed]
71. Ramachandran, A.K.; Das, S.; Joseph, A.; Shenoy, G.G.; Alex, A.T.; Mudgal, J. Neurodegenerative Pathways in Alzheimer's Disease: A Review. *Curr. Neuropharmacol.* **2021**, *19*, 679–692. [CrossRef]
72. Wetering, J.V.; Geut, H.; Bol, J.J.; Galis, Y.; Timmermans, E.; Twisk, J.W.R.; Hepp, D.H.; Morella, M.L.; Pihlstrom, L.; Lemstra, A.W.; et al. Neuroinflammation is associated with Alzheimer's disease co-pathology in dementia with Lewy bodies. *Acta Neuropathol. Commun.* **2024**, *12*, 73. [CrossRef]
73. Subramanian, J.; Savage, J.C.; Tremblay, M.È. Synaptic Loss in Alzheimer's Disease: Mechanistic Insights Provided by Two-Photon in vivo Imaging of Transgenic Mouse Models. *Front. Cell. Neurosci.* **2020**, *14*, 592607. [CrossRef] [PubMed]
74. Manuello, J.; Min, J.; McCarthy, P.; Alfaro-Almagro, F.; Lee, S.; Smith, S.; Elliott, L.T.; Winkler, A.M.; Douaud, G. The effects of genetic and modifiable risk factors on brain regions vulnerable to ageing and disease. *Nat. Commun.* **2024**, *15*, 2576. [CrossRef] [PubMed]
75. Xiao, X.; Liu, H.; Liu, X.; Zhang, W.; Zhang, S.; Jiao, B. *APP*, *PSEN1*, and *PSEN2* Variants in Alzheimer's Disease: Systematic Re-evaluation According to ACMG Guidelines. *Front. Aging Neurosci.* **2021**, *13*, 695808. [CrossRef] [PubMed]
76. Goldsmith, H.S. Alzheimer's Disease: A Decreased Cerebral Blood Flow to Critical Intraneuronal Elements Is the Cause. *J. Alzheimers Dis.* **2022**, *85*, 1419–1422. [CrossRef] [PubMed]

77. Tamagno, E.; Guglielmotto, M.; Vasciaveo, V.; Tabaton, M. Oxidative Stress and Beta Amyloid in Alzheimer's Disease. Which Comes First: The Chicken or the Egg? *Antioxidants* **2021**, *10*, 1479. [CrossRef] [PubMed]
78. Roy, R.G.; Mandal, P.K.; Maroon, J.C. Oxidative Stress Occurs Prior to Amyloid Aβ Plaque Formation and Tau Phosphorylation in Alzheimer's Disease: Role of Glutathione and Metal Ions. *ACS Chem. Neurosci.* **2023**, *14*, 2944–2954. [CrossRef]
79. Xia, W.; Yu, H.; Wen, P. Meta-analysis on GLP-1 mediated modulation of autophagy in islet β-cells: Prospectus for improved wound healing in type 2 diabetes. *Int. Wound, J.* **2024**, *21*, e14841. [CrossRef]
80. Dave, B.P.; Shah, Y.B.; Maheshwari, K.G.; Mansuri, K.A.; Prajapati, B.S.; Postwala, H.I.; Chorawala, M.R. Pathophysiological Aspects and Therapeutic Armamentarium of Alzheimer's Disease: Recent Trends and Future Development. *Cell. Mol. Neurobiol.* **2023**, *43*, 3847–3884. [CrossRef] [PubMed]
81. Arnold, S.E.; Arvanitakis, Z.; Macauley-Rambach, S.L.; Koenig, A.M.; Wang, H.Y.; Ahima, R.S.; Craft, S.; Gandy, S.; Buettner, C.; Stoeckel, L.E.; et al. Brain insulin resistance in type 2 diabetes and Alzheimer disease: Concepts and conundrums. *Nat. Rev. Neurol.* **2018**, *14*, 168–181. [CrossRef]
82. Baker, L.D.; Cross, D.J.; Minoshima, S.; Belongia, D.; Watson, G.S.; Craft, S. Insulin resistance and Alzheimer-like reductions in regional cerebral glucose metabolism for cognitively normal adults with prediabetes or early type 2 diabetes. *Arch. Neurol.* **2011**, *68*, 51–57. [CrossRef]
83. Currais, A.; Prior, M.; Lo, D.; Jolivalt, C.; Schubert, D.; Maher, P. Diabetes exacerbates amyloid and neurovascular pathology in aging-accelerated mice. *Aging Cell* **2012**, *11*, 1017–1026. [CrossRef] [PubMed]
84. Owen, M.; Bose, N.; Nisenbaum, L.; Partrick, K.A.; Fillit, H.M. The Critical Role of Biomarkers for Drug Development Targeting the Biology of Aging. *J. Prev. Alzheimers Dis.* **2023**, *10*, 729–742. [CrossRef] [PubMed]
85. Nørgaard, C.H.; Friedrich, S.; Hansen, C.T.; Gerds, T.; Ballard, C.; Møller, D.V.; Knudsen, L.B.; Kvist, K.; Zinman, B.; Holm, E.; et al. Treatment with glucagon-like peptide-1 receptor agonists and incidence of dementia: Data from pooled double-blind randomized controlled trials and nationwide disease and prescription registers. *Alzheimers Dement.* **2022**, *8*, e12268. [CrossRef]
86. Muriach, M.; Flores-Bellver, M.; Romero, F.J.; Barcia, J.M. Diabetes and the brain: Oxidative stress, inflammation, and autophagy. *Oxid. Med. Cell Longev.* **2014**, *2014*, 102158. [CrossRef] [PubMed]
87. Butterfield, D.A.; Halliwell, B. Oxidative stress, dysfunctional glucose metabolism and Alzheimer disease. *Nat. Rev. Neurosci.* **2019**, *20*, 148–160. [CrossRef] [PubMed]
88. Simon, C.; Soga, T.; Okano, H.J.; Parhar, I. α-Synuclein-mediated neurodegeneration in Dementia with Lewy bodies: The pathobiology of a paradox. *Cell Biosci.* **2021**, *11*, 196. [CrossRef] [PubMed]
89. Borghammer, P.; Okkels, N.; Weintraub, D. Parkinson's Disease and Dementia with Lewy Bodies: One and the Same. *J. Park. Dis.* **2024**, *14*, 383–397. [CrossRef] [PubMed]
90. Kouli, A.; Spindler, L.R.B.; Fryer, T.D.; Hong, Y.T.; Malpetti, M.; Aigbirhio, F.I.; White, S.R.; Camacho, M.; O'Brien, J.T.; Williams-Gray, C.H. Neuroinflammation is linked to dementia risk in Parkinson's disease. *Brain* **2024**, *147*, 923–935. [CrossRef]
91. Wang, Y.; Shi, X.; Yin, Y.; Yang, F.; Zhang, Y.; He, X.; Wen, D.; Li, B.X.; Ma, K. Association Between Neuroinflammation and Parkinson's Disease: A Comprehensive Mendelian Randomization Study. *Mol. Neurobiol.* **2024**, 1–11. [CrossRef]
92. Payne, T.; Burgess, T.; Bradley, S.; Roscoe, S.; Sassani, M.; Dunning, M.J.; Hernandez, D.; Scholz, S.; McNeill, A.; Taylor, R.; et al. Multimodal assessment of mitochondrial function in Parkinson's disease. *Brain* **2024**, *147*, 267–280. [CrossRef]
93. Blagov, A.; Postnov, A.; Sukhorukov, V.; Popov, M.; Uzokov, J.; Orekhov, A. Significance of Mitochondrial Dysfunction in the Pathogenesis of Parkinson's Disease. *Front. Biosci. (Landmark Ed.)* **2024**, *29*, 36. [CrossRef]
94. Bhore, N.; Bogacki, E.C.; O'Callaghan, B.; Plun-Favreau, H.; Lewis, P.A.; Herbst, S. Common genetic risk for Parkinson's disease and dysfunction of the endo-lysosomal system. *Philos. Trans. R. Soc. Lond. B Biol. Sci.* **2024**, *379*, 20220517. [CrossRef]
95. Hull, A.; Atilano, M.L.; Gergi, L.; Kinghorn, K.J. Lysosomal storage, impaired autophagy and innate immunity in Gaucher and Parkinson's diseases: Insights for drug discovery. *Philos. Trans. R. Soc. Lond. B Biol. Sci.* **2024**, *379*, 20220381. [CrossRef]
96. Volta, M. Roles of neuronal lysosomes in the etiology of Parkinson's disease. *Neural Regen. Res.* **2024**, *19*, 1981–1983. [CrossRef]
97. Poupon-Bejuit, L.; Hughes, M.P.; Liu, W.; Geard, A.; Faour-Slika, N.; Whaler, S.; Massaro, G.; Rahim, A.A. A GLP1 receptor agonist diabetes drug ameliorates neurodegeneration in a mouse model of infantile neurometabolic disease. *Sci. Rep.* **2022**, *12*, 13825. [CrossRef]
98. Cerroni, C.; Steiner, A.; Seanez, L.; Kwon, S.; Lewis, A.S. Effects of repeated developmental GLP-1R agonist exposure on young adult behavior and hippocampal structure in mice. *Neurosci. Lett.* **2023**, *808*, 137299. [CrossRef] [PubMed]
99. Loh, J.S.; Mak, W.Q.; Tan, L.K.S.; Ng, C.X.; Chan, H.H.; Yeow, S.H.; Foo, J.B.; Ong, Y.S.; How, C.W.; Khaw, K.Y. Microbiota-gut-brain axis and its therapeutic applications in neurodegenerative diseases. *Signal Transduct. Target. Ther.* **2024**, *9*, 37. [CrossRef] [PubMed]
100. Battini, V.; Barbieri, M.A.; Carnovale, C.; Spina, E.; Clementi, E.; Sessa, M. Comparing major and mild cognitive impairment risks in older type-2 diabetic patients: A Danish register-based study on dipeptidyl peptidase-4 inhibitors vs. glucagon-like peptide-1 analogues. *J. Neurol.* **2024**, *271*, 3417–3425. [CrossRef] [PubMed]
101. Dei Cas, A.; Micheli, M.M.; Aldigeri, R.; Gardini, S.; Ferrari-Pellegrini, F.; Perini, M.; Messa, G.; Antonini, M.; Spigoni, V.; Cinquegrani, G.; et al. Long-acting exenatide does not prevent cognitive decline in mild cognitive impairment: A proof-of-concept clinical trial. *J. Endocrinol. Investig.* **2024**, 1–11. [CrossRef]

102. Husain, M.; Bain, S.C.; Jeppesen, O.K.; Lingvay, I.; Sørrig, R.; Treppendahl, M.B.; Vilsbøll, T. Semaglutide (SUSTAIN and PIONEER) Reduces Cardiovascular Events in Type 2 Diabetes Across Varying Cardiovascular Risk. *Diabetes Obes. Metab.* **2020**, *22*, 442–451. [CrossRef]
103. Zhang, L.; Zhang, L.; Li, L.; Hölscher, C. Semaglutide is Neuroprotective and Reduces α-Synuclein Levels in the Chronic MPTP Mouse Model of Parkinson's Disease. *J. Park. Dis.* **2019**, *9*, 157–171. [CrossRef] [PubMed]

current issues in molecular biology

MDPI

Article

Neurotransmission Sex Dichotomy in the Rat Hypothalamic Paraventricular Nucleus in Healthy and Infantile Spasm Model

Dumitru Andrei Iacobas [1,*], Jana Veliskova [2], Tamar Chachua [3], Chian-Ru Chern [3], Kayla Vieira [3], Sanda Iacobas [4] and Libor Velíšek [5]

1 Personalized Genomics Laboratory, Undergraduate Medical Academy, School of Public and Allied Health, Prairie View A&M University, Prairie View, TX 77446, USA
2 Departments of Cell Biology & Anatomy, Obstetrics and Gynecology, and Neurology, New York Medical College, Valhalla, NY 10595, USA; jana_veliskova@nymc.edu
3 Department of Cell Biology & Anatomy, New York Medical College, Valhalla, NY 10595, USA; tamarchachua@gmail.com (T.C.); chianru_chern@nymc.edu (C.-R.C.); kvieira2@student.nymc.edu (K.V.)
4 Department of Pathology, New York Medical College, Valhalla, NY 10595, USA; sandaiacobas@gmail.com
5 Departments of Cell Biology & Anatomy, Pediatrics, and Neurology, New York Medical College, Valhalla, NY 10595, USA; libor_velisek@nymc.edu
* Correspondence: daiacobas@pvamu.edu

Abstract: We profiled the gene expressions in the hypothalamic paraventricular nuclei of 12 male and 12 female pups from a standard rat model of infantile spasms to determine the sex dichotomy of the neurotransmission genomic fabrics. Infantile spasms were triggered in rat pups prenatally primed with two doses of betamethasone followed by the postnatal repeated administration of N-methyl-D-aspartic acid to induce spasms. Publicly available microarray data were used to characterize each gene in each condition for both sexes by the independent transcriptomic features: average expression level, control of the transcript abundance, and expression correlation with every other gene. This study revealed substantial sex differences in the expression level, control, and inter-coordination of the investigated genes among the studied groups. The transcriptomic differences assist in providing a molecular explanation of the behavioral differences and development of infantile epilepsy spasm syndrome in the two sexes.

Keywords: Adcy5; cholinergic synapse; dopaminergic synapse; GABAergic synapse; glutamatergic synapse; serotonergic synapse; synaptic vesicle cycle; transcriptomic network

1. Introduction

This report presents an analysis of experimental data on the hypothalamic paraventricular nucleus (PVN) and complements a large study aiming to determine the consequences of infantile spasms (infantile epilepsy spasm syndrome; IESS) on the neurotransmission transcriptome within the hypothalamic nuclei in a male and female rat model of IESS. The analyses encompassed the KEGG-constructed pathways: the synaptic vesicle cycle (SVC) [1] and glutamatergic (GLU) [2], GABAergic (GABA) [3], cholinergic (ACh) [4], dopaminergic (DA) [5], and serotonergic (5HT) [6] synapses. Previously, we have shown that prenatal priming with betamethasone increases the occurrence of clinical spasms in the prenatal betamethasone–postnatal N-methyl-D-aspartic acid (NMDA) model and identified the activation of several hypothalamic nuclei (i.e., arcuate nucleus and paraventricular nucleus) during the spasms [7,8]. Thus, we first studied the spasm-induced transcriptomic alterations in the hypothalamic arcuate nucleus (ARC) and the efficacy of two anti-IESS treatments [9,10].

IESS (formerly infantile spasms, also West Syndrome) represents a unique and devastating seizure syndrome of infancy [11,12]. IESS affects one out of each 3200–3400 infants with a yearly occurrence of approximately 1700 new cases in the US [13]. The syndrome consists of (1) characteristic epileptic spasms during infancy (3–24 months of age), (2) interictal hypsarrhythmia (large amplitude and asynchronous waves) on the electroencephalogram (EEG), and (3) developmental or psychomotor arrest/delay [13]. IESS-specific FDA-approved first-line therapy is hormonal (adrenocorticotropin; ACTH, or corticosteroids such as prednisone, prednisolone, or methylprednisolone) or vigabatrin [14–16]. However, these treatments neither fully alleviate the condition nor are they free of serious side effects [17,18]. Many patients with IESS may die within the first years of life or suffer from permanent developmental deficits [19]. This poor prognosis necessitates a search for novel treatment targets. Interestingly, IESS has sex preponderance affecting more boys than girls (from 1.5:1.0 to 1.1:1.0) [20–22].

We have developed a model of IESS in infant rats, which includes prenatal priming with betamethasone and an early postnatal trigger of spasms by NMDA [7], which can be repetitive [23]. The spasms triggered by NMDA in the betamethasone-primed rat brain are tightly linked to early development, are semiologically similar to spasms observed in human patients with IESS, share similar EEG patterns, and respond to ACTH, corticosteroids (methylprednisolone), or vigabatrin treatment [23–25]. This model has been independently reproduced and validated [26–28]. The disorganized EEG recordings seen in this model, as well as in the human condition of IESS [12], indicate altered brain circuitry, presumably caused by impaired inter-neuronal communication via neurotransmitters [9]. Our previous imaging studies indicated that the hypothalamus represents a critical hub that may participate in the control of spasms [7].

Among the brain regions, the hypothalamus is responsible for performing numerous neuroendocrine functions through the neuronal networks located in its specialized nuclei [15]. The paired paraventricular nuclei of the hypothalamus, located in the anterior hypothalamus adjacent to the sides of the third ventricle, are central to regulating the stress response and emotions leading to addictive behavior [14–16], as well as to promoting satiety [17,18] through excitatory synaptic transmission circuits [17,18]. The PVN is also critical for the synthesis of vasopressin to regulate blood pressure and oxytocin for the control of stress responses and has connections to the brain stem to control sympathetic circuitry [19,29].

The PVN consists of an intricate network of neurons interconnected by cholinergic [20], dopaminergic [21], GABAergic [22], glutamatergic [7], and serotonergic [23] synapses, each classified according to the neurotransmitter used in the synaptic vesicle cycle [24]. GLU is a primary excitatory neurotransmitter [26] and GABA is the most abundant inhibitory [27] synapse in the mammalian central nervous system, and thus, both are associated with the fundamental functions of the nervous system [28,29]. Other neurotransmitters and their corresponding synapses also play important roles in behavior. Accordingly, the ACh synapse facilitates learning, memory, and attention [30,31], the DA synapse controls learning, memory, motivation, and reward [32–34], and the 5HT synapse is involved in learning and memory, emotion, abnormal mood, and cognition [35–37].

Given the inextricable link between synaptic sex-specific brain organization and behavior, the development of neurological diseases suggests potentially distinct brain neuronal wiring, most likely related to the organizational effects of sex hormones [38–40]. Among others, we have previously reported a substantial sex dichotomy in the gene networking and topology of the rat hypothalamic cytoskeleton [41], as well as in the myelination [41] and GLU and GABA synapse genomic fabrics. We defined the genomic fabric of a functional pathway as the most inter-coordinated and stably expressed gene network whose encoded proteins are responsible for that function [8].

In the present study, at the time of the animal sacrifice on postnatal day (P) 16, their developmentally programmed sex differences are already irreversible. Although the gonads become active in males and females around P28-P30 (rat puberty), the males are exposed to gonadal steroid surges prenatally, and most importantly, to the neonatal testosterone surge between P0 and P5. The role of sex hormones in modulating brain activity in epilepsy is well documented (e.g., [30,31,42,43])

2. Materials and Methods

2.1. Animals, Treatments, and Tissue Collection

We used the offspring of timed-pregnant Sprague Dawley rats (Taconic Farms, Germantown, NY, USA), purchased on gestational day 8 (G8). Dams were housed in our AAALAC-accredited animal facility with free access to chow and water on a 12 h light–dark cycle (lights on at 7:00 a.m.). All experiments were approved by the New York Medical College Institutional Animal Care and Use Committee (IACUC) and conform to the NIH Guide for the Care and Use of Laboratory Animals, 8th edition.

On their G15, 10 pregnant females were injected twice with either saline or 0.4 mg/kg of betamethasone phosphate (Sigma-Aldrich, St. Louis, MO, USA). After birth on G23 (designated as P0), pups were weighed and sexed. Some of the prenatal betamethasone-primed male and female pups received N-methyl-D-aspartic acid (NMDA) on P12, P13, and P15 to trigger spasms. Spasms were followed for 60 min after the trigger. The remainder of the betamethasone-primed male and female pups were injected with the corresponding volume of saline for control (no spasms). Animals were euthanized on P16 under deep CO_2 inhalation anesthesia, the pups were quickly perfused with ice-cold saline, the brains were removed, and the PVNs were dissected. The tissue was immediately snap frozen in dry ice for further processing. There were 6 groups labeled by three letters where the first is the sex (M/F), the second is the priming saline/betamethasone (S/B), and the third is the presence (Y/N) of spasms: MSN, FSN, MBN, FBN, MBY, and FBY (or analogously SN, BN, and BY for each sex). No more than two male and two female pups from each litter entered the experiments so that each group was composed of pups collected from two mothers.

2.2. Microarray and Data Processing

Profiling the gene expressions of technical replicates convinced us that Agilent microarrays (Agilent, Santa Clara, CA, USA) were not only better priced but, with our improved wet protocol, had a lower technical noise than the Illumina MiSeq and NextSeq 550 (Illumina, San Diego, CA, USA) available to us at the time. Most genomists use 3 biological replicas per condition, and we used 4 ($\times$3 conditions = 12 per sex), which considerably increased the statistical relevance. However, more than 4 replicas would only increase the experiment costs without improving the statistical significance because of the inherent technical noise of the method.

Total RNA was extracted with the Qiagen RNeasy mini-kit (Qiagen, Venlo, Netherlands), the concentration was determined with a NanoDrop ND-2000 Spectrophotometer (ThermoFisher Scientific, Thessalonikis, Greece), and purity was determined with the Agilent RNA 6000 Nano kit in an Agilent 2100 Bioanalyzer. Total RNA was reverse transcribed in the presence of Cy3/Cy5 dUTP, and the incorporation of the fluorescent tags was determined with the NanoDrop. Fluorescently labeled RNAs were hybridized with the dual-mode Agilent-028282 Whole Rat Genome Microarray 4x44K v3, printed with 4 arrays of 45,220 spots with a total of 37,520 sequences, out of which 30,100 were mapped to at least one gene (16,066 unigenes). The arrays were scanned and primarily analyzed with an Agilent G4900DA SureScan Microarray Scanner Bundle (dual laser scanner + PC data system + Feature Extraction Software G4464AA). The wet protocol and the raw data were deposited in the publicly accessible Gene Expression Omnibus databases [44–46]. All spots affected by local corruption or with foreground fluorescence less than twice the background in one microarray were disregarded, and background-subtracted foreground fluorescence signals were normalized to the median, and the results were averaged for every set of spots redundantly probing the same gene. Normalization to the median gene expression provides a comparable expression of individual genes across biological replicas, otherwise affected by the errors in sizing the samples.

According to our Genomic Fabric Paradigm [47], the expression of each quantifiable gene is characterizable by three independent measures: *AVE* = average expression level (1), *REC* = Relative Expression Control (2), and *COR* = expression correlation with each other gene (3). *AVE* shows how much the gene is expressed with respect to all other genes, *REC* indicates the influence of the homeostatic mechanisms, while *COR* justifies the gene networking in functional pathways. Together, *AVE*, *REC*, and *COR*, defined by the below formulas, provide the most theoretically possible comprehensive characterization of the transcriptome topology:

$$\forall i,j = 1 \div N \;\&\; \forall s = MSN,\ FSN,\ MBN,\ FBN,\ MBY, FBY$$

$$AVE_i^{(s)} \equiv \frac{1}{4}\sum_{k=1}^{4}\left(\frac{\alpha_{i;k}^{(c)}}{\left\langle \alpha_{i;k}^{(c)} \right\rangle_{i;k}}^{(c)}\right) \; with\; a_i^{(c)} = \frac{1}{4}\sum_{k=1}^{4} \alpha_{i;k}^{(c)} \tag{1}$$

$\alpha_{i;k}^{(c)}$ is the background-subtracted fluorescence of the spot probing for which the gene in replica k (=1, 2, 3, 4) of sample s, $\left\langle \alpha_{i;k}^{(c)} \right\rangle$ is the net fluorescence of the median gene, and $a_i^{(c)}$ is the average net fluorescence over all biological replicas.

$$REC_i^{(c)} \equiv log_2\left(\frac{\left\langle REV_i^{(c)} \right\rangle}{REV_i^{(c)}}\right), \tag{2}$$

where

$$RCS_i^{(c)} \equiv \frac{\left\langle REV_i^{(c)} \right\rangle}{REV_i^{(c)}} = \text{the relative control strength} \tag{2a}$$

$$\left\langle REV_i^{(c)} \right\rangle \text{ is the median } REV \tag{2b}$$

$$REV_i^{(c)} \equiv \frac{\sigma_i^{(c)}}{2AVE_i^{(c)}}\left(\sqrt{\frac{r_i}{\chi^2(\beta; r_i)}} - \sqrt{\frac{r_i}{\chi^2(1-\beta; r_i)}}\right) \tag{2c}$$

REV is computed using the midinterval of the χ^2 distribution of the coefficient of variation in the normalized expression levels across biological replicas. *REV* shows how spread the expression levels are across the biological replicas of that particular type of sample. The expression controls in two conditions of the same sex or one condition in both sexes were compared through the fold-change (*FC*), negative for down-regulation:

$$FC_i^{(compared\ vs\ reference)} = \begin{cases} \frac{RCS_i^{(compared)}}{RCS_i^{(reference)}}, & if\ RCS_i^{(compared)} > RCS_i^{(reference)} \\ -\frac{RCS_i^{(reference)}}{RCS_i^{(compared)}}, & if\ RCS_i^{(compared)} \leq RCS_i^{(reference)} \end{cases} \tag{2d}$$

COR is the pair-wise Pearson correlation coefficient of the (log_2) of the normalized expression levels of the two genes [48].

$$COR_{i,j}^{(c)} \equiv correl\left(log_2\left(\frac{\alpha_{i;k}^{(c)}}{\left\langle \alpha_{i;k}^{(c)} \right\rangle_{i;k}} \right)^{(c)}, log_2\left(\frac{\alpha_{j;k}^{(c)}}{\left\langle \alpha_{j;k}^{(c)} \right\rangle_{i;k}} \right)^{(c)} \right) \tag{3}$$

COR analysis [48] was used to identify the $p < 0.05$ significant inter-gene synergistic/antagonistic/independent expressions. This analysis is the prerequisite to determine the most active transcriptomic networks interlinking (here) the genes involved in neurotransmission. It is important to remember that the statistically significant positive correlation means that the expression of either gene stimulates the expression of the other, the negative correlation points out the opposite tendency, while independence reveals the total decoupling of the encoded products of the two genes. *COR* analysis can also be used to test the validity of the wiring in the KEGG-constructed pathways under normal conditions (M/F)SN and quantify their remodeling in the imposed conditions (M/F)BN and (M/F)BY. Moreover, by comparing the results in males and females, one can find whether the documented effects of the sex hormones on neurotransmission [49–51] should include the differences in the expression control and organization of gene transcriptomic networks beyond differential expression levels.

The transcriptomic influential powers of individual genes computed using the measure termed "Gene Commanding Height", *GCH*, that combines the expression control and the median of the expression coordination with all other genes:

$$GCH_i^{(c)} \equiv exp\left(REC_i^{(c)} + \left\langle \left(2COR_{i,j}^{(c)} \right)^2 \right\rangle_j \right) \tag{4}$$

The top gene (highest GCH) in each condition was termed the Gene Master Regulator (GMR). Pending of the type of genetic manipulation, the GMR might be the most legitimate target for the gene therapy aiming to destroy or to stimulate the proliferation of the most abundant clone in that condition [52].

The expression of a gene is considered significantly regulated when comparing BN with SN and BY with BN for each sex or significantly different when comparing the two sexes within the same condition if it satisfies the composite criterion (4). For the absolute fold-change $|x|$ and the *p*-value of the heteroscedastic *t*-test of means' equality [53],

$$\begin{cases} \left| x_i^{(compared\ vs\ reference)} \right| > CUT_i^{(compared\ vs\ reference)} \\ p_i^{(compared\ vs\ reference)} < 0.05 \end{cases} \tag{5}$$

where

$$x_i^{(compared\ vs\ reference)} = \begin{cases} \frac{AVE_i^{(compared)}}{AVE_i^{(reference)}}, & if\ AVE_i^{(compared)} > AVE_i^{(reference)} \\ -\frac{AVE_i^{(reference)}}{AVE_i^{(compared)}}, & if\ AVE_i^{(compared)} \leq AVE_i^{(reference)} \end{cases} \tag{5a}$$

$$CUT_i^{(compared\ vs\ reference)} = 1 + \sqrt{\frac{2}{100}\left(\left(REV_i^{(compared)} \right)^2 + \left(REV_i^{(reference)} \right)^2 \right)} \tag{5b}$$

2.3. KEGG-Constructed Functional Neurotransmission Pathways

The analyses were directed toward genes associated with the KEGG (Kyoto Encyclopedia of Genes and Genomes, [54])-constructed pathways: synaptic vesicle cycle (SVC, denoted by "0" in the column "Path" of tables below), and glutamatergic (GLU, "1"), GABAergic (GABA, "2"), cholinergic (ACh, "3"), dopaminergic (DA, "4"), and serotonergic (5HT, "5") synapse [1–6]. We were able to quantify properly in all samples: 69 out of 80 of the KEGG-listed SVC genes, 90 out of 115 GLU genes, 67 out of 90 GABA genes, 80 out of 113 ACh genes, 111 out of 132 DA genes, and 71 out of 130 5HT genes. The pathways are partially overlapping, with several genes shared by two or more pathways. For instance, *Gnai2* is part of all five types of synapses and *Mapk3* of the glutamatergic, cholinergic, and serotonergic synapses.

3. Results

3.1. There Is Little Sex Dichotomy of the Most Highly Expressed Neurotransmission Genes

Table 1 presents the top five genes associated with the functional pathways, SVC ("0"), GLU ("1"), GABA ("2"), ACh ("3"), DA ("4"), and 5HT ("5"), which exhibited the largest expression levels in each sex in all three conditions. Of note is the almost unchanged gene hierarchy according to their normalized (to the median gene) expression levels, although their expression was a little higher in females (see Table S1 in Supplementary Materials for the ratio "×" of the (M/F) expression levels according to definition (5a)). For instance, with respect to the median gene expression, the DA gene *Caly* has 126× more transcripts than the median gene in male SN (but 195× in female SN), 139× in male BN (but 143× in female BN), and 126× in male BY (but 155× in female BY). For comparison, the table also includes the non-neurotransmission genes (no number in the "Path" column) with the largest expression levels (*Cst3* and *Rpl41*), indicating that the neurotransmission genes are among the most highly expressed in the PVN transcriptome. However, although these top five genes in the analyzed neurotransmission functional pathways were practically not differentially expressed, other neurotransmission genes presented statistically significant differential expression between the two sexes. However, it is interesting to note the differences among the three conditions for each sex.

3.2. Sex Dichotomy in the Expression Control and Alteration by IESS

Tables 2 and 3 present the most and the least controlled neurotransmission genes in the paraventricular nodes of both sexes in all three conditions as quantified by the Relative Expression Control (*REC*) score. Positive *REC*s indicate how many times a gene is under stricter control than the median gene, while a negative *REC* indicates how many times the gene is less controlled than the median of that group of samples.

The most controlled genes (highest positive *REC*s) are most likely critical for cell survival and phenotypic expression, while the least controlled genes might be essential for the cell adaptation to the slight environmental changes like those differentiating the biological replicas. Supplementary Tables S2 and S3 list the ratios of the relative control strength (*RCS*) scores of the same genes between the two sexes in all three conditions.

One of the most controlled neurotransmission genes in the IESS female PVN, *Gng10*, is part of all five types of synapses analyzed in this study. Of note are the substantial differences between the two sexes in all three conditions, as well as the switch from very controlled in (M/F)SN to less controlled in (M/F)BN of *Atp6v0b*, *Calml4*, and *Atp6v1b*. Interestingly, the dopaminergic gene, *Th*, with a very loose control in male SN, became strictly controlled in the condition of spasms.

Table 1. The top five most expressed neurotransmission genes in the PVNs of the two sexes subjected to each of the three conditions. Numbers in the MALE and FEMALE SN, BN, and BY columns are the average expression levels normalized to the expression level of the median gene in that condition for each sex. For instance, the expression of *Caly* in male SN is 126 times larger than that of the median gene in the PVNs of the saline-primed rats without infantile spasms. Note the similarity of the gene hierarchy in each group of samples.

	Top 5 Expressed Neurotransmission Genes		Male			Female		
Gene	**Description**	**PATH**	**SN**	**BN**	**BY**	**SN**	**BN**	**BY**
Caly	calcyon neuron-specific vesicular protein	4	126	139	126	195	143	155
Gabarapl1	GABA(A) receptor-associated protein like 1	2	104	112	80	69	108	129
Ap2m1	adaptor-related protein complex 2, mu 1 subunit	0	96	110	89	125	112	122
Calm2	calmodulin 2	4	72	70	60	60	75	72
Hap1	huntingtin-associated protein 1	2	63	63	67	73	72	73
Caly	calcyon neuron-specific vesicular protein	4	126	139	126	195	143	155
Ap2m1	adaptor-related protein complex 2, mu 1 subunit	0	96	110	89	125	112	122
Mapk3	mitogen activated protein kinase 3	135	59	64	67	85	68	68
Gnai2	guanine nucleotide binding protein (G protein), alpha inhibiting activity polypeptide 2	12345	57	64	57	75	64	74
Hap1	huntingtin-associated protein 1	2	63	63	67	73	72	73
Caly	calcyon neuron-specific vesicular protein	4	126	139	126	195	143	155
Gabarapl1	GABA(A) receptor-associated protein like 1	2	104	112	80	69	108	129
Ap2m1	adaptor-related protein complex 2, mu 1 subunit	0	96	110	89	125	112	122
Calm2	calmodulin 2	4	72	70	60	60	75	72
Gnai2	guanine nucleotide binding protein (G protein), alpha inhibiting activity polypeptide 2	12345	57	64	57	75	64	74
Caly	calcyon neuron-specific vesicular protein	4	126	139	126	195	143	155
Ap2m1	adaptor-related protein complex 2, mu 1 subunit	0	96	110	89	125	112	122
Gabarapl1	GABA(A) receptor-associated protein like 1	2	104	112	80	69	108	129
Calm2	calmodulin 2	4	72	70	60	60	75	72
Hap1	huntingtin-associated protein 1	2	63	63	67	73	72	73
Caly	calcyon neuron-specific vesicular protein	4	126	139	126	195	143	155
Ap2m1	adaptor-related protein complex 2, mu 1 subunit	0	96	110	89	125	112	122
Gabarapl1	GABA(A) receptor-associated protein like 1	2	104	112	80	69	108	129
Mapk3	mitogen activated protein kinase 3	135	59	64	67	85	68	68
Hap1	huntingtin-associated protein 1	2	63	63	67	73	72	73
Caly	calcyon neuron-specific vesicular protein	4	126	139	126	195	143	155
Gabarapl1	GABA(A) receptor-associated protein like 1	2	104	112	80	69	108	129
Ap2m1	adaptor-related protein complex 2, mu 1 subunit	0	96	110	89	125	112	122
Gnai2	guanine nucleotide binding protein (G protein), alpha inhibiting activity polypeptide 2	12345	57	64	57	75	64	74
Hap1	huntingtin-associated protein 1	2	63	63	67	73	72	73

Table 2. The most controlled neurotransmission genes in the PVNs of the two sexes subjected to each of the three conditions. Numbers in the MALE and FEMALE SN, BN, and BY columns are the Relative Expression Control (*REC*) scores. Note the alteration of the normal hierarchy of controlled genes in (M/F)SN and (M/F)BY conditions and the substantial differences between the two sexes in all three conditions. For comparison, the table includes the *REC*s of the most controlled non-neurotransmission genes (no number in the "Path" column): *Erg88*, *Erap1*, *Tmem238*, *Cul7*, *Oxsr1*, and *Tsc2*.

	Top 5 Most Controlled Neurotransmission Genes		**Male**			**Female**		
Gene	**Description**	**PATH**	**SN**	**BN**	**BY**	**SN**	**BN**	**BY**
Pik3r2	phosphoinositide-3-kinase, regulatory subunit 2 (beta)	3	3.52	1.04	0.82	0.83	0.75	0.73
Atp6v0b	ATPase, H+ transporting, lysosomal V0 subunit B	0	2.40	−0.59	1.22	1.01	0.12	−0.02
Calml4	calmodulin-like 4	4	2.15	−0.61	0.65	−0.56	−0.02	−0.71
Ppp1ca	protein phosphatase 1, catalytic subunit, alpha isozyme	4	2.13	0.55	1.12	1.16	2.00	1.32
Atp6v1g2	ATPase, H+ transporting, lysosomal V1 subunit G2	0	1.95	−0.32	0.67	0.06	0.87	1.39
Abat	4-aminobutyrate aminotransferase	2	0.38	1.52	1.63	3.58	1.81	0.33
Gabbr1	gamma-aminobutyric acid (GABA) B receptor 1	2	−0.26	0.72	0.75	2.87	0.15	1.23
Slc6a7	solute carrier family 6 (neurotransmitter transporter), member 7	0	1.08	−0.01	1.01	2.82	−0.08	1.63
Chrnb4	cholinergic receptor, nicotinic, beta 4 (neuronal)	3	0.87	0.09	0.40	2.75	0.60	0.11
Gnal	GTP-binding protein Golf alpha subunit	4	0.83	−0.98	−0.45	2.66	−0.28	−0.48
Pik3r5	phosphoinositide-3-kinase, regulatory subunit 5	3	−0.25	2.42	1.25	0.94	−1.19	1.17
Atp2a2	ATPase, Ca++ transporting, cardiac muscle, slow twitch 2	0	0.60	2.18	0.81	−0.60	1.53	0.94
Ppp2r5e	protein phosphatase 2, regulatory subunit B′, epsilon isoform	4	0.76	2.04	2.08	−0.44	0.85	0.47
Ppp2r3c	protein phosphatase 2, regulatory subunit B″, gamma	4	1.70	1.85	0.72	−0.32	0.10	1.20
Slc38a5	solute carrier family 38, member 5	2	1.94	1.81	0.50	−0.09	−0.88	0.94
Grm8	glutamate receptor, metabotropic 8	1	0.25	−0.24	1.81	0.47	2.70	0.70
Cpne3	copine III	0	0.23	0.68	0.58	−0.98	2.39	−0.20
Atp6v1h	ATPase, H+ transporting, lysosomal V1 subunit H	0	0.80	1.55	0.50	−0.24	2.30	0.57
Gls	glutaminase (Gls), nuclear gene encoding mitochondrial protein	12	0.04	1.07	1.27	−1.34	2.19	0.76
Gabarapl2	GABA(A) receptor-associated protein like 2	2	0.66	0.62	1.10	−1.40	2.09	1.43
Th	tyrosine hydroxylase	4	−1.77	−0.50	3.71	0.05	−0.14	−0.16
Maoa	monoamine oxidase A	45	0.59	0.53	2.62	1.17	0.93	−0.42
Mapk10	mitogen activated protein kinase 10	4	0.97	0.30	2.35	−1.84	−0.04	0.44
Scn1a	sodium channel, voltage-gated, type I, alpha	4	−0.30	0.69	2.29	1.00	−0.67	0.30
Gabrg1	gamma-aminobutyric acid (GABA) A receptor, gamma 1	2	0.24	0.04	2.22	0.79	1.76	−0.87
Trpc1	transient receptor potential cation channel, subfamily C, member 1	15	0.57	0.98	1.87	−1.06	0.64	4.87
Gng10	guanine nucleotide binding protein (G protein), gamma 10	12345	0.56	1.08	0.11	0.05	1.38	2.79
Gng8	guanine nucleotide binding protein (G protein), gamma 8	1245	0.20	0.37	0.40	0.78	−0.18	2.58
Raf1	v-raf-leukemia viral oncogene 1	5	1.05	1.68	0.68	0.98	−0.64	2.21
Atp6v0a1	ATPase, H+ transporting, lysosomal V0 subunit A1	0	−0.21	0.11	1.68	−0.69	2.06	2.04

Table 3. The least controlled neurotransmission genes in the PVNs of the two sexes subjected to all three conditions. Numbers in the MALE and FEMALE SN, BN, and BY columns are the Relative Expression Control (*REC*) scores. Note the alteration of the normal hierarchy of controlled genes in the BNS and BYS conditions and the substantial differences between the two sexes in all three conditions. For comparison, the table also includes the least controlled non-neurotransmission genes in each group of samples: *C11h21orf91*, *Snx5*, *Pddc1*, *Mobp*, *Pfk1*, and *Ptgds*.

	Top 5 Least Controlled Neurotransmission Genes		**Male**			**Female**		
Gene	**Description**	**PATH**	**SN**	**BN**	**BY**	**SN**	**BN**	**BY**
Calm1	calmodulin 1	4	−2.05	−0.87	−1.41	−1.27	−0.56	−0.30
Alox15	arachidonate 15-lipoxygenase	5	−2.04	−0.40	−1.20	−0.03	−1.23	−1.47
Th	tyrosine hydroxylase	4	−1.77	−0.50	3.71	0.05	−0.14	−0.16
Plcb1	phospholipase C, beta 1 (phosphoinositide-specific)	1345	−1.73	−1.61	−1.06	−0.27	−1.28	−1.58
Clock	clock circadian regulator	4	−1.48	−2.33	−1.76	−1.10	−1.61	−1.80
Mapk10	mitogen activated protein kinase 10	4	0.97	0.30	2.35	−1.84	−0.04	0.44
Gna11	guanine nucleotide binding protein, alpha 11	3	−0.54	−1.47	−1.16	−1.76	−0.62	−1.41
Gabarapl1	GABA(A) receptor-associated protein like 1	2	−0.72	−0.64	−0.90	−1.74	−0.66	−0.53
Rims1	regulating synaptic membrane exocytosis 1	0	−1.17	−1.73	−1.37	−1.69	−1.41	−1.67
Map2k1	mitogen activated protein kinase kinase 1	35	−0.51	0.19	0.57	−1.64	1.03	−0.19
Drd2	dopamine receptor D2	4	−0.63	−2.45	−1.42	−0.74	−1.59	−1.74
Slc6a12	solute carrier family 6 (neurotransmitter transporter), member 12	02	−0.58	−2.35	−1.35	−0.61	−1.29	−1.62
Clock	clock circadian regulator	4	−1.48	−2.33	−1.76	−1.10	−1.61	−1.80
Alox12b	arachidonate 12-lipoxygenase, 12R type	5	−1.16	−2.25	−1.39	−0.27	−1.53	−1.66
Gnb3	guanine nucleotide binding protein (G protein), beta polypeptide 3	12345	−0.88	−2.24	−1.57	−0.96	−1.56	−1.81
Creb3	cAMP responsive element binding protein 3	34	0.47	0.61	0.33	0.41	−2.71	0.13
Gng5	guanine nucleotide binding protein (G protein), gamma 5	12345	0.65	0.52	1.23	0.40	−2.22	1.47
Camk2b	calcium/calmodulin-dependent protein kinase II beta	34	0.90	−0.60	0.39	−1.08	−2.15	−0.05
Akt1	v-akt murine thymoma viral oncogene homolog 1	34	0.46	−0.23	0.29	−0.46	−2.15	−0.87
Slc1a3	solute carrier family 1 (glial high affinity glutamate transporter), member 3	01	−0.23	−0.48	−0.77	0.23	−2.07	−0.17
Clock	clock circadian regulator	4	−1.48	−2.33	−1.76	−1.10	−1.61	−1.80
Gria2	glutamate receptor, ionotropic, AMPA 2	14	0.28	−0.51	−1.64	−1.18	0.77	−0.32
Htr7	5-hydroxytryptamine (serotonin) receptor 7, adenylate cyclase-coupled	5	−0.94	−2.17	−1.60	−0.78	−1.66	−1.71
Unc13b	unc-13 homolog B (C. elegans)	0	−1.07	−2.22	−1.60	−0.24	−1.63	−1.78
Akt2	v-akt murine thymoma viral oncogene homolog 2	34	−0.94	−2.14	−1.57	−1.08	−1.29	−1.65
Grin1	glutamate receptor, ionotropic, N-methyl D-aspartate 1	1	−0.79	−1.87	−1.40	−0.45	−1.41	−1.87
Gnaq	guanine nucleotide binding protein (G protein), q polypeptide	1345	−1.04	−1.89	−1.46	−0.21	−1.19	−1.87
Chrna7	cholinergic receptor, nicotinic, alpha 7 (neuronal)	3	−1.38	−2.01	−1.57	−0.91	−1.36	−1.87
Cyp2c11	cytochrome P450, subfamily 2, polypeptide 11	5	0.54	−1.33	−0.99	0.15	−1.04	−1.86
Gnb3	guanine nucleotide binding protein (G protein), beta polypeptide 3	12345	−0.88	−2.24	−1.57	−0.96	−1.56	−1.81

We believe that the reason why the expressions of some genes were left free to fluctuate is to provide adaptation to the changes in the environmental conditions. Thus, *Gnb3* and *Gng5* were the most flexibly expressed genes in the BN condition of both male and female PVNs five synapse pathways.

Figure 1 illustrates the substantial sex differences in the gene expression control by plotting the *REC*s of the most (1a) and the least (1b) controlled genes in the three conditions of the hypothalamic paraventricular nuclei of rat pups subjected to the three conditions. It is remarkable that genes such as *Pik3r5*, *ThTrpc1*, *Erg28*, *Mapk10*, and *Creb3* are over-controlled in some conditions and less controlled in others, indicating differences in the regulatory homeostatic mechanisms.

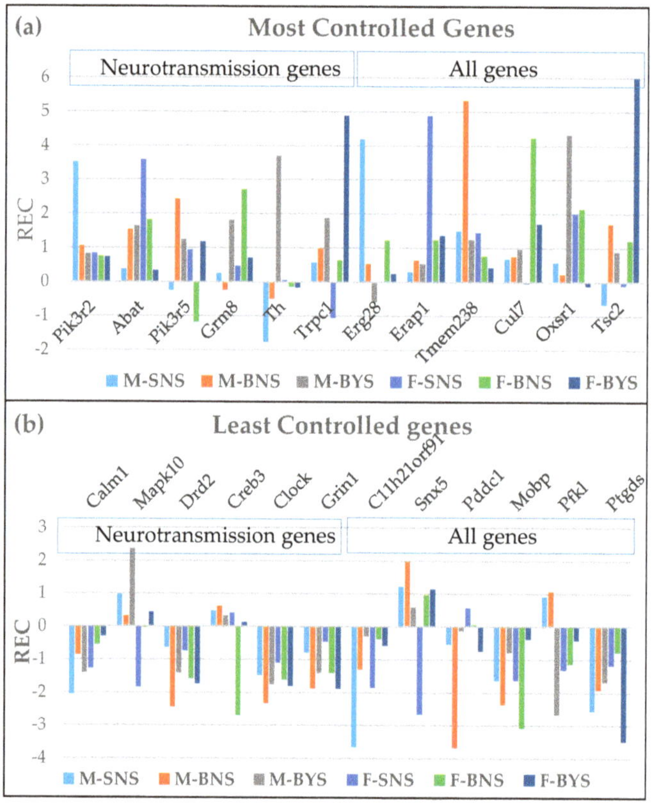

Figure 1. Relative Expression Control (*REC*) of the extremely controlled and extremely flexibly expressed neurotransmission genes in comparison with all other genes in the male and female paraventricular nuclei of rats with/without betamethasone priming, with/without ISEE NMDA triggering. (**a**) Top controlled (highest REC). (**b**) Most flexibly expressed genes. Note the substantial differences among the three conditions in each sex as well as between the two sexes in each condition.

3.3. Sex Differences in the Unaltered State of the Six Neurotransmission Pathways

Figure 2 presents the statistically significant (i.e., satisfying the composite criterion of $p < 0.05$ + absolute expression ratio > CUT) differential expression of the SVC (a), GLU (b), GABA (c), ACh (d), DA (e), and 5HT (f) pathways' genes between males and females in the unaltered state (SN) of the paraventricular hypothalamic nucleus. In this figure, the female transcriptome is the reference and the male is the referred, so that the red background indicates a significantly higher expression in males while a green background specifies higher expression in females.

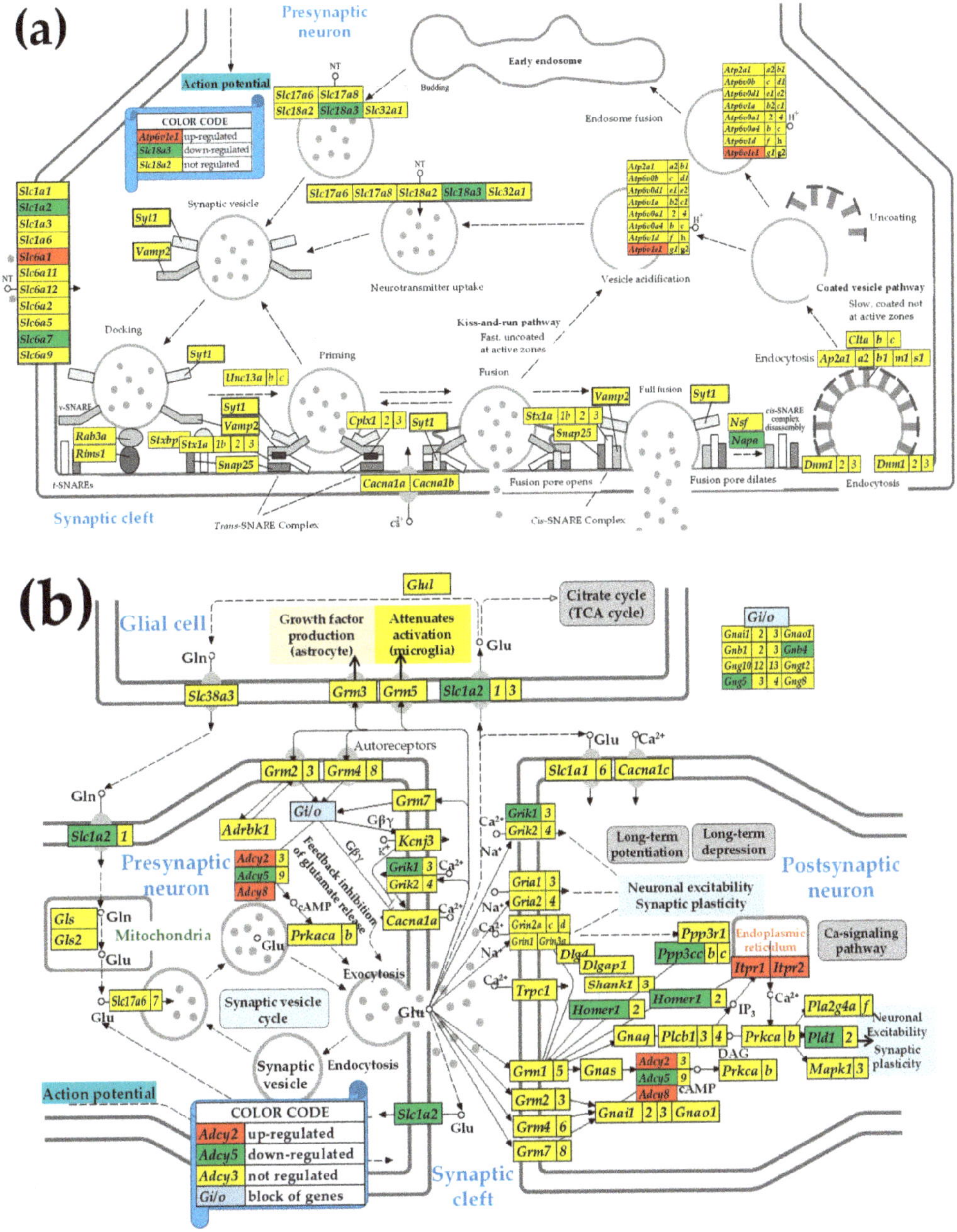

Figure 2. *Cont.*

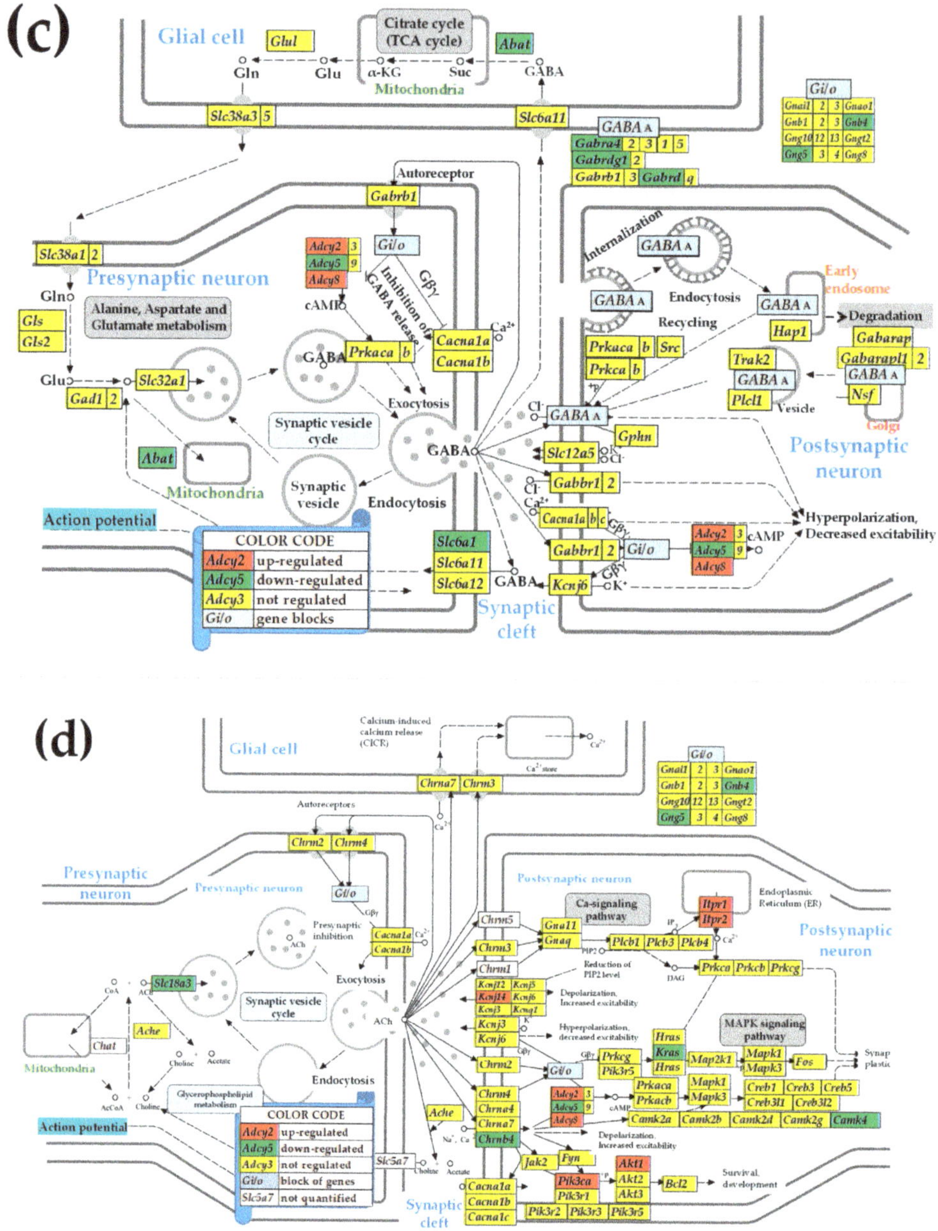

Figure 2. *Cont.*

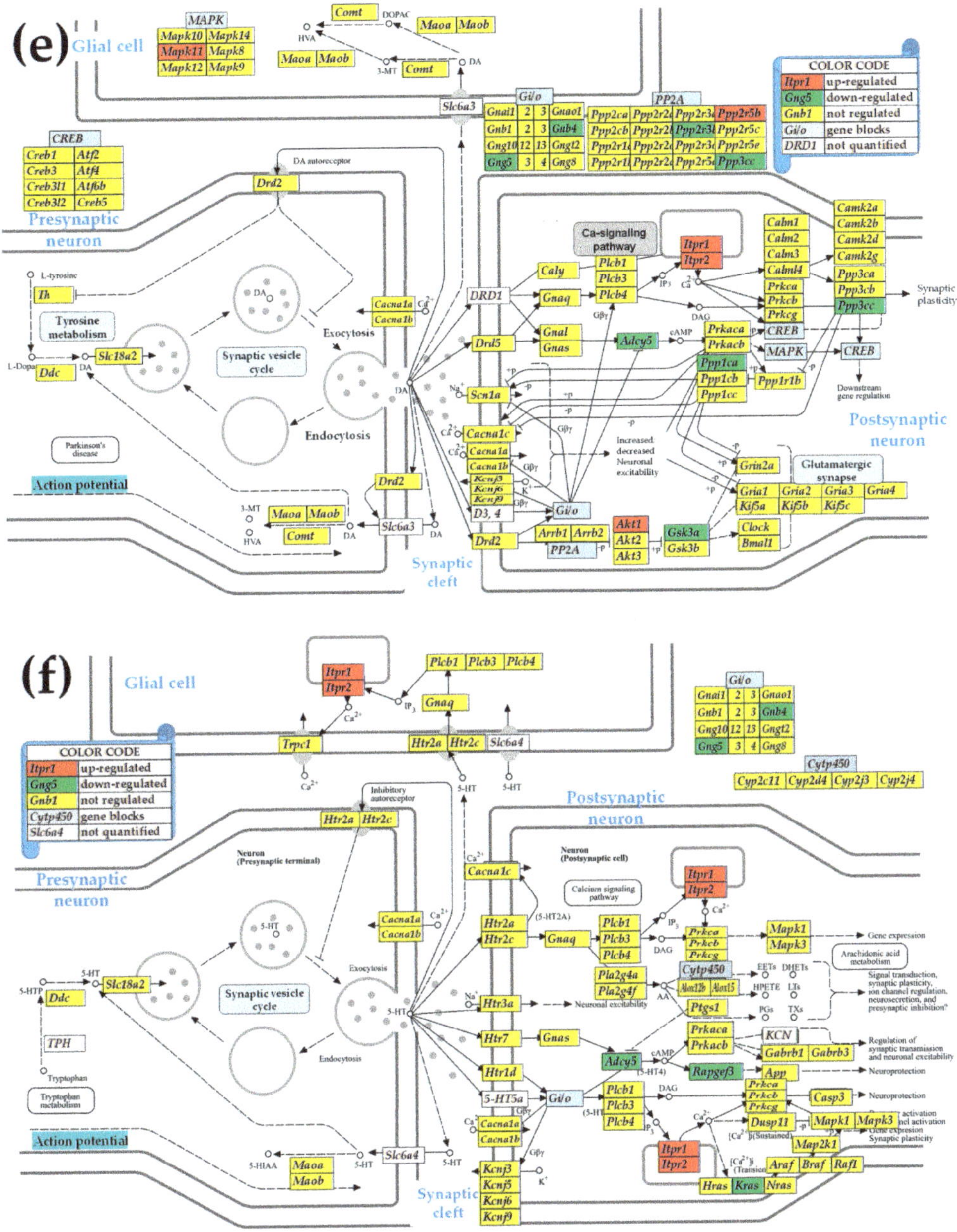

Figure 2. Sex differences in the unaltered (SN) state of the KEGG-constructed pathways: (**a**) synaptic vesicle cycle, (**b**) Glutamatergic Synapse, (**c**) GABAergic, (**d**) cholinergic, (**e**) dopaminergic, and (**f**) serotonergic synapses in the PVNs of males and females. The red/green background of the gene symbols indicates whether that gene was significantly over/underexpressed in the males with respect to the females' tissue, while the yellow background indicates that the expression difference was not significant. Differentially expressed genes: *Abat* (4-aminobutyrate aminotransferase), *Adcy2/5/8* (adenylate cyclase 2/5/8), *Akt1* (v-akt murine thymoma viral oncogene homolog 1), *Atp6v1c1* (ATPase, H+ transporting, lysosomal V1 subunit C1), *Chrnb4* (cholinergic receptor, nicotinic, beta 4 (neuronal)),

Gabra4/d/g1 (gamma-aminobutyric acid (GABA) A receptor, alpha 4/delta/gamma1), *Gnb4* (guanine nucleotide-binding protein (G protein), beta polypeptide 4), *Gng5* (guanine nucleotide-binding protein (G protein), gamma 5), *Grik1* (glutamate receptor, ionotropic, kainate 1), *Homer1* (homer homolog 1 (Drosophila)), *Itpr1/2* (inositol 1,4,5-trisphosphate receptor, type 1/2), *Kcnj14* (potassium inwardly rectifying channel, subfamily J, member 14), *Kras* (Kirsten rat sarcoma viral oncogene), *Mapk11* (mitogen-activated protein kinase 11), *Napa* (N-ethylmaleimide-sensitive factor attachment protein, alpha), *Pik3ca* (phosphoinositide-3-kinase, catalytic, alpha polypeptide), *Pld1* (phospholipase D1), *Ppp1ca* (protein phosphatase 1, catalytic subunit, alpha isozyme), *Ppp3cc* (protein phosphatase 3, catalytic subunit, gamma isozyme), *Slc18a3* (solute carrier family 18 (vesicular acetylcholine transporter), member 3), *Rapgef3* (Rap guanine nucleotide exchange factor (GEF) 3), *Slc1a2* (solute carrier family 1 (glial high-affinity glutamate transporter), member 2), *Slc18a3* (solute carrier family 18 (vesicular acetylcholine transporter), member 3, and *Slc6a1/7* (solute carrier family 6 (neurotransmitter transporter), member 1/7).

3.4. Sex Differences Between the Significantly Regulated SVC Genes in the PVNs by the Induction of Spasms in the Betamethasone-Primed Rats

Figure 3 presents the statistically significant ($p < 0.05$, absolute fold-change > CUT) regulations in the SVC functional pathway following the induction of the spasms in the betamethasone-primed state (BYS/BNS) of the PVNs of male and female rats.

Out of the sixty-nine quantified SVC genes, one was up-regulated in males while four were up-regulated in females. Three SVC genes were down-regulated in males versus two in females. Interestingly, two down-regulated genes in males, *Atp2a2* and *Cplx2*, were up-regulated in females, indicating opposite effects of triggering the infantile spasms in the two sexes.

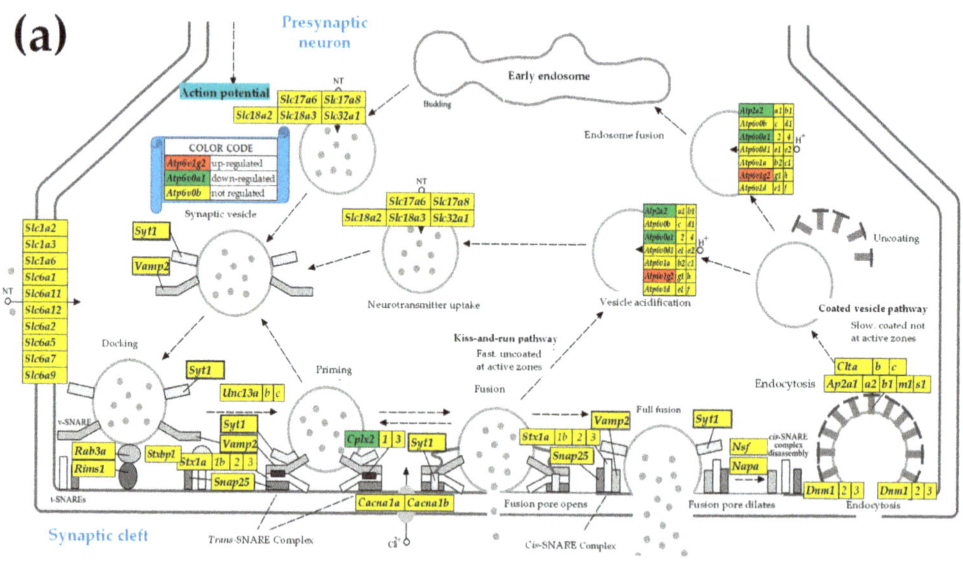

Figure 3. *Cont.*

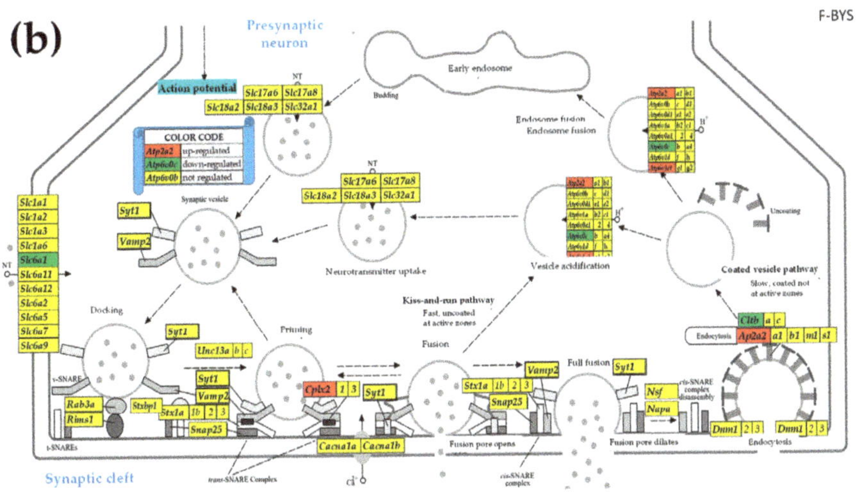

Figure 3. Sex differences in the regulome of the KEGG-constructed synaptic vesicle cycle (SVC) of the betamethasone-primed PVN following the induction of the spasms. (**a**) Male rats. (**b**) Female rats. The red/green background of the gene symbols indicates whether that gene was significantly over/underexpressed in the males with respect to the females' tissue, while the yellow background indicates that the expression difference was not significant. Differentially expressed genes: *Ap2a2* (adaptor-related protein complex 2, alpha 2 subunit), *Atp2a2* (ATPase, Ca++ transporting, cardiac muscle, slow twitch 2), *Atp6v0c* (ATPase, H+ transporting, lysosomal V0 subunit C), *Atp6v1c1/g2*, *Cplx2* (complexin 2), and *Slc6a1*.

3.5. Sex Differences Between the Significantly Regulated GLU Genes in the PVN by the Induction of Infantile Spasms in the Betamethasone-Primed Rats

Figure 4 presents the statistically significant ($p < 0.05$, absolute fold-change > CUT) regulations in the GLU functional pathway following the induction of the spasms in the betamethasone-primed state (BYS/BNS) of the PVNs of male and female rats. Out of the ninety quantified GLU genes, four genes were up-regulated and three were down-regulated in males, compared to two up-regulated and one down-regulated in females. Interestingly, *Adcy5*, included in all five synaptic pathways, was down-regulated by IS in males but up-regulated in females, indicating opposite effects of IS on the two sexes.

3.6. Sex Differences Between the Significantly Regulated GABA Genes in the PVN by the Induction of Infantile Spasms in the Betamethasone-Primed Rats

Figure 5 presents the statistically significant ($p < 0.05$, absolute fold-change > CUT) regulations in the GABA functional pathway following the induction of the infantile spasms in the betamethasone-primed state (BYS/BNS) of the PVNs of male and female rats. Out of the sixty-nine quantified GABA genes, four were up-regulated and two were down-regulated in males, compared to one up-regulated and four down-regulated in females, with *Adcy5* being down-regulated in males but up-regulated in females.

3.7. Sex Dichotomy of the Genes' Transcriptomic Networks

Figure 6 shows the significant differences between the two sexes in the correlated expressions of SVC genes. Panel (a) presents the SVC gene pairs that are oppositely correlated in the two sexes, while, as shown in panels (b) and (c), several independently expressed gene pairs in one sex became significantly synergistically or antagonistically expressed in the other.

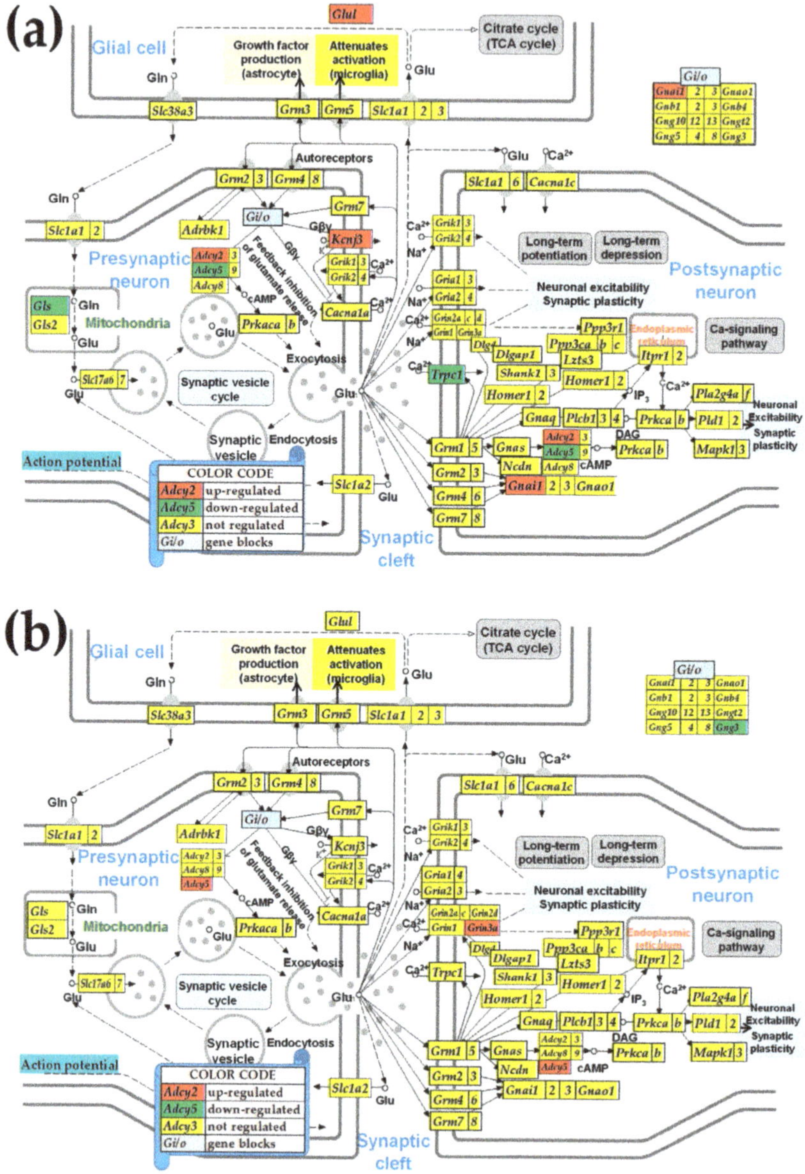

Figure 4. Significantly regulated genes in the KEGG-constructed Glutamatergic Synapse (GLU) pathway of the betamethasone-primed PVNs of male (**a**) and female (**b**) rats following the induction of the infantile spasms. The red/green background of the gene symbols indicates whether that gene was significantly up/down-regulated by the induction of spasms in the betamethasone-primed animals, while the yellow background indicates not significant regulation. Regulated genes: *Adcy2/5*, *Gls* (glutaminase (Gls), nuclear gene encoding mitochondrial protein), *Glul* (glutamate-ammonia ligase), *Gnai1* (guanine nucleotide-binding protein (G protein), alpha inhibiting activity polypeptide 1), *Kcnj3* (potassium inwardly rectifying channel, subfamily J, member 3), and *Trpc1* (transient receptor potential cation channel, subfamily C, member 1).

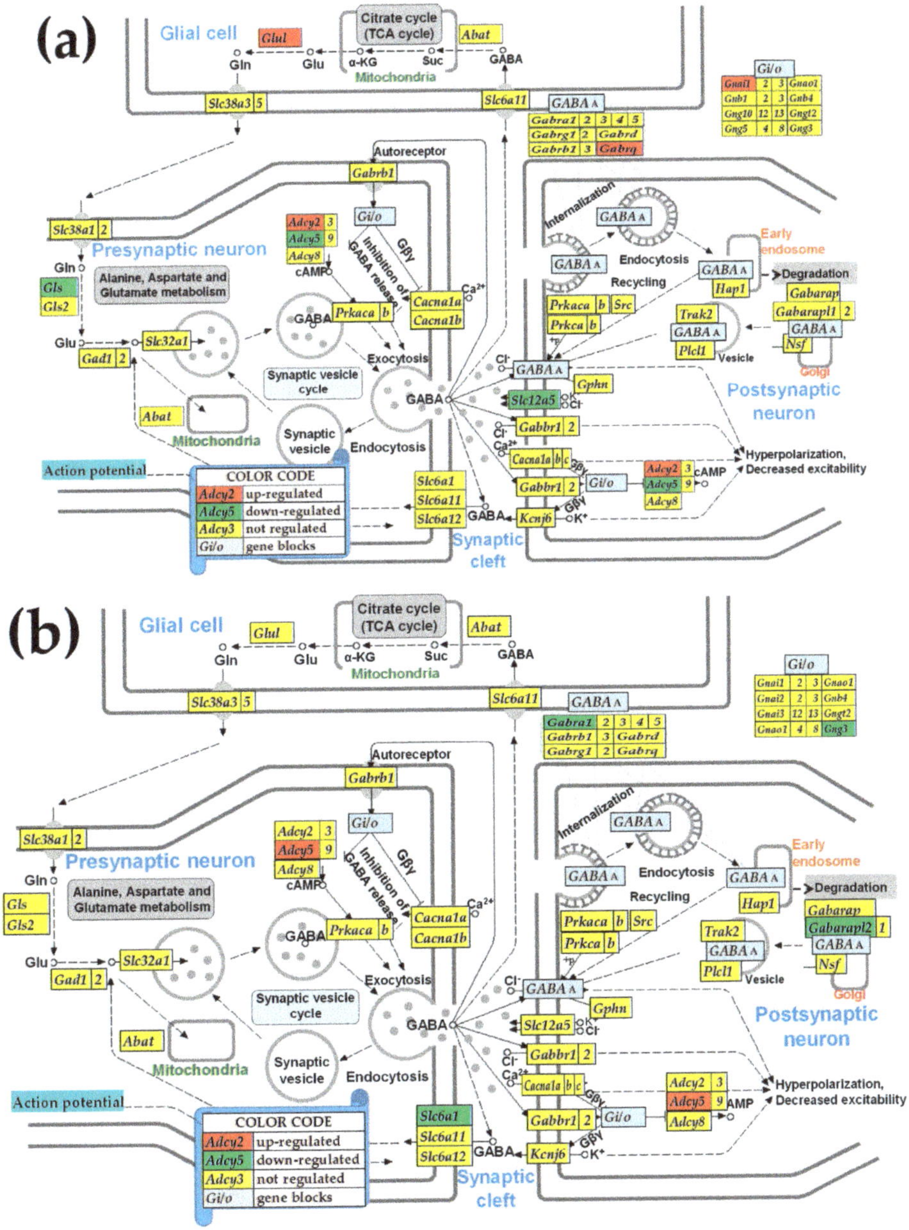

Figure 5. Significantly regulated genes in the KEGG-constructed GABA synapse (GABA) pathway of the betamethasone-primed PVNs of male (**a**) and female (**b**) rats following the induction of the infantile spasms. The red/green background of the gene symbols indicates whether that gene was significantly up/down-regulated by the induction of spasms in the betamethasone-primed animals, while the yellow background indicates not significant regulation. Regulated genes: *Adcy2/5*, *Gabra1*, *Gabrq*, *Gabarapl2* (GABA(A) receptor-associated protein like 2), *Gls*, *Glul*, *Gnai1*, *Gng3*, *Slc12a5*, and *Slc6a1* (solute carrier family 6 (neurotransmitter transporter), member 1).

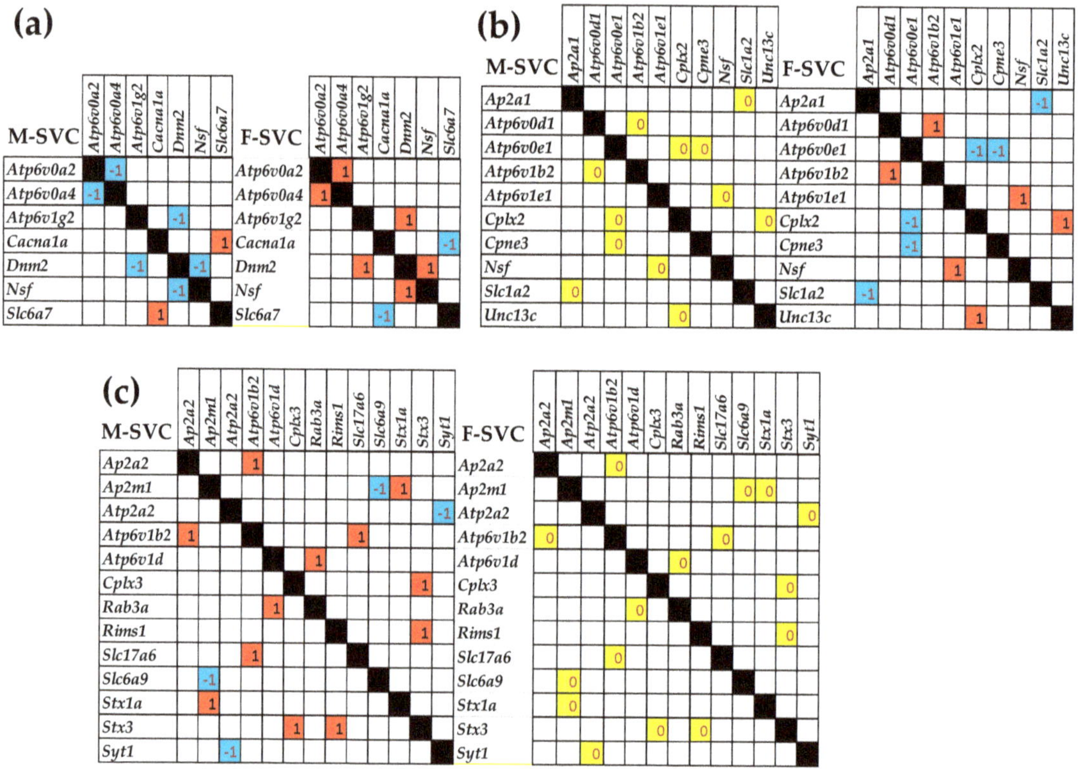

Figure 6. Significant sex dichotomy in the expression correlations among the SVC genes. (**a**) Gene pairs that switch their significant synergistic (red square) or antagonistic (blue square) correlation from male to the opposite in female. (**b**) Independently expressed gene pairs (yellow square) in males that became significantly synergistically (red square) or antagonistically (blue square) correlated in females. (**c**) Significantly correlated gene pairs in males that are independently expressed in females. Interesting genes: *Ap2a1/m1* (adaptor-related protein complex 2, alpha 1/m1 subunit), *Atp2a2* (ATPase, Ca++ transporting, cardiac muscle, slow twitch 2), *Atpv0a2/4* (ATPase, H+ transporting, lysosomal V0 subunit A2/4), *Atp6v0d1/e1* (ATPase, H+ transporting, lysosomal V0 subunit D1/e1), *Atp6v1b2/e1/g2* (ATPase, H+ transporting, lysosomal V1 subunit B2/E1/G2), *Cacna1a* (calcium channel, voltage-dependent, P/Q type, alpha 1A subunit), *Cplx2* (complexin 2), *Cpne3* (copine III), *Dnm2* (dynamin 2), *Nsf* (N-ethylmaleimide-sensitive factor), *Rab3a* (RAB3A, member RAS oncogene family), *Slc1a2* (solute carrier family 1 (glial high-affinity glutamate transporter)), and *Unc13c* (unc-13 homolog C).

Figure 7 shows the significant differences between the two sexes in the correlated expressions of GLU genes. Panel (a) presents the genes that are oppositely correlated in the two sexes. Thus, four antagonistically expressed gene pairs in males were switched to synergistically expressed in females (*Gls2—Gng13*, *Gnao1—Gria2*, *Gng5—Itpr1*, *Grm2—Slc38a2*), while two others (*Gnao1—Gng8*, *Izts3—Prkcg*) were switched from synergistically expressed in males to antagonistically expressed in females. Moreover, as shown in panels (b) and (c), several independently expressed gene pairs in one sex became significantly synergistically/antagonistically expressed in the other. All these differences indicate distinct molecular mechanisms involved in the glutamatergic synaptic transcription.

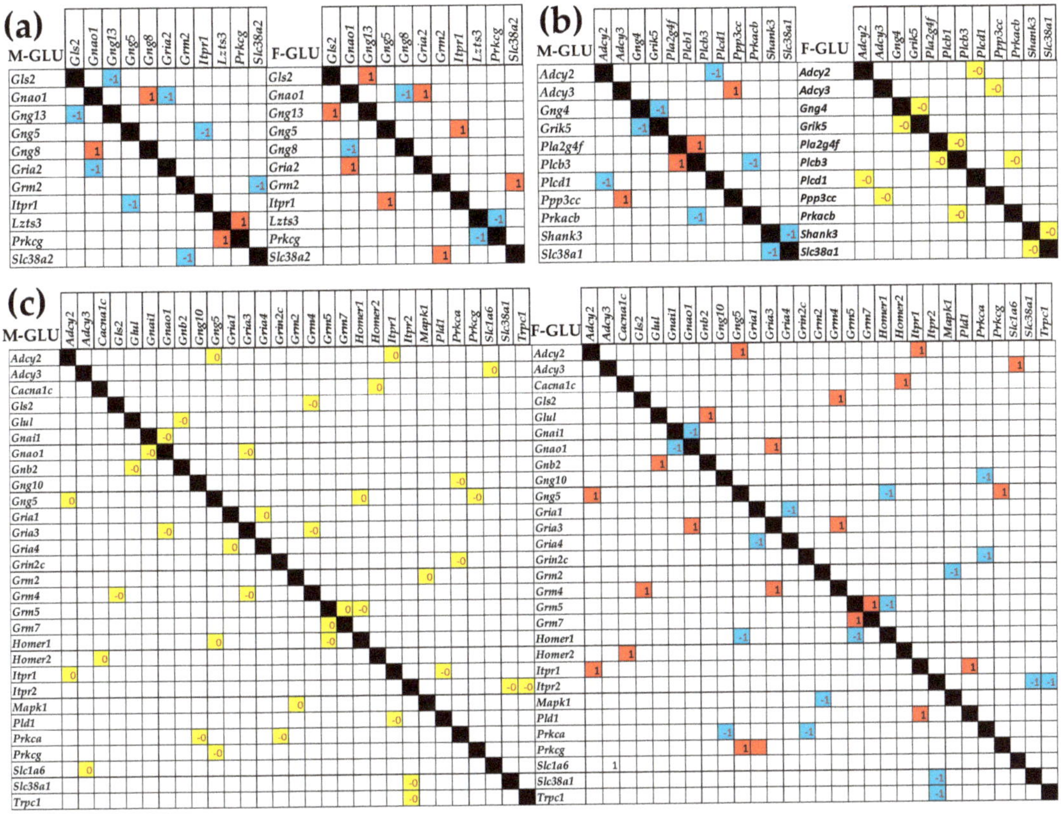

Figure 7. Significant sex dichotomy in the expression correlations among the GLU genes. (**a**) Gene pairs that switch their significant synergistic (red square) or antagonistic (blue square) correlation in one sex to the opposite in the other. (**b**) Significantly synergistically (red square) and antagonistically (blue square) correlated gene pairs in males that were independently (yellow square) expressed in females. (**c**) Significantly independently (yellow square) expressed genes in males that were significantly synergistically (red square) or antagonistically (blue square) expressed in females.

3.8. Sex Dichotomy of the Genes' Hierarchy

Table 4 lists the most influential neurotransmission genes (higher GCH) and the Gene Master Regulators in all six groups of the profiled samples. The relevant neurotransmission genes, *Gnb4*, *Gng10*, and *Gng12*, are part of all five synaptic pathways. *GCHs* were computed using the software #GENE COMMANDING HEIGHT# [52]. Of note is the substantially lower GCH scores of the top neurotransmission genes with respect to the corresponding GMRs in the six groups: *Erg28* (40 vs. 20 for *Pik3r2* in MSN), *Erap1* (70 vs. 26 for *Abat* in FSN), *Tmem238* (162 vs. 16 for *Gphn* in MBN), *Taf8* (38 vs. 14 for *Grm8* in FBN), and *Tmem134* (78 vs. 19 for *Mapk10* in MBY, respectively, 78 vs. Homer1 in F-BYS).

Table 4. The Gene Commanding Height (CGH) scores of the most influential neurotransmission genes compared to those of the Gene Master Regulators in all six groups of profiled samples.

Gene	Description	PATH	Male			Female		
			SN	BN	BY	SN	BN	BY
Pik3r2	phosphoinositide-3-kinase, regulatory subunit 2	3	20	4	1	2	3	1
Gng12	guanine nucleotide binding protein (G protein), gamma 12	12345	8	2	8	5	1	8
Ppp1ca	protein phosphatase 1, catalytic subunit, alpha isozyme	4	7	9	4	2	6	4
Ppp2r1a	protein phosphatase 2, regulatory subunit A, alpha	4	7	3	2	3	1	2
Calml4	calmodulin-like 4	4	6	2	3	2	1	3
Abat	4-aminobutyrate aminotransferase	2	3	4	5	26	6	5
Pld1	phospholipase D1	1	1	1	2	17	1	2
Slc6a7	solute carrier family 6 (neurotransmitter transporter), member 7	0	4	1	4	11	1	4
Gabra1	gamma-aminobutyric acid (GABA) A receptor, alpha 1	2	1	2	4	8	2	4
Homer1	homer homolog 1	1	1	2	13	8	2	13
Gphn	gephyrin	2	3	16	0	3	2	0
Ap2a2	adaptor-related protein complex 2, alpha 2 subunit	0	1	16	3	2	2	3
Creb3l1	cAMP responsive element binding protein 3-like 1	34	1	14	4	3	1	4
Gng10	guanine nucleotide binding protein (G protein), gamma 10	12345	2	11	4	2	3	4
Gabbr1	gamma-aminobutyric acid (GABA) B receptor 1	2	1	10	5	5	2	5
Grm8	glutamate receptor, metabotropic 8	1	2	1	5	3	14	5
Cpne3	copine III	0	2	2	2	1	14	2
Atp6v1h	ATPase, H+ transporting, lysosomal V1 subunit H	0	4	3	6	2	12	6
Atp6v0e1	ATPase, H+ transporting, lysosomal, V0 subunit e1	0	3	1	1	3	12	1
Gabarapl2	GABA(A) receptor-associated protein like 2	2	3	8	7	1	10	7
Mapk10	mitogen activated protein kinase 10	4	2	6	19	1	1	19
Homer1	homer homolog 1	1	1	2	13	8	2	13
Th	tyrosine hydroxylase	4	1	1	11	2	1	11
Gnb4	guanine nucleotide binding protein (G protein), beta polypeptide 4	12345	3	5	10	6	1	10
Glul	glutamate-ammonia ligase	12	1	1	10	3	5	10
Mapk10	mitogen activated protein kinase 10	4	2	6	19	1	1	19
Homer1	homer homolog 1	1	1	2	13	8	2	13
Th	tyrosine hydroxylase	4	1	1	11	2	1	11
Gnb4	guanine nucleotide binding protein (G protein), beta polypeptide 4	12345	3	5	10	6	1	10
Glul	glutamate-ammonia ligase	12	1	1	10	3	5	10
Erg28	ergosterol biosynthesis 28 homolog		40	6	1	3	7	1
Erap1	endoplasmic reticulum aminopeptidase 1		2	2	2	70	2	2
Tmem238	transmembrane protein 238		4	162	3	3	4	3
Taf8	TAF8 RNA polymerase II, TATA box binding protein (TBP)-associated factor		1	1	3	5	38	3
Tmem134	transmembrane protein 134		2	7	78	5	2	78
Tmem134	transmembrane protein 134		2	7	78	5	2	78

4. Discussion

While a certain sex-specific prevalence of IESS in boys was discovered in large cohort studies [22], and we also saw trends to increased susceptibility in males, this never reached statistical significance in our relatively small experimental cohorts (<20 per sex group) on an IESS rat model. Nevertheless, the very sensitive and unbiased transcriptomic analyses were able to provide a glimpse of the significant sex dichotomy in the genomic molecular machinery.

The analyses of six neurotransmission pathways in the PVNs of male and female rats at P16 revealed substantial transcriptomic differences between the two sexes, which extend, although at different levels, to the betamethasone prenatally primed pups with and without NMDA-triggered spasms.

Beyond traditional gene expression studies that are limited to quantifying the expression profile, our approach incorporates two additional independent measures of the individual genes: the control of transcripts' abundances and the inter-coordination of their expression. Together, the three independent measures provide the most comprehensive characterization of the two sexes' PVN transcriptomic topologies and their differential remodeling in infantile spasms.

Although the tissue pieces were very small, they were still heterocellular, which is one major limitation of this study. In the worst scenario, the non-significant change in genes, when comparing different conditions for the same sex or different sexes for the same condition, might result from up-regulation in a particular phenotype and down-regulation in another. However, taking a particular type of cell from its natural environment would have a larger effect on the transcriptome, as we proved by profiling cortical astrocytes and precursor oligodendrocytes when co-cultured and cultured separately [55–57].

We found (Table 1) few sex differences between the expression levels of the top neurotransmission genes. For instance, the active regulator of intracellular Ca^{2+} release, *Caly,* has the largest expression level among all neurotransmission genes in the PVNs of both sexes in all three investigated conditions. An abundance of *Cali* transcripts was between 126 and 195 times larger than the expression level of the median gene in the respective group, close enough to *Cst3* and *Rpl41*, the top-expressed genes in the entire transcriptome. *Cali*, localized in the neuron dendritic spines, is related to D1 dopaminergic transmission and schizophrenia [31,32]. However, the expression of *Caly* (Table 2) was less controlled than the median gene in all groups, $REC = -0.98$ in MSN, −0.41 in FSN, −1.26 in MBN, −0.90 in FBN, −0.85 in MBY, and −0.69 in FBY, indicating remarkable flexibility.

As seen in Table 2, the most controlled neurotransmission genes are as follows: *Pik3r2* and *Abat* in the two SN groups, *Pik3r5* and *Grm8* in BNSs, and *Th* and *Trpc1* in BYSs. Interestingly, a mutation of *Pik3R2* was associated with familial temporal lobe epilepsy [58], and its overexpression may reduce cell viability and boost autophagy and apoptosis [59]. GABA transaminase deficiency caused by a mutation of *Abat* leads to neonatal epilepsy [60], while activation through the FOXA2/ABAT/GABA axis mediates the development of brain metastasis in lung cancer [61]. Therefore, the high control of these two genes in the normal condition (SN) prevents neurotransmission alterations associated with IEES in the corresponding sex.

Moreover (see Supplementary Table S2 for the M/F ratios of RCS), neurogenes like *Mapk10* in SN, *Pik3r5* (BN), and *Th* (BY) are strictly controlled in males but allowed to fluctuate in females in the corresponding conditions. In contrast, genes like *Abat* and *Gabbr1* in SN and *Trpc1* (BY) are flexibly expressed in males but strictly controlled in females in the corresponding conditions. Both *Mapk10* and *Gabbr1* are considered potential targets for vascular dementia treatment [62,63]. The differences are even larger for the top controlled genes in each condition, with *Erg28, Tmem238,* and *Oxsr1* very strictly controlled in males but much less controlled in females, while the opposite is observed for *Erap1*, *Cul7*, and *Tac2*. All these differences point to distinct homeostatic mechanisms that control the transcripts' abundances.

The effect of IEES triggering in betamethasone primed rats (BY condition) has distinct sex-dependent effects on genes' RCSs (Supplementary Table S3). While the RCSs of *Pik3r2* are increased by IEES in males (by 6.49×), with little effect on females, that of *Gnal* is increased in females (by 8.84×). *Gnal* having greater effects on female than on male dystonia was recently documented in a population study [64].

There are also substantial sex differences among the most flexibly expressed neurotransmission genes (Table 3) in all three conditions: *Calml1* vs. *Mapk10* in SN, *Drd2* vs. *Creb3* in BN, and *Clock* vs. *Grin1* in BY. Interestingly, all the top flexible genes are included in the dopaminergic synapse pathway. Although several other reports discussed sex differences in the expressions of neurotransmission genes and their encoded proteins (e.g., [65–69]), here, we report, for the first time, the sex dichotomy in gene expression control.

Th, a rate-limiting enzyme (tyrosine hydroxylase) in dopamine, epinephrine, and norepinephrine biosynthesis [70], has a spectacular (by 44.51×) RCS increase in IESS with respect to the healthy counterpart in males (Supplementary Table S3), which is also 14.58× larger than in females' BYSs. Therefore, we consider that *Th* might be a potential gene therapy target for future research for a male with IESS but not for a female with IESS.

In contrast, the control strength of *Creb3* in females decreased significantly (by 8.68×) in both BN and BY conditions (Supplementary Table S3). The *Creb3* protein tethers chromatin to the cell's inner nuclear membrane and prevents karyoptosis, a type of cell death caused by DNA release into the cytosol [71]. Therefore, the high expression flexibility of the encoding gene makes both cholinergic and dopaminergic transmission more adaptable to prenatal corticosteroids, even in the absence of IS.

Figure 2a shows a higher synaptic vesicle acidification following endocytosis but a lower neurotransmission uptake in male versus female PVNs. Apparently, these differences indicate that in males, there is a higher efficiency in recycling the synaptic vesicles, yet a decreased release of neurotransmitters compared to females. However, as demonstrated in Figure 3a,b, IESS induction does not cause an overall imbalance of the synaptic vesicle cycle in either sex. Interestingly, reports by others demonstrated that some factors, such as exposure to diazepam [72] or maternal immune activation [73], affect the synaptic vesicle cycle pathway. We further found substantial differences between the significantly regulated genes by IESS in males (Figure 2a) and in females (Figure 2b). For instance, while in males, the ATPase *Atp2a2* (also known as. *Serca2*), is involved in actively pumping Ca^{2+} from the cytosol into the endoplasmic reticulum and is a candidate gene for IESS [74] is down-regulated, it is up-regulated in females. We can speculate that this calcium homeostasis regulator [75] may be responding to different cytosolic calcium conditions after betamethasone/spasm exposure in males and females. While *ATP2A2* is a monogenic cause of Darier disease (a skin disorder with neuropsychiatric abnormalities), the prevalence of epilepsy in this condition is higher than in the general population [76]. Interestingly, our unpublished in vitro data (not stratified for sex) indicate that hippocampal LTP is diminished after prenatal betamethasone exposure, and this effect is independent of NMDA-induced spasms, and increasing the number of subjects and stratification by sex may fully reveal the biological importance of this finding.

Figure 2b indicates lower glutamatergic transmission in control saline-injected (i.e., SN) males compared to the female PVNs, caused by the underexpression of *Grik1* and Slc1a2 in the presynaptic neuron. The higher expression of *Grik1* in women relative to that in men was also detected in patients with depression [77]. Through the underexpression of *Gabra4, Gabrd,* and *Gabrdg1,* Figure 2c confirms the report [78] of male rats lagging behind females in the development of the ionotropic of GABA-A receptors. The underexpression of the G proteins *Gnb4* and *Gng5* in males with respect to their female counterparts was common to all five investigated synapse pathways (Figure 2b–f). These G proteins are involved in the presynaptic inhibition, diminishing the release of glutamate, GABA, and Ach release in the synaptic cleft [79,80]. However, the effect of the reduced expression of the G proteins is compensated by the increased expression of the inositol 1,4,5-trisphosphate receptors *Itpr1* and *Itpr2* (*Itpr3* was not quantified). The activation of these receptors releases Ca^{2+} (which controls almost all important cellular processes [81]) from the intracellular IP_3-sensitive storage [82].

The differences between the two sexes also appear in the regulomes of SVC (Figure 3), GLU (Figure 4), and GABA (Figure 5) pathways after the induction of IESS. For instance, the presynaptic synaptic vesicle regulatory protein *Cplx2* (complexin 2), whose variants affect cognition and memory in schizophrenic patients [83,84], is down-regulated in males (Figure 3a) but up-regulated in females (Figure 3b). A very recent study looking at the percentage reads of new isoforms identified new *CPLX2* isoforms not only in patients with schizophrenia but also in patients with epilepsy [85]. Our finding of altered *Cplx2* expression indirectly corroborates a study on chronic mild stress that links *Cplx2* to the anxiety-susceptible experimental rat group [86]. The expression of several genes (e.g., Kcnj3 and *Trpc1*) was not affected in one sex (female) but was significantly regulated in the other. These findings suggest that dissimilar pathological processes affected the neurotransmission in the two sexes. Among others, our result explains why the suppression of the potassium channel encoded by *Kcnj3* impairs prelimbic cortical function in male but not female mice [87].

Figure 6 presents the spectacular differences between the male and female statistically significant SVC pathway transcriptome networks. Thus, three antagonistically expressed gene pairs in males (*Atp6v0a2–Atp6v0a4, Atp6v1g2–Dnm2, Dnm2-Nsf*) were switched to synergistically expressed pairs in females, while the pair *Cacna1a–Slc6a7* was switched from synergistically expressed in males to antagonistically expressed in females (Figure 6a). Moreover, six independently expressed gene pairs in males were significantly synergistically or antagonistically correlated in females (Figure 6b), and eight synergistically or antagonistically expressed in males were independently expressed in females (Figure 6c).

Given the roles of v-ATPase subunits in phagocytosis, endocytosis, and autophagy [88], it would be interesting to study the functional consequences of the opposite expression coordination of *Atp6v0a2* and *Atp6v0a4* in the two sexes. Of note is the sex discrepancy in the expression correlation of the dynamin *Dnm2*, responsible for vesicle recovery after releasing the neurotransmitters into the synaptic cleft, with the v-ATPase *Atp6v1g2* involved in vesicle acidification needed for neurotransmitter uptake. Also surprising is the antagonistic expression of *Nsf* (which removes the cis-SNARE complex [89]) and *Dnm2* in males, while they are supposed to stimulate each other's expression (as it happens in females).

Likewise, we found substantial sex differences in the transcriptomic networks of the GLU pathway. Thus, the antagonistically expressed pairs in males, *Gng13-Gls2, Gria2-Gnao1, Itpr1-Gng5,* and *Slc38a2-Grm2,* are synergistically expressed in females, while the synergistically expressed pairs in males, *Gng8-Gnao1,* and *Prkcg-Lzts3,* are antagonistically expressed in females (Figure 6a). In addition, six significantly correlated gene pairs in males are independently expressed in females, and 20 (*sic!*) independently expressed pairs in males are significantly correlated in females. The opposite expression correlations of *Gng13* with *Gls2* in the two sexes suggest an opposite relationship between mitophagy and the feedback inhibition of glutamate release. Such coordination might have consequences on the epilepsy occurrence [90], where *Gls2* is down-regulated (as we also found, Figure 4a).

All these transcriptomic network differences indicate distinct molecular mechanisms responsible for the formation of synaptic vesicles, the release of neurotransmitters, and the response by the post-synaptic neurons in the PVNs of the two sexes. The neurotransmission differences are most likely responsible for different brain circuitries in males and females (e.g., [91–93]).

Interestingly, we observed that the genes involved in neurotransmission are not among the most influential in both male and female rats subjected to each of the three conditions. Yet, the most prominent genes in the IESS condition, *Grm8* (male) and *Mapk10* (female), have documented implications in epilepsy (e.g., [94–96]). However, the present study pinpoints *Tmem134*, a protein located in the perinuclear region of the cytoplasm, involved in RNA splicing [97] and associated with obesity [98], as the best target for the gene therapy of IESS in rats of both sexes based on symmetrical expression change in both sexes. Additionally, our model suggests a significant involvement of hypothalamic nuclei, such as the arcuate nucleus [7], also participating in the control of food intake. *Tmem134* is also involved in the regulation of the NF-kappaB pathway [33]. Activity in this pathway is increased after seizures, and the down-regulation of this pathway attenuates seizures [99]. Hence, affecting this pathway through Tmem134 may provide a feasible way for the control of spasms. In previous reports, we assumed and verified [52,100] that the manipulation of genes with higher *GCHs* has greater consequences on the transcriptome, the top gene, named the Gene Master Regulator (GMR), being the most influential, whose silence might be lethal for the cell.

There are several limitations of this study. First, a sample size of 12 is too low to provide reliable stratification by sex, especially if biological variables such as spasms or body weight are considered. Second, our transcriptomic data were not further validated in a proteomic experiment. This may discount the observed effects only to the transcriptome without translation to the effector proteins. Since, in addition to translation, protein abundance is affected by several post-translational modifications, and the genes' expression correlations do not exactly overlap the protein–protein interactions, our results are relevant only at the transcriptomic level, and integration with epigenetic and proteomic data is needed to strengthen the conclusion. However, our electrophysiology data [101], as well as a behavioral study [102], indicate electrophysiological as well as behavioral effects of prenatal betamethasone exposure, though larger sample sizes would be required for proper stratification by sex. Finally, the effects of repetitive spasms during development (P12, P13, P15) on behaviors and delayed seizure susceptibility are still being investigated and therefore are missing as comparators.

5. Conclusions

Our transcriptomic analysis of six neurotransmission pathways in the PVNs of P16 12 male and 12 female rats revealed substantial sex differences, persisting even in prenatally betamethasone-primed pups, regardless of NMDA triggering of IESS. By integrating expression level, transcript abundance control, and expression inter-coordination, we provide the most theoretically possible comprehensive transcriptomic characterization of these differences. Nonetheless, because transcript abundances and protein content are not proportional [103,104] (gene transcription is triggered by the necessity to maintain a certain level of proteins), our results cannot be automatically translated into sex-dependent proteome topology and remodeling by IESS.

Sex-specific transcriptomic shifts in synaptic vesicle cycling, glutamatergic, and GABAergic pathways suggest distinct pathological mechanisms, influenced by the sex hormones [105–107]. We found that gene co-expression patterns differed, highlighting the fundamental sex-dependent synaptic organization that determines brain circuits (e.g., [108–110]). This study extends our previous findings of sex transcriptomic dichotomy in regions of the brain [8–10], heart [111,112], and kidneys [113].

Finally, in our rat model, *Tmem134* (encoding cytosolic and membrane proteins likely involved in the cytokine pathway [33]) emerged as the most influential gene for IESS pathology in both sexes. Nevertheless, the dominance of *Tmem134* is surprising and deserves to be tested in further experiments on the same IEES rat model.

Supplementary Materials: The following supporting information can be downloaded at: https://www.mdpi.com/article/10.3390/cimb47050380/s1.

Author Contributions: Conceptualization, D.A.I. and L.V.; methodology, D.A.I., T.C. and C.-R.C.; software, D.A.I.; validation, S.I., D.A.I., T.C., C.-R.C., K.V., J.V. and L.V.; formal analysis, D.A.I.;

investigation, S.I., L.V., J.V. and K.V.; resources, D.A.I. and L.V.; data curation, D.A.I.; writing—original draft preparation, D.A.I., J.V., T.C., C.-R.C., K.V. and L.V.; writing—review and editing, D.A.I., J.V., T.C., C.-R.C., K.V. and L.V.; visualization, S.I.; supervision, D.A.I. and L.V.; project administration, D.A.I.; funding acquisition, L.V. All authors have read and agreed to the published version of the manuscript.

Funding: Supported by the NIH awards RC4 NS072966, R21 NS118337, by the CURE Epilepsy Infantile Spasms Consortium Award, and by the Graduate School of Biomedical Sciences at the New York Medical College.

Institutional Review Board Statement: The animal study protocol was approved by the IACUC of New York College of Medicine, #52-1-0913 approved on 25 September 2013 for 3 years.

Informed Consent Statement: Not applicable.

Data Availability Statement: The wet protocol and the microarray raw data were deposited in the publicly accessible Gene Ex-pression Omnibus: https://www.ncbi.nlm.nih.gov/gds/?term=gse123721, https://www.ncbi.nlm.nih.gov/gds/?term=gse124613, https://www.ncbi.nlm.nih.gov/gds/?term=gse128091 (accessed on 1 April 2025).

Conflicts of Interest: The authors declare no conflict of interest.

References

1. Synaptic Vesicle Cycle. Available online: https://www.genome.jp/kegg-bin/show_pathway?rno04721 (accessed on 12 December 2024).
2. Glutamatergic Synapse. Available online: https://www.genome.jp/pathway/rno04724 (accessed on 12 December 2024).
3. GABAergic Synapse. Available online: https://www.genome.jp/kegg-bin/show_pathway?rno04727 (accessed on 12 December 2024).
4. Cholinergic Synapse. Available online: https://www.genome.jp/kegg-bin/show_pathway?rno04725 (accessed on 12 December 2024).
5. Dopaminergic Synapse. Available online: https://www.genome.jp/kegg-bin/show_pathway?rno04728 (accessed on 12 December 2024).
6. Serotonergic Synapse. Available online: https://www.genome.jp/kegg-bin/show_pathway?rno04726 (accessed on 12 December 2024).
7. Velíšek, L.; Jehle, K.; Asche, S.; Velíšková, J. Model of infantile spasms induced by N-methyl-D-aspartic acid in prenatally impaired brain. *Ann. Neurol.* **2007**, *61*, 109–119. [CrossRef] [PubMed]
8. Iacobas, D.A.; Iacobas, S.; Chachua, T.; Goletiani, C.; Sidyelyeva, G.; Veliskova, J.; Velisek, L. Prenatal corticosteroids modify glutamatergic and GABAergic synapse genomic fabric: Insights from a novel animal model of infantile spasms. *J. Neuroendocrinol.* **2013**, *25*, 964–979. [CrossRef] [PubMed]
9. Iacobas, D.A.; Chachua, T.; Iacobas, S.; Benson, M.J.; Borges, K.; Veliskova, J.; Velisek, L. ACTH and PMX53 recover synaptic transcriptome alterations in a rat model of infantile spasms. *Sci. Rep.* **2018**, *8*, 5722. [CrossRef]
10. Iacobas, D.A.; Velisek, L. Regeneration of neurotransmission transcriptome in a model of epileptic encephalopathy after antiinflammatory treatment. *Neural Regen. Res.* **2018**, *13*, 1715–1718. [CrossRef]
11. Hrachovy, R.A. West's syndrome (infantile spasms). Clinical description and diagnosis. *Adv. Exp. Med. Biol.* **2002**, *497*, 33–50.
12. Dulac, O.; Soufflet, C.; Chiron, C.; Kaminska, A. What is West syndrome? *Int. Rev. Neurobiol.* **2002**, *49*, 1–22.
13. Hrachovy, R.A.; Frost, J.D., Jr. Infantile spasms. In *Handbook of Clinical Neurology*; Elsevier: Amsterdam, The Netherlands, 2013; Volume 111, pp. 611–618. [CrossRef]
14. Pavone, P.; Striano, P.; Falsaperla, R.; Pavone, L.; Ruggieri, M. Infantile spasms syndrome, West syndrome and related phenotypes: What we know in 2013. *Brain Dev.* **2014**, *36*, 739–751. [CrossRef]
15. Mackay, M.T.; Weiss, S.K.; Adams-Webber, T.; Ashwal, S.; Stephens, D.; Ballaban-Gill, K.; Baram, T.Z.; Duchowny, M.; Hirtz, D.; Pellock, J.M.; et al. Practice parameter: Medical treatment of infantile spasms: Report of the American Academy of Neurology and the Child Neurology Society. *Neurology* **2004**, *62*, 1668–1681. [CrossRef]
16. Go, C.Y.; Mackay, M.T.; Weiss, S.K.; Stephens, D.; Adams-Webber, T.; Ashwal, S.; Snead, O.C., 3rd; Child Neurology Society; American Academy of Neurology. Evidence-based guideline update: Medical treatment of infantile spasms: Report of the Guideline Development Subcommittee of the American Academy of Neurology and the Practice Committee of the Child Neurology Society. *Neurology* **2012**, *78*, 1974–1980. [CrossRef]
17. Riikonen, R. The latest on infantile spasms. *Curr. Opin. Neurol.* **2005**, *18*, 91–95. [CrossRef]

18. Lux, A.L.; Edwards, S.W.; Hancock, E.; Johnson, A.L.; Kennedy, C.R.; Newton, R.W.; O'Callaghan, F.J.; Verity, C.M.; Osborne, J.P. The United Kingdom Infantile Spasms Study (UKISS) comparing hormone treatment with vigabatrin on developmental and epilepsy outcomes to age 14 months: A multicentre randomised trial. *Lancet Neurol.* **2005**, *4*, 712–717. [CrossRef]
19. Riikonen, R. Long-term outcome of patients with West syndrome. *Brain Dev.* **2001**, *23*, 683–687. [CrossRef]
20. Luthvigsson, P.; Olafsson, E.; Sigurthardottir, S.; Hauser, W.A. Epidemiologic features of infantile spasms in Iceland. *Epilepsia* **1994**, *35*, 802–805. [CrossRef]
21. Harini, C.; Nagarajan, E.; Bergin, A.M.; Pearl, P.; Loddenkemper, T.; Takeoka, M.; Morrison, P.F.; Coulter, D.; Harappanahally, G.; Marti, C.; et al. Mortality in infantile spasms: A hospital-based study. *Epilepsia* **2020**, *61*, 702–713. [CrossRef]
22. Hancock, E.C.; Osborne, J.P.; Edwards, S.W. Treatment of infantile spasms. *Cochrane Database Syst. Rev.* **2013**, CD001770. [CrossRef]
23. Chachua, T.; Yum, M.-S.; Velíšková, J.; Velíšek, L. Validation of the rat model of cryptogenic infantile spasms. *Epilepsia* **2011**, *52*, 1666–1677. [CrossRef]
24. Mareš, P.; Velíšek, L. N-methyl-D-aspartate (NMDA)-induced seizures in developing rats. *Dev. Brain Res.* **1992**, *65*, 185–189. [CrossRef]
25. Yum, M.S.; Chachua, T.; Velíšková, J.; Velíšek, L. Prenatal stress promotes development of spasms in infant rats. *Epilepsia* **2012**, *53*, e46–e49. [CrossRef]
26. Tsuji, M.; Takahashi, Y.; Watabe, A.M.; Kato, F. Enhanced long-term potentiation in mature rats in a model of epileptic spasms with betamethasone-priming and postnatal N-methyl-d-aspartate administration. *Epilepsia* **2016**, *57*, 495–505. [CrossRef]
27. Baek, H.; Yi, M.H.; Pandit, S.; Park, J.B.; Kwon, H.H.; Zhang, E.; Kim, S.; Shin, N.; Kim, E.; Lee, Y.H.; et al. Altered expression of KCC2 in GABAergic interneuron contributes prenatal stress-induced epileptic spasms in infant rat. *Neurochem. Int.* **2016**, *97*, 57–64. [CrossRef]
28. Janicot, R.; Shao, L.R.; Stafstrom, C.E. 2-deoxyglucose and beta-hydroxybutyrate fail to attenuate seizures in the betamethasone-NMDA model of infantile spasms. *Epilepsia Open* **2022**, *7*, 181–186. [CrossRef] [PubMed]
29. Savic, B.; Murphy, D.; Japundzic-Zigon, N. The Paraventricular Nucleus of the Hypothalamus in Control of Blood Pressure and Blood Pressure Variability. *Front. Physiol.* **2022**, *13*, 858941. [CrossRef]
30. Velíšková, J. Sex matters in epilepsy. In *Developmental Epilepsy: From Clinical Medicine to Neurobiological Mechanisms*; Stafstrom, C.E., Velíšek, L., Eds.; World Scientific Publishing: Singapore, 2019; pp. 387–405.
31. Koh, P.O.; Bergson, C.; Undie, A.S.; Goldman-Rakic, P.S.; Lidow, M.S. Up-regulation of the D1 dopamine receptor-interacting protein, calcyon, in patients with schizophrenia. *Arch. Gen. Psychiatry* **2003**, *60*, 311–319. [CrossRef]
32. Ha, C.M.; Park, D.; Han, J.K.; Jang, J.I.; Park, J.Y.; Hwang, E.M.; Seok, H.; Chang, S. Calcyon forms a novel ternary complex with dopamine D1 receptor through PSD-95 protein and plays a role in dopamine receptor internalization. *J. Biol. Chem.* **2012**, *287*, 31813–31822. [CrossRef]
33. Tian, Y.; Huang, W.; Yang, J.; Wen, Z.; Geng, Y.; Zhao, C.; Zhang, H.; Wang, Y. Systematic identification of hepatitis E virus ORF2 interactome reveals that TMEM134 engages in ORF2-mediated NF-kappaB pathway. *Virus Res.* **2017**, *228*, 102–108. [CrossRef]
34. Gold, M.S.; Blum, K.; Oscar-Berman, M.; Braverman, E.R. Low dopamine function in attention deficit/hyperactivity disorder: Should genotyping signify early diagnosis in children? *Postgrad. Med.* **2014**, *126*, 153–177. [CrossRef]
35. Puig, M.V.; Gulledge, A.T. Serotonin and prefrontal cortex function: Neurons, networks, and circuits. *Mol. Neurobiol.* **2011**, *44*, 449–464. [CrossRef]
36. Lei, S. Serotonergic modulation of Neural activities in the entorhinal cortex. *Int. J. Physiol. Pathophysiol. Pharmacol.* **2012**, *4*, 201–210.
37. Seyedabadi, M.; Fakhfouri, G.; Ramezani, V.; Mehr, S.E.; Rahimian, R. The role of serotonin in memory: Interactions with neurotransmitters and downstream signaling. *Exp. Brain Res.* **2014**, *232*, 723–738. [CrossRef]
38. Bakker, J. The role of steroid hormones in the sexual differentiation of the human brain. *J. Neuroendocrinol.* **2022**, *34*, e13050. [CrossRef]
39. Cutia, C.A.; Christian-Hinman, C.A. Mechanisms linking neurological disorders with reproductive endocrine dysfunction: Insights from epilepsy research. *Front. Neuroendocrinol.* **2023**, *71*, 101084. [CrossRef]
40. Akman, O.; Moshe, S.L.; Galanopoulou, A.S. Sex-specific consequences of early life seizures. *Neurobiol. Dis.* **2014**, *72 Pt B*, 153–166. [CrossRef]
41. Iacobas, S.; Neal-Perry, G.; Iacobas, D.A. Analyzing the Cytoskeletal Transcriptome: Sex Differences in Rat Hypothalamus. In *The Cytoskeleton*; Neuromethods Series; Dermietzel, R., Ed.; Humana Press: Totowa, NJ, USA, 2013; Volume 79.
42. Velíšková, J.; Iacobas, D.; Iacobas, S.; Sidyelyeva, G.; Chachua, T.; Velíšek, L. Oestradiol Regulates Neuropeptide Y Release and Gene Coupling with the GABAergic and Glutamatergic Synapses in the Adult Female Rat Dentate Gyrus. *J. Neuroendocrinol.* **2015**, *27*, 911–920. [CrossRef]

43. Bakker, J. The Sexual Differentiation of the Human Brain: Role of Sex Hormones Versus Sex Chromosomes. *Curr. Top. Behav. Neurosci.* **2019**, *43*, 45–67. [CrossRef]
44. Sex Differences in the Synaptic Genomic Fabrics of the Rat Hypothalamic Paraventricular Node. Available online: https://www.ncbi.nlm.nih.gov/geo/query/acc.cgi?acc=GSE123721 (accessed on 1 April 2025).
45. Prenatal Betamethasone Remodels the Genomic Fabrics of the Synaptic Transmission in the Rat Hypothalamic Paraventricular Nucleus. Available online: https://www.ncbi.nlm.nih.gov/geo/query/acc.cgi?acc=GSE124613 (accessed on 1 April 2025).
46. Remodeling of Synaptic Transmission Genomic Fabrics in the Hypothalamic Paraventricular Nucleus of a Rat Model of Autism. Available online: https://www.ncbi.nlm.nih.gov/geo/query/acc.cgi?acc=GSE128091 (accessed on 1 April 2025).
47. Iacobas, D.A. The Genomic Fabric Perspective on the Transcriptome Between Universal Quantifiers and Personalized Genomic Medicine. *Biol. Theory* **2016**, *11*, 123–137. [CrossRef]
48. Iacobas, D.A.; Iacobas, S.; Lee, P.R.; Cohen, J.E.; Fields, R.D. Coordinated Activity of Transcriptional Networks Responding to the Pattern of Action Potential Firing in Neurons. *Genes* **2019**, *10*, 754. [CrossRef]
49. Bicknell, R.J. Sex-steroid actions on neurotransmission. *Curr. Opin. Neurol.* **1998**, *11*, 667–671. [CrossRef]
50. Foster, T.C.; Kumar, A. Sex, senescence, senolytics, and cognition. *Front. Aging Neurosci.* **2025**, *17*, 1555872. [CrossRef]
51. Sinclair, D.; Purves-Tyson, T.D.; Allen, K.M.; Weickert, C.S. Impacts of stress and sex hormones on dopamine neurotransmission in the adolescent brain. *Psychopharmacology* **2014**, *231*, 1581–1599. [CrossRef]
52. Iacobas, S.; Ede, N.; Iacobas, D.A. The Gene Master Regulators (GMR) Approach Provides Legitimate Targets for Personalized, Time-Sensitive Cancer Gene Therapy. *Genes* **2019**, *10*, 560. [CrossRef]
53. Krishna, S.; Cheng, B.; Sharma, D.R.; Yadav, S.; Stempinski, E.S.; Mamtani, S.; Shah, E.; Deo, A.; Acherjee, T.; Thomas, T.; et al. PPAR-gamma activation enhances myelination and neurological recovery in premature rabbits with intraventricular hemorrhage. *Proc. Natl. Acad. Sci. USA* **2021**, *118*, e2103084118. [CrossRef] [PubMed]
54. Kanehisa, M. The KEGG database. In *Silico'Simulation of Biological Processes: Novartis Foundation Symposium 247*; John Wiley & Sons, Ltd.: Chichester, UK, 2002; pp. 91–101; discussion 101–103, 119–128, 244–252.
55. Iacobas, S.; Iacobas, D.A. Astrocyte proximity modulates the myelination gene fabric of oligodendrocytes. *Neuron Glia Biol.* **2010**, *6*, 157–169. [CrossRef] [PubMed]
56. Iacobas, S.; Thomas, N.M.; Iacobas, D.A. Plasticity of the myelination genomic fabric. *Mol. Genet. Genom.* **2012**, *287*, 237–246. [CrossRef]
57. Iacobas, D.A.; Iacobas, S.; Stout, R.F.; Spray, D.C. Cellular Environment Remodels the Genomic Fabrics of Functional Pathways in Astrocytes. *Genes* **2020**, *11*, 520. [CrossRef]
58. Wang, Y.; Peng, J.; Bai, S.; Yu, H.; He, H.; Fan, C.; Hao, Y.; Guan, Y. A PIK3R2 Mutation in Familial Temporal Lobe Epilepsy as a Possible Pathogenic Variant. *Front. Genet.* **2021**, *12*, 596709. [CrossRef]
59. Ge, J.; Jiao, X.; Li, H. MicroRNA-126-3P targets PIK3R2 to ameliorate autophagy and apoptosis of cortex in hypoxia-reoxygenation treated neonatal rats. *Cell. Mol. Biol.* **2023**, *69*, 210–217. [CrossRef]
60. Feng, Y.; Wei, Z.H.; Liu, C.; Li, G.Y.; Qiao, X.Z.; Gan, Y.J.; Zhang, C.C.; Deng, Y.C. Genetic variations in GABA metabolism and epilepsy. *Seizure* **2022**, *101*, 22–29. [CrossRef]
61. Xie, M.; Qin, H.; Liu, L.; Wu, J.; Zhao, Z.; Zhao, Y.; Fang, Y.; Yu, X.; Su, C. GABA regulates metabolic reprogramming to mediate the development of brain metastasis in non-small cell lung cancer. *J. Exp. Clin. Cancer Res.* **2025**, *44*, 61. [CrossRef]
62. Wang, J.; Wang, X.; Yang, J.; Zhen, Y.; Ban, W.; Zhu, G. Molecular profiling of a rat model of vascular dementia: Evidences from proteomics, metabolomics and experimental validations. *Brain Res.* **2025**, *1846*, 149254. [CrossRef]
63. Zheng, C.; Zhao, Y.; Hu, C.; Zhang, L.; Li, G.; Yang, C. Transcriptomic and network analysis identifies shared pathways across Alzheimer's disease and vascular dementia. *Brain Res.* **2025**, *1854*, 149548. [CrossRef] [PubMed]
64. Kilic-Berkmen, G.; Scorr, L.M.; McKay, L.; Thayani, M.; Donsante, Y.; Perlmutter, J.S.; Norris, S.A.; Wright, L.; Klein, C.; Feuerstein, J.S.; et al. Sex Differences in Dystonia. *Mov. Disord. Clin. Pract.* **2024**, *11*, 973–982. [CrossRef] [PubMed]
65. Abeledo-Machado, A.; Peña-Zanoni, M.; Bornancini, D.; Camilletti, M.A.; Faraoni, E.Y.; Marcial, A.; Rulli, S.; Alhenc-Gelas, F.; Díaz-Torga, G.S. Sex-specific Regulation of Prolactin Secretion by Pituitary Bradykinin Receptors. *Endocrinology* **2022**, *163*, bqac108. [CrossRef] [PubMed]
66. Smith, B.S.; Diaguarachchige De Silva, K.H.; Hashemi, A.; Duncan, R.E.; Grapentine, S.; Bakovic, M.; Lu, R. Transcription factor CREB3 is a potent regulator of high-fat diet-induced obesity and energy metabolism. *Int. J. Obes.* **2022**, *46*, 1446–1455. [CrossRef]
67. Deluca, A.; Bascom, B.; Key Planas, D.A.; Kocher, M.A.; Torres, M.; Arbeitman, M.N. Contribution of neurons that express fruitless and Clock transcription factors to behavioral rhythms and courtship. *iScience* **2025**, *28*, 112037. [CrossRef]
68. Towers, E.B.; Kilgore, M.; Bakhti-Suroosh, A.; Pidaparthi, L.; Williams, I.L.; Abel, J.M.; Lynch, W.J. Sex differences in the neuroadaptations associated with incubated cocaine-craving: A focus on the dorsomedial prefrontal cortex. *Front. Behav. Neurosci.* **2023**, *16*, 1027310. [CrossRef]

69. Eskow Jaunarajs, K.L.; Scarduzio, M.; Ehrlich, M.E.; McMahon, L.L.; Standaert, D.G. Diverse Mechanisms Lead to Common Dysfunction of Striatal Cholinergic Interneurons in Distinct Genetic Mouse Models of Dystonia. *J. Neurosci.* **2019**, *39*, 7195–7205. [CrossRef]
70. Daubner, S.C.; Le, T.; Wang, S. Tyrosine hydroxylase and regulation of dopamine synthesis. *Arch. Biochem. Biophys.* **2011**, *508*, 1–12. [CrossRef]
71. Chen, W.; Byun, J.; Kang, H.C.; Lee, H.S.; Lee, J.Y.; Kwon, Y.J.; Cho, Y.Y. Karyoptosis as a novel type of UVB-induced regulated cell death. *Free Radic. Res.* **2024**, *58*, 796–810. [CrossRef]
72. Zhang, Y.; Shi, Y.; Tang, J.; Chen, K.; Wu, M.; Wu, X.; Qiu, X. A transcriptomics-based analysis of mechanisms involved in the sex-dependent effects of diazepam on zebrafish. *Aquat. Toxicol.* **2024**, *275*, 107063. [CrossRef]
73. Yotova, A.Y.; Li, L.L.; O'Leary, A.; Tegeder, I.; Reif, A.; Courtney, M.J.; Slattery, D.A.; Freudenberg, F. Synaptic proteome perturbations after maternal immune activation: Identification of embryonic and adult hippocampal changes. *Brain Behav. Immun.* **2024**, *121*, 351–364. [CrossRef]
74. Peng, J.; Wang, Y.; He, F.; Chen, C.; Wu, L.W.; Yang, L.F.; Ma, Y.P.; Zhang, W.; Shi, Z.Q.; Chen, C.; et al. Novel West syndrome candidate genes in a Chinese cohort. *CNS Neurosci. Ther.* **2018**, *24*, 1196–1206. [CrossRef] [PubMed]
75. Nakajima, K.; Ishiwata, M.; Weitemier, A.Z.; Shoji, H.; Monai, H.; Miyamoto, H.; Yamakawa, K.; Miyakawa, T.; McHugh, T.J.; Kato, T. Brain-specific heterozygous loss-of-function of ATP2A2, endoplasmic reticulum Ca^{2+} pump responsible for Darier's disease, causes behavioral abnormalities and a hyper-dopaminergic state. *Hum. Mol. Genet.* **2021**, *30*, 1762–1772. [CrossRef]
76. Gordon-Smith, K.; Jones, L.A.; Burge, S.M.; Munro, C.S.; Tavadia, S.; Craddock, N. The neuropsychiatric phenotype in Dari-er disease. *Br. J. Dermatol.* **2010**, *163*, 515–522. [CrossRef]
77. Gray, A.L.; Hyde, T.M.; Deep-Soboslay, A.; Kleinman, J.E.; Sodhi, M.S. Sex differences in glutamate receptor gene expression in major depression and suicide. *Mol. Psychiatry* **2015**, *20*, 1057–1068. [CrossRef]
78. Kipnis, P.A.; Sullivan, B.J.; Kadam, S.D. Sex-Dependent Signaling Pathways Underlying Seizure Susceptibility and the Role of Chloride Cotransporters. *Cells* **2019**, *8*, 448. [CrossRef]
79. Philibert, C.E.; Garcia-Marcos, M. Smooth operator(s): Dialing up and down neurotransmitter responses by G-protein regulators. *Trends Cell Biol.* **2024**, *35*, 330–340. [CrossRef]
80. Gonzalez-Hernandez, A.J.; Munguba, H.; Levitz, J. Emerging modes of regulation of neuromodulatory G protein-coupled receptors. *Trends Neurosci.* **2024**, *47*, 635–650. [CrossRef]
81. Berridge, M.J.; Lipp, P.; Bootman, M.D. The versatility and universality of calcium signalling. *Nat. Rev. Mol. Cell Biol.* **2000**, *1*, 11–21. [CrossRef]
82. Iacobas, D.A.; Suadicani, S.O.; Spray, D.C.; Scemes, E. A stochastic two-dimensional model of intercellular Ca2+ wave spread in glia. *Biophys. J.* **2006**, *90*, 24–41. [CrossRef]
83. Zakharyan, R.; Atshemyan, S.; Boyajyan, A. Risk and protective effects of the complexin-2 gene and gene-environment interactions in schizophrenia. *Recent Adv. DNA Gene Seq.* **2014**, *8*, 30–34. [CrossRef]
84. Hass, J.; Walton, E.; Kirsten, H.; Turner, J.; Wolthusen, R.; Roessner, V.; Sponheim, S.R.; Holt, D.; Gollub, R.; Calhoun, V.D.; et al. Complexin2 modulates working memory-related neural activity in patients with schizophrenia. *Eur. Arch. Psychiatry Clin. Neurosci.* **2015**, *265*, 137–145. [CrossRef] [PubMed]
85. Aguzzoli Heberle, B.; Brandon, J.A.; Page, M.L.; Nations, K.A.; Dikobe, K.I.; White, B.J.; Gordon, L.A.; Fox, G.A.; Wadsworth, M.E.; Doyle, P.H.; et al. Mapping medically relevant RNA isoform diversity in the aged human frontal cortex with deep long-read RNA-seq. *Nat. Biotechnol.* **2025**, *43*, 635–646. [CrossRef]
86. Liao, W.; Liu, Y.; Wang, L.; Cai, X.; Xie, H.; Yi, F.; Huang, R.; Fang, C.; Xie, P.; Zhou, J. Chronic mild stress-induced protein dysregulations correlated with susceptibility and resiliency to depression or anxiety revealed by quantitative pro-teomics of the rat prefrontal cortex. *Transl. Psychiatry* **2021**, *11*, 143. [CrossRef]
87. Anderson, E.M.; Loke, S.; Wrucke, B.; Engelhardt, A.; Demis, S.; O'Reilly, K.; Hess, E.; Wickman, K.; Hearing, M.C. Suppression of pyramidal neuron G protein-gated inwardly rectifying K^+ channel signaling impairs prelimbic cortical function and underlies stress-induced deficits in cognitive flexibility in male, but not female, mice. *Neuropsychopharmacology* **2021**, *46*, 2158–2169. [CrossRef]
88. Chen, Q.; Kou, H.; Demy, D.L.; Liu, W.; Li, J.; Wen, Z.; Herbomel, P.; Huang, Z.; Zhang, W.; Xu, J. The different roles of V-ATPase a subunits in phagocytosis/endocytosis and autophagy. *Autophagy* **2024**, *20*, 2297–2313. [CrossRef]
89. Prinslow, E.A.; Stepien, K.P.; Pan, Y.Z.; Xu, J.; Rizo, J. Multiple factors maintain assembled trans-SNARE complexes in the presence of NSF and alphaSNAP. *eLife* **2019**, *8*, e38880. [CrossRef]
90. Gao, Y.; Ma, L.; Yuan, J.; Huang, Y.; Ban, Y.; Zhang, P.; Tan, D.; Liang, M.; Li, Z.; Gong, C.; et al. GLS2 reduces the occurrence of epilepsy by affecting mitophagy function in mouse hippocampal neurons. *CNS Neurosci. Ther.* **2024**, *30*, e70036. [CrossRef]

91. Gauthier, M.; Hebert, L.P.; Dugast, E.; Lardeux, V.; Letort, K.; Thiriet, N.; Belnoue, L.; Balado, E.; Solinas, M.; Belujon, P. Sex-dependent effects of stress on aIC-NAc circuit neuroplasticity: Role of the endocannabinoid system. *Prog. Neuropsychopharmacol. Biol. Psychiatry* **2025**, *138*, 111335. [CrossRef]
92. Sazhina, T.; Tsurugizawa, T.; Mochizuki, Y.; Saito, A.; Joji-Nishino, A.; Ouchi, K.; Yagishita, S.; Emoto, K.; Uematsu, A. Time- and sex-dependent effects of juvenile social isolation on mouse brain morphology. *Neuroimage* **2025**, *310*, 121117. [CrossRef]
93. Wei, A.; Zhao, A.; Zheng, C.; Dong, N.; Cheng, X.; Duan, X.; Zhong, S.; Liu, X.; Jian, J.; Qin, Y.; et al. Sexually dimorphic dopaminergic circuits determine sex preference. *Science* **2025**, *387*, eadq7001. [CrossRef]
94. Sangu, N.; Shimojima, K.; Takahashi, Y.; Ohashi, T.; Tohyama, J.; Yamamoto, T. A 7q31.33q32.1 microdeletion including LRRC4 and GRM8 is associated with severe intellectual disability and characteristics of autism. *Hum. Genome Var.* **2017**, *4*, 17001. [CrossRef]
95. Friedman, D.; Kannan, K.; Faustin, A.; Shroff, S.; Thomas, C.; Heguy, A.; Serrano, J.; Snuderl, M.; Devinsky, O. Cardiac arrhythmia and neuroexcitability gene variants in resected brain tissue from patients with sudden unexpected death in epilepsy (SUDEP). *NPJ Genom. Med.* **2018**, *3*, 9. [CrossRef] [PubMed]
96. Liu, J.; Tang, F.; Hu, D.; Zhang, Z.; Yan, Y.; Ma, Y. TMT-based proteomics profile reveals changes of the entorhinal cortex in a kainic acid model of epilepsy in mice. *Neurosci. Lett.* **2023**, *800*, 137127. [CrossRef] [PubMed]
97. Wu, B.; Chen, X.; Pan, X.; Deng, X.; Li, S.; Wang, Z.; Wang, J.; Liao, D.; Xu, J.; Chen, M.; et al. Single-cell transcriptome analyses reveal critical roles of RNA splicing during leukemia progression. *PLoS Biol.* **2023**, *21*, e3002088. [CrossRef] [PubMed]
98. Keustermans, G.C.; Kofink, D.; Eikendal, A.; de Jager, W.; Meerding, J.; Nuboer, R.; Waltenberger, J.; Kraaijeveld, A.O.; Jukema, J.W.; Sels, J.W.; et al. Monocyte gene expression in childhood obesity is associated with obesity and complexity of atherosclerosis in adults. *Sci. Rep.* **2017**, *7*, 16826. [CrossRef]
99. Cai, M.; Lin, W. The Function of NF-Kappa B During Epilepsy, a Potential Therapeutic Target. *Front. Neurosci.* **2022**, *16*, 851394. [CrossRef]
100. Iacobas, D.A.; Tuli, N.Y.; Iacobas, S.; Rasamny, J.K.; Moscatello, A.; Geliebter, J.; Tiwari, R.K. Gene master regulators of papillary and anaplastic thyroid cancers. *Oncotarget* **2018**, *9*, 2410–2424. [CrossRef]
101. Benson, M.J.; Laukova, M.; Borges, K.; Velíšková, J.; Velíšek, L. Prenatal betamethasone exposure increases corticotro-pin-releasing hormone expression along with increased hippocampal slice excitability in the developing hippo-campus. *Epilepsy Res.* **2020**, *160*, 106276. [CrossRef]
102. Velíšek, L. Prenatal exposure to betamethasone decreases anxiety in developing rats: Hippocampal neuropeptide Y as a target molecule. *Neuropsychopharmacology* **2006**, *31*, 2140–2149. [CrossRef]
103. Schwehn, P.M.; Falter-Braun, P. Inferring protein from transcript abundances using convolutional neural networks. *BioData Min.* **2025**, *18*, 18. [CrossRef]
104. Mekic, R.; Zolotovskaia, M.A.; Sorokin, M.; Mohammad, T.; Shaban, N.; Musatov, I.; Buzdin, A. Number of human protein interactions correlates with structural, but not regulatory conservation of the respective genes. *Front. Genet.* **2024**, *15*, 1472638. [CrossRef] [PubMed]
105. Xie, J.; Wang, J.; Cui, X. Research progress on estrogen and estrogen receptors in the occurrence and progression of autoimmune thyroid diseases. *Autoimmun. Rev.* **2025**, *24*, 103803. [CrossRef]
106. Aten, S.; Ramirez-Plascencia, O.; Blake, C.; Holder, G.; Fishbein, E.; Vieth, A.; Zarghani-Shiraz, A.; Keister, E.; Howe, S.; Appo, A.; et al. A time for sex: Circadian regulation of mammalian sexual and reproductive function. *Front. Neurosci.* **2025**, *18*, 1516767. [CrossRef]
107. Iacobas, D.A.; Iacobas, S.; Nebieridze, N.; Velíšek, L.; Velíšková, J. Estrogen Protects Neurotransmission Transcriptome During Status Epilepticus. *Front. Neurosci.* **2018**, *12*, 332. [CrossRef]
108. Huang, S.; Shi, C.; Tao, D.; Yang, C.; Luo, Y. Modulating reward and aversion: Insights into addiction from the paraventricular nucleus. *CNS Neurosci. Ther.* **2024**, *30*, e70046. [CrossRef]
109. Xing, M.; Li, Y.; Zhang, Y.; Zhou, J.; Ma, D.; Zhang, M.; Tang, M.; Ouyang, T.; Zhang, F.; Shi, X.; et al. Paraventricular hypothalamic RUVBL2 neurons suppress appetite by enhancing excitatory synaptic transmission in distinct neurocircuits. *Nat. Commun.* **2024**, *15*, 8939. [CrossRef]
110. Griffin, H.; Hanson, J.; Phelan, K.D.; Baldini, G. MC4R Localizes at Excitatory Postsynaptic and Peri-Postsynaptic Sites of Hypothalamic Neurons in Primary Culture. *Cells* **2024**, *13*, 1235. [CrossRef]
111. Iacobas, D.A.; Iacobas, S.; Thomas, N.; Spray, D.C. Sex-dependent gene regulatory networks of the heart rhythm. *Funct. Integr. Genom.* **2010**, *10*, 73–86. [CrossRef]

112. Iacobas, S.; Amuzescu, B.; Iacobas, D.A. Transcriptomic uniqueness and commonality of the ion channels and transporters in the four heart chambers. *Sci. Rep.* **2021**, *11*, 2743. [CrossRef]
113. Iacobas, D.A.; Fan, C.; Iacobas, S.; Spray, D.C.; Haddad, G.G. Transcriptomic changes in developing kidney exposed to chronic hypoxia. *Biochem. Biophys. Res. Commun.* **2006**, *349*, 329–338. [CrossRef]

current issues in molecular biology

MDPI

Article

Hypomyelination Leukodystrophy 16 (HLD16)-Associated Mutation p.Asp252Asn of TMEM106B Blunts Cell Morphological Differentiation

Sui Sawaguchi [1], Miki Ishida [1], Yuki Miyamoto [1,2] and Junji Yamauchi [1,2,3,*]

1 Laboratory of Molecular Neurology, Tokyo University of Pharmacy and Life Sciences, Tokyo 192-0392, Japan; miyamoto-y@ncchd.go.jp (Y.M.)
2 Laboratory of Molecular Pharmacology, National Research Institute for Child Health and Development, Tokyo 157-8535, Japan
3 Diabetic Neuropathy Project, Tokyo Metropolitan Institute of Medical Science, Tokyo 156-8506, Japan
* Correspondence: yamauchi@toyaku.ac.jp; Tel.: +81-42-676-7164; Fax: +81-42-676-8841

Abstract: Transmembrane protein 106B (TMEM106B), which is a type II transmembrane protein, is believed to be involved in intracellular dynamics and morphogenesis in the lysosome. TMEM106B is known to be a risk factor for frontotemporal lobar degeneration and has been recently identified as the receptor needed for the entry of SARS-CoV-2, independently of angiotensin-converting enzyme 2 (ACE2). A missense mutation, p.Asp252Asn, of TMEM106B is associated with hypomyelinating leukodystrophy 16 (HLD16), which is an oligodendroglial cell-related white matter disorder causing thin myelin sheaths or myelin deficiency in the central nervous system (CNS). However, it remains to be elucidated how the mutated TMEM106B affects oligodendroglial cells. Here, we show that the TMEM106B mutant protein fails to exhibit lysosome distribution in the FBD-102b cell line, an oligodendroglial precursor cell line undergoing differentiation. In contrast, wild-type TMEM106B was indeed localized in the lysosome. Cells harboring wild-type TMEM106B differentiated into ones with widespread membranes, whereas cells harboring mutated TMEM106B failed to differentiate. It is of note that the output of signaling through the lysosome-resident mechanistic target of rapamycin (mTOR) was greatly decreased in cells harboring mutated TMEM106B. Furthermore, treatment with hesperetin, a citrus flavonoid known as an activator of mTOR signaling, restored the molecular and cellular phenotypes induced by the TMEM106B mutant protein. These findings suggest the potential pathological mechanisms underlying HLD16 and their amelioration.

Keywords: TMEM106B; oligodendrocyte; differentiation; hesperetin; mTOR

1. Introduction

Transmembrane protein 106B (TMEM106B) is a type II transmembrane protein [1] whose membrane protein family generally plays a key role not only in sustaining various organelle functions but also in cell morphogenesis and, in turn, tissue development [1–4]. TMEM106B is specifically localized in the late endosome and lysosome membranes [1,2].

Detailed studies using mice illustrate that TMEM106B is expressed primarily in oligodendroglial precursor cells and early maturating oligodendroglial cells in the central nervous system (CNS) [2]. The expression profiles of TMEM106B are preserved in humans and TMEM106B exhibits high expression levels in oligodendroglial lineage cells [2]. Interestingly, the overexpression of TMEM106B in mouse oligodendroglial cells enlarges the lysosomal size, leading to dysfunction in the endosomal and lysosomal system and abnormal cell morphologies [3,4], underscoring the critical relationship between TMEM106B and oligodendroglial cell morphogenesis.

On the other hand, in rat hippocampal and cortical neurons, the decreased expression of the TMEM106B protein results in enhanced retrograde lysosomal trafficking in neuronal dendrites, reducing their branching [5]. In this context, the knockdown of microtubule-associated protein 6 (MAP6) restores the balance of anterograde and retrograde lysosomal trafficking, preventing dendrite loss [5]. It is therefore thought that TMEM106B regulates lysosome morphologies, cell morphologies, and putative cellular functions in both oligodendroglial and neuronal cells [5,6].

Hypomyelinating leukodystrophies (HLDs) are a group of hereditary neuropathies involving thin and aberrant oligodendroglial cell plasma membrane-derived myelin membranes in the CNS [7–12]. Oligodendroglial cells are a type of glial cell in the CNS and are responsible for the formation of myelin sheaths, which are essential in controlling saltatory conduction and protecting nerve axons [13–16]. HLDs are rare, occurring in 1 in 250,000 to 500,000 people. Typical clinical features include impaired motor development, progressive limb spasticity, nystagmus, and a gradual decline in cognitive function [7–12]. The responsible genes have been identified following advances in nucleotide sequencing technologies, including next-generation sequencing (NGS) techniques [9,10]. TMEM106B is the gene product identified by such NGS techniques as being responsible for HLD type 16 (HLD16) [2]. The missense mutation p.Asp252Asn (an Asp252-to-Asn mutation) is associated with HLD16 [2]. Brain magnetic resonance imaging (MRI) demonstrates that HLD16 has many typical HLD symptoms, with thin myelin sheaths or some brain regions exhibiting complete myelin deficiency. In addition, many cases display common clinical symptoms, including nystagmus and motor impairment, as well as characteristic symptoms such as hypotonia [2,17–19]. There are no known treatments for HLD16, including thin myelin sheath-related dementia associated with TMEM106B [2,17–20].

Herein, we report that the HLD16-associated TMEM106B mutant protein fails to exhibit lysosome distribution in the FBD-102b cell line, a mouse oligodendroglial cell line involved in the formation of myelin-like widespread membranes [21–24]. In contrast, the wild-type TMEM106B was indeed localized in the lysosome. While cells harboring the wild-type TMEM106B exhibited morphologically differentiated phenotypes, those harboring TMEM106B p.Asp252Asn failed to differentiate. Decreased levels of phosphorylation of lysosome-related mechanistic target of rapamycin (mTOR) signaling output molecules, such as the ribosomal S6 and translational 4E-BP1 proteins, were observed in cells harboring mutated TMEM106B. Hesperetin, a citrus flavonoid, is known for its role as an mTOR signaling activator [25,26] and for its neuronal and glial protective effects [27,28]. Hesperetin resulted in the retention of these phenotypic defects. These results suggest that the HLD16-associated mutation of TMEM106B may contribute to blunted morphological differentiation through the decreased phosphorylation of the ribosomal S6 protein and 4E-BP1.

2. Materials and Methods

2.1. Antibodies, Plasmids, and siRNAs

The key antibodies and plasmids are listed in Table 1.

Table 1. Key materials used in this study.

Anti-lysosomal-associated membrane protein 1 (LAMP1)	Santa Cruz Biotechnology	sc-20011	J0919	IF, 1:100
Anti-Rab5	Santa Cruz Biotechnology	sc-46692	B2124	Immunoprecipitation (IP), 0.5 μg per 500 μg of cell extracts; immunoblotting (IB), 1:50
Anti-Rab7	Santa Cruz Biotechnology	sc-376362	F1023	IP, 0.5 μg per 500 μg of cell extracts; IB, 1:50

Table 1. *Cont.*

Anti-Arf6	Santa Cruz Biotechnology	sc-7971	E0919	IP, 0.5 µg per 500 µg of cell extracts; IB, 1:50
Anti-green fluorescent protein (GFP)	MBL	598	084	IF, 1:100,000; IB, 1:1000
Anti-myelin proteolipid protein 1 (PLP1)	Atlas Antibodies	HPA004128	8115828	IB, 1:1000
Anti-myelin basic protein (MBP)	BioLegend	836506	B225469	IB, 1:500; IF, 1:100
Anti-Sox10	Santa Cruz Biotechnology	sc-365692	J0720	IB, 1:500
Anti-actin (also called pan-bata-type actin)	MBL	M177-3	007	IB, 1:500
Anti-eIF4EBP1 (phosphorylated T37-specific)	abcam	ab75767	GR88680-14	IB, 1:2500
Anti-elF4EBP1	abcam	ab32024	GR239794-12	IB, 1:5000
Anti-ribosomal protein S6 (phosphorylated S240 and S244)	abcam	ab215214	GR3205097-3	IB, 1:10,000
Anti-ribosomal protein S6	Santa Cruz Biotechnology	sc-74459	D2921	IB, 1:500
Anti-IgG (H+L chain) (mouse) pAb-HRP	MBL	330	366	IB, 1:5000
Anti-IgG (H+L chain) (rabbit) pAb-HRP	MBL	458	354	IB, 1:5000
Alexa Fluor TM 488 goat anti-mouse IgG (H+L)	Thermo Fisher Scientific	A11001	774904	IF, 1:500
Alexa Fluor TM 594 goat anti-mouse IgG (H+L)	Thermo Fisher Scientific	A11005	2179228	IF, 1:500
Alexa Fluor TM 488 goat anti-rabbit IgG (H+L)	Thermo Fisher Scientific	A11008	751094	IF, 1:500
Alexa Fluor TM 594 goat anti-rabbit IgG (H+L)	Thermo Fisher Scientific	A11012	2018240	IF, 1:500
Hesperetin	Santa Cruz Biotechnology	sc-202647	D1921	Final concentration, 10 µm
Dimethyl sulfoxide (DMSO)	FUJIFILM Wako Pure Chemical Corporation	047-29353	CDN0170	Final concentration, less than 0.1%
pEGFP-C1-human TMEM106B	Synthesized by GeneScript	n.d.	n.d.	1.25 µg of DNA per 3.5 cm dish or 6 cm dish
pEGFP-C1-human TMEM106B (D252N)	Synthesized by GeneScript	n.d.	n.d.	1.25 µg of DNA per 3.5 cm dish or 6 cm dish
pEGFP-C1 (for mock transfection)	Isolated from pEGFP-C1-TMEM106B	n.d.	n.d.	1.25 µg of DNA per 3.5 cm dish or 6 cm dish

2.2. Cell Culture, Differentiation, and Image Capture

The FBD-102b cell line is a mouse oligodendroglial precursor cell line (Riken, Saitama, Japan). Cells were cultured on Nunc cell culture dishes (Thermo Fisher Scientific, Waltham, MA, USA) in Dulbecco's modified Eagle medium (DMEM)/F-12 medium (Nacalai Tesque, Kyoto, Japan; Fujifilm, Tokyo, Japan)/10% heat-inactivated fetal bovine serum (FBS)/Pen-Strep mixture (Thermo Fisher Scientific) in 5% CO_2 at 37 °C.

In order to induce differentiation, polylysine (Nacalai Tesque)-coated cell culture dishes were cultured in medium with 1% fetal bovine serum for several days in 5% CO_2 at

37 °C in the presence or absence of hesperetin. Cells with secondary branches from primary ones or with myelin membrane-like widespread membranes (cells large enough to contain a circle with a diameter of more than 50 μm) were considered to represent differentiated phenotypes [23,24].

The number of attached cells incorporating trypan blue (Nacalai Tesque) was estimated to be less than 5% under these conditions [23,24]. Cell morphologies were captured and preserved using microscopic systems equipped with i-NTER LENS (Micronet, Saitama, Japan). The images in the figures are representative of multiple images and were analyzed with the Image J software ver. 1.54j (https://imagej.nih.gov/, accessed on 1 March 2024).

2.3. Transient and Stable Transfection

In accordance with the manufacturer's instructions, the respective plasmids were transfected using the ScreenFect A or ScreenFect A Plus transfection kit (Fujifilm). The medium was replaced 4 h after transfection and generally used for more than 48 h after transfection for experiments.

Stable clones were collected in the presence of 1 mg/mL of G418 (Nacalai Tesque) in accordance with the manufacturer's instructions. Under these conditions, the number of attached cells incorporating trypan blue was estimated to be less than 5% in each experiment at 48 h after transfection.

2.4. Fluorescence Images

Cells on coverslips were fixed with 4% paraformaldehyde (Nacalai Tesque) or 100% cold methanol (Nacalai Tesque) and blocked with Blocking One (Nacalai Tesque). Slides were incubated with primary specific antibodies preloaded with fluorescent dye-conjugated secondary antibodies. The coverslips were mounted using the Vectashield mixture (Vector Laboratories, Burlingame, CA, USA). Fluorescent images were collected and merged with a microscopic system, FV3000 or FV4000, equipped with a laser scanning Fluoview apparatus (both from Olympus, Tokyo, Japan), or the BZ-X700 microscopic system equipped with a fluorescence apparatus (Keyence, Tokyo, Japan). The images in the figures are representative of multiple images and were analyzed using the Image J software. Merged percentages are statistically depicted using merged image pixel values (yellow fluorescence) relative to the image values showing TMEM106B (green fluorescence).

2.5. Cell Lysis and Polyacrylamide Gel Electrophoresis

Lysis buffer (50 mM HEPES-NaOH, pH 7.5, 150 mM NaCl, 3 mM $MgCl_2$, 1 mM dithiothreitol, 1 mM phenylmethane sulfonylfluoride, 1 μg/mL leupeptin, 1 mM EDTA, 1 mM Na_3VO_4, 10 mM NaF, and 0.5% NP-40) was used for lysing [23,24]. Cell lysates were denatured in pre-made sample buffers (Nacalai Tesque or Fujifilm). The denatured samples were separated on pre-made sodium dodecyl sulfate–polyacrylamide gel (Nacalai Tesque or Fujifilm).

2.6. Immunoblotting

The electrophoretically separated proteins were transferred to polyvinylidene fluoride membranes (Fujifilm). The membranes were blocked with Blocking One. They were immunoblotted using primary specific antibodies and in turn using peroxidase enzyme-conjugated secondary antibodies. The immunoreactive bands in the membranes were captured and preserved using the CanoScan LiDE 400 system (Canon, Tokyo, Japan). Multiple sets of experiments were conducted in the immunoblotting studies, and the quantification of the immunoreactive bands, using another sample's immunoreactive band as 100%, was performed with the Image J software.

2.7. Immunoprecipitation of Intact Intracellular Components

Cells were extracted in an isotonic extraction buffer (50 mM HEPES-NaOH, pH 7.5, 125 mM NaCl, 3 mM $MgCl_2$, 1 mM phenylethane sulfonylfluoride, 1 μg/mL leupeptin,

1 mM EDTA, 1 mM Na_3VO_4, and 10 mM NaF) with short-term sonication. Cell extracts were used for immunoprecipitation with the respective antibodies against intact intracellular components [29,30]. The denatured, immunoprecipitated samples containing intracellular components were separated on pre-made sodium dodecyl sulfate–polyacrylamide gel for subsequent immunoblots using specific antibodies.

2.8. Statistical Analysis

Values are means ± standard deviation (SD) from separate experiments. Intergroup comparisons were performed using the unpaired *t*-test with Student's or Welch's correction in the Excel software (Microsoft, Redmond, WA, USA).

Differences were considered significant at less than 0.05. For all analyses, the investigator was blinded to the sample conditions.

2.9. Ethics Statement

In accordance with a protocol approved by the Tokyo University of Pharmacy and Life Sciences Gene and Animal Care Committee (Approval Nos. LS28-20 and LSR3-011), techniques using genetically modified cells and related techniques were performed.

3. Results

3.1. Mutated TMEM106B Fails to Be Localized around the Lysosome, Whereas Wild-Type TMEM106B Is Localized around the Lysosome

To explore whether mutated TMEM106B changes its intracellular localization, we transfected the plasmid encoding GFP-tagged mutated *TMEM106B* in FBD-102b cells. Transfected wild-type TMEM106B exhibited lysosome organelle-like punctate structures in cells [2–4], whereas mutated TMEM106B failed to be distributed primarily in punctate structures (Figure 1A,B). Overall, 90% of the cells expressing mutated TMEM106B exhibited abnormal localization (Figure 1C).

Thus, we investigated whether mutated TMEM106B was preferentially localized in the lysosome. We stained cells transfected with mutated TMEM106B with the respective organelle antibodies. Mutated TMEM106B did not primarily colocalize with antibodies against endoplasmic reticulum (ER)-specific Lys-Asp-Asn-Leu (KDEL) antigen, 130 kDa Golgi body protein GM130 antigen, and lysosomal-associated membrane protein 1 (LAMP1) antigen (Figure 2A–C), suggesting that mutated TMEM106B is mostly unable to localize to the lysosome.

To investigate whether mutated TMEM106B was present in other small vesicular intracellular components, we prepared extracts from cells transfected with the plasmid encoding EGFP-tagged *TMEM106B* or the mutant protein in an isotonic solution. Immunoprecipitation data using antibodies against Arf6 as the vesicular marker protein around the plasma membrane, the early endosome marker Rab5, and the late endosome marker Rab7 [29–32] illustrated that the mutant protein, but not the wild-type version, was present in a Rab7-positive intracellular component (Figure S1). The expression levels of transfected proteins and marker proteins were comparable in cells expressing mutated and wild-type TMEM106B.

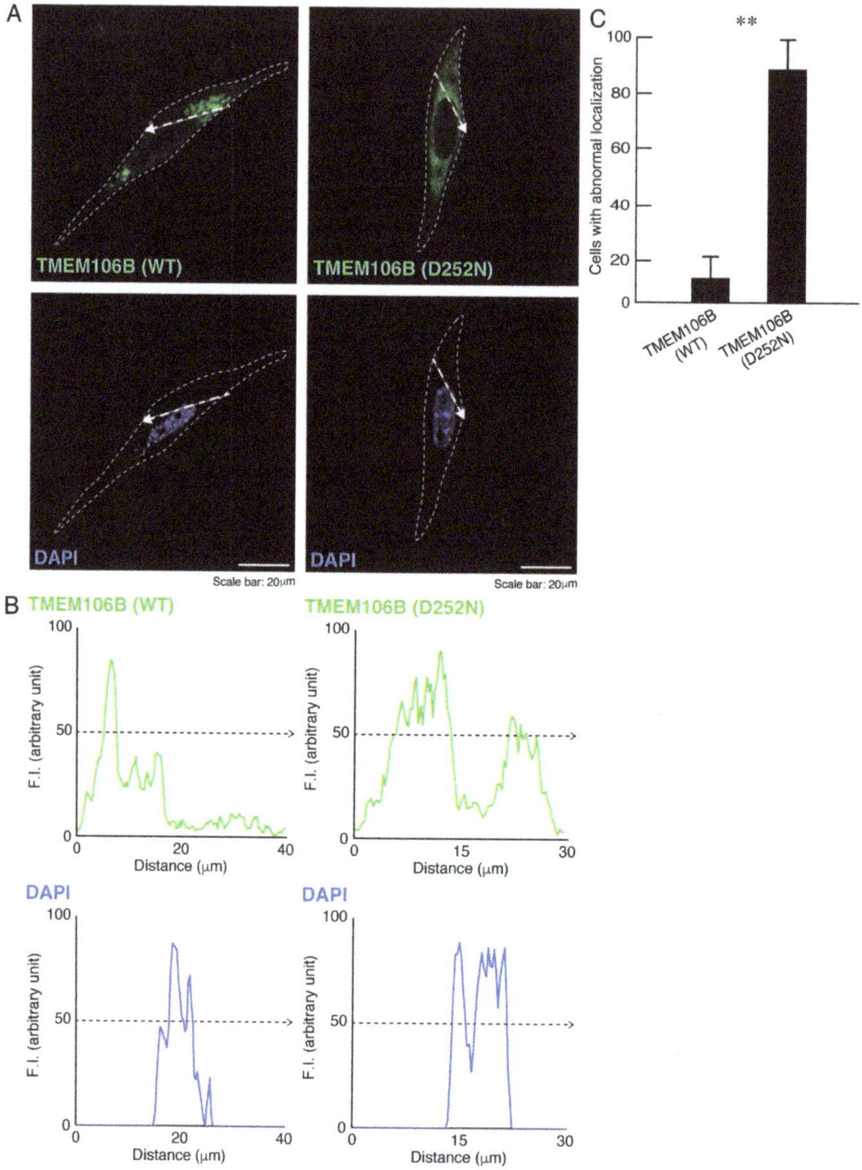

Figure 1. TMEM106B protein with the HLD16-associated D252N mutation is widely distributed throughout the cytoplasmic regions. (**A**) FBD-102b cells (surrounded by white dotted lines) were transfected with the plasmid encoding wild-type (WT) TMEM106B tagged with EGFP at its C-terminus or EGFP-tagged TMEM106B with the D252N mutation. Transfected cells were stained with DAPI for nuclear staining. Scan plots were created along the white dotted lines in the direction of the arrows in the images. (**B**) Graphs showing fluorescence intensities (F.I., arbitrary units) along the white dotted lines in the direction of the arrows are presented at the bottom of the representative fluorescence images. (**C**) Cells with abnormal, widely distributed structures were counted and statistically depicted (** $p < 0.01$; $n = 10$ fields).

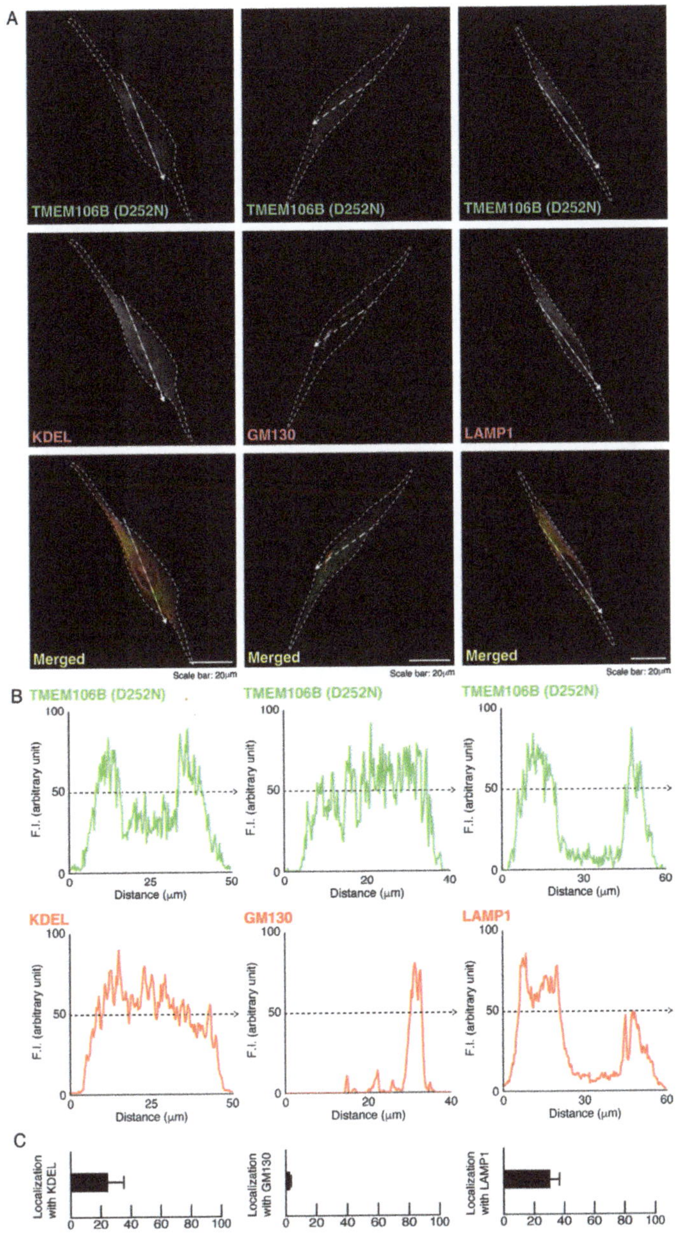

Figure 2. Mutated TMEM106B is present in the lysosome. (**A**) Cells (surrounded by white dotted lines) were transfected with the plasmid encoding mutated TMEM106B (D252N). Transfected cells were stained with the respective antibodies against ER-specific KDEL, Golgi body-specific GM130, and lysosome-resident LAMP1. Scan plots were created along the white dotted lines in the direction of the arrows in the images. (**B**) Graphs showing fluorescence intensities (F.I., arbitrary units) along the white dotted lines in the direction of the arrows are presented at the bottom of the representative fluorescence images. (**C**) The respective merged percentages are depicted in bar graphs (n = 3 fields).

3.2. Cells Harboring Mutated TMEM106B Fail to Exhibit Differentiated Phenotypes, Whereas Cells Harboring Wild-Type TMEM106B Can Exhibit Them

Since mutated TMEM106B is unable to localize to lysosomes, we examined whether it also affected the morphological differentiation in FBD-102b cells. Following the induction of differentiation, cells harboring mutated TMEM106B failed to exhibit differentiating phenotypes with widespread membranes; in contrast, cells harboring wild-type TMEM106B achieved differentiation (Figure 3A,B). These phenotypes were consistent with the decreased expression levels of oligodendrocyte differentiation/myelination marker proteins proteolipid protein 1 (PLP1) and myelin basic protein (MBP) in cells harboring mutated TMEM106B (Figure 3C,D). Oligodendrocyte lineage Sox10 and internal control actin proteins were comparable in cells harboring mutated and wild-type TMEM106B. To confirm the effect of mutated TMEM106B on the differentiating morphologies, we stained the cells with an antibody against MBP. Mutated TMEM106B resulted in decreased differentiation phenotypes (Figure S2A,B).

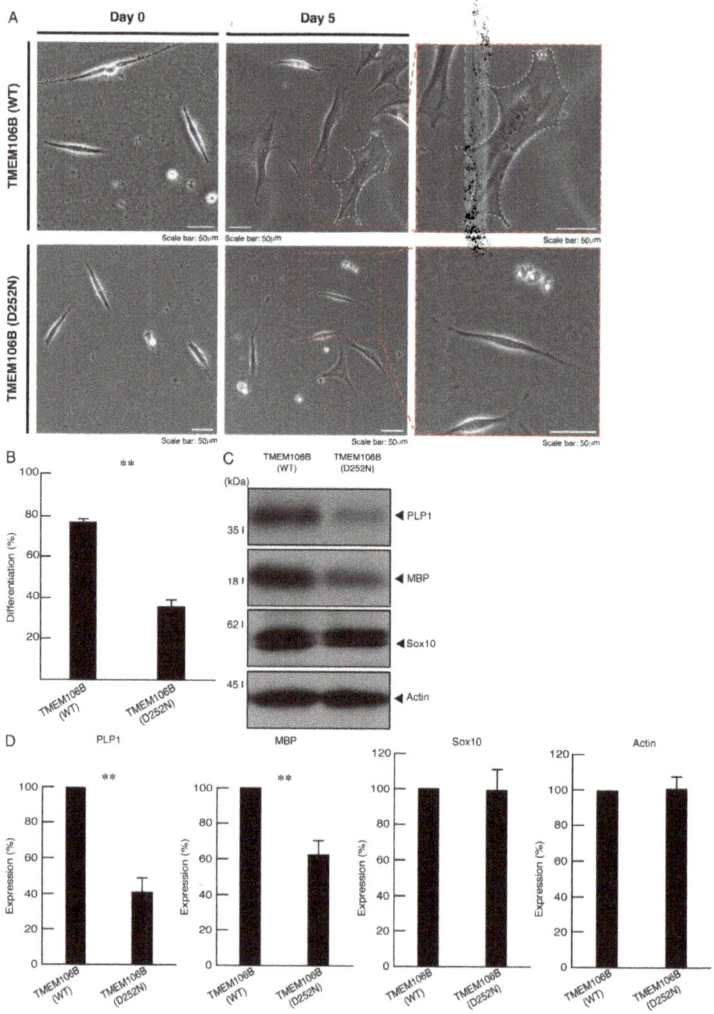

Figure 3. Cells harboring mutated TMEM106B show decreased cell differentiation abilities. (**A**) Cells harboring wild-type (WT) or mutated (D252N) TMEM106B were allowed to differentiate for 0 or 5 days.

Cells surrounded with dotted red lines in the middle panels are magnified in the right panels. The cell surrounded by a white dotted line is a typically differentiated one with widespread membranes. (**B**) Differentiated cells are statistically depicted (** $p < 0.01$; $n = 10$ fields). (**C**) The lysates of cells at 5 days following the induction of differentiation were immunoblotted with the respective antibodies against differentiation markers PLP1 and MBP, cell lineage marker Sox10, and internal control actin. (**D**) Quantification of immunoreactive bands, using control immunoreactive bands as 100%, is depicted in the respective graphs of PLP1, MBP, Sox10, and actin (** $p < 0.01$; $n = 3$ blots).

Next, we checked the phosphorylation levels of the ribosomal S6 and translational 4E-BP1 proteins as the output molecules of mTOR signaling, which is essential for oligodendrocyte differentiation/myelination [15,16]. As expected, their phosphorylation levels were greatly decreased in cells harboring mutated TMEM106B, whereas the protein expression levels of ribosomal S6 and translational 4E-BP1 were comparable in cells harboring mutated and wild-type TMEM106B (Figure 4A,B), indicating that mutated TMEM106B has the ability to decrease morphological differentiation.

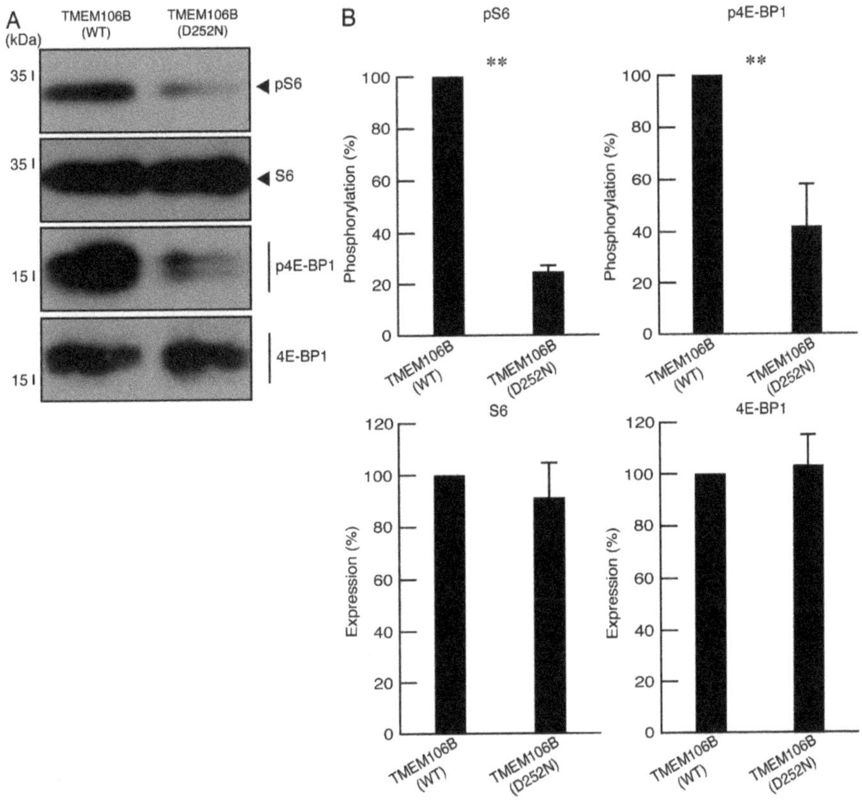

Figure 4. Cells harboring mutated TMEM106B show decreased phosphorylation levels of ribosomal S6 and translational 4E-BP1 proteins. (**A**) The lysates of cells at 5 days following the induction of differentiation were immunoblotted with the respective antibodies against phosphorylated ribosomal S6 and translational 4E-BP1 proteins (pS6 and p4E-BP1). Total ribosomal S6 and translational 4E-BP1 protein (S6 and 4E-BP1) bands are also presented. (**B**) Quantification of immunoreactive bands, using control immunoreactive bands as 100%, is depicted in the respective graphs of pS6, S6, p4E-BP1, and 4E-BP1 (** $p < 0.01$; $n = 3$ blots).

3.3. Hesperetin Recovers Phenotypes in Cells Harboring Mutated TMEM106B

We investigated whether hesperetin, a citrus flavonoid known as an mTOR signaling activator with cell-protective effects [25,26], recovered the phenotypes in cells harboring mutated TMEM106B. When we treated the cells harboring mutated TMEM106B with hesperetin, the cellular phenotypes were recovered (Figure 5A,B). Consistently, the expression levels of oligodendrocyte differentiation/myelination marker proteins were recovered (Figure 5C,D). To confirm the effect of hesperetin on the differentiating morphologies, we stained cells with an antibody against MBP. Hesperetin resulted in increased differentiation phenotypes (Figure S2C,D). Similarly, the phosphorylation levels of the ribosomal S6 and translational 4E-BP1 proteins in cells harboring mutated TMEM106B were also recovered (Figure 6A,B).

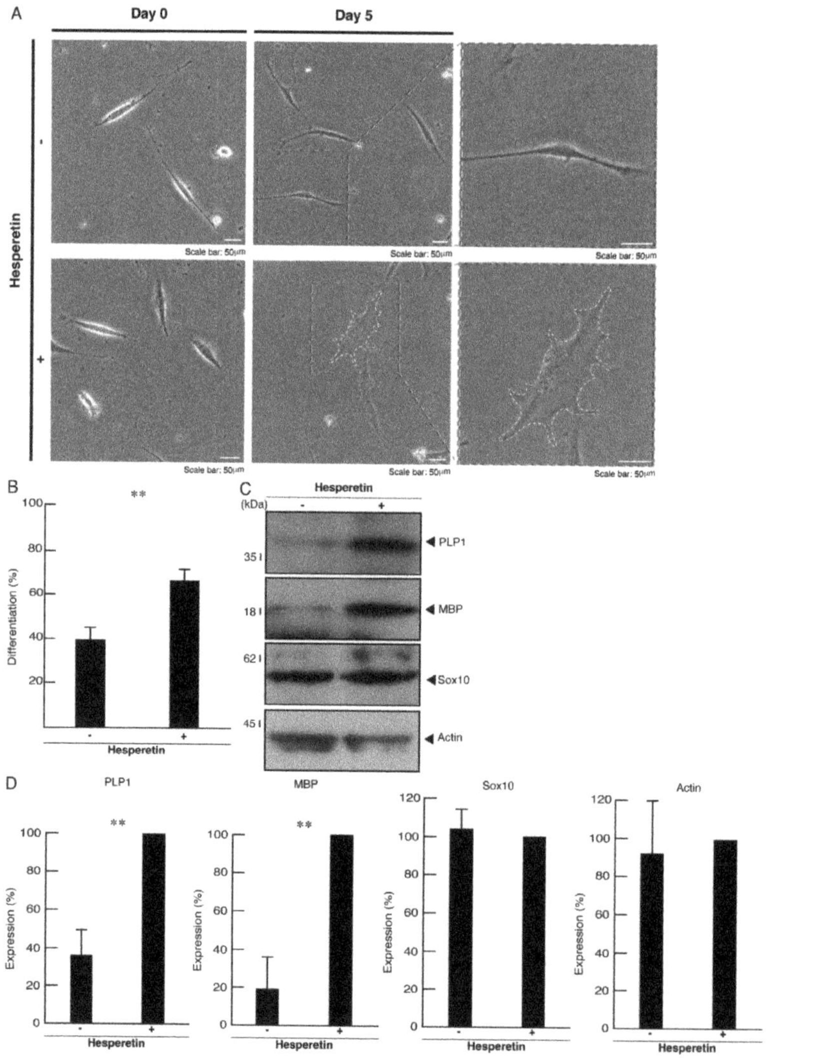

Figure 5. Hesperetin recovers phenotypes of cells harboring mutated TMEM106B. (**A**) Cells harboring mutated TMEM106B were allowed to differentiate for 0 or 5 days in the presence or absence of

10 μm hesperetin (DMSO as the vehicle). Cells surrounded with dotted red lines in the middle panels are magnified in the right panels. The cell surrounded by a white dotted line is a typically differentiated one with widespread membranes. (**B**) Differentiated cells are statistically depicted (** $p < 0.01$; $n = 10$ fields). (**C**) The lysates of cells at 5 days following the induction of differentiation were immunoblotted with the respective antibodies against differentiation markers PLP1 and MBP, cell lineage marker Sox10, and internal control actin. (**D**) Quantification of immunoreactive bands, using hesperetin plus immunoreactive bands as 100%, is depicted in the respective graphs of PLP1, MBP, Sox10, and actin (** $p < 0.01$; $n = 3$ blots).

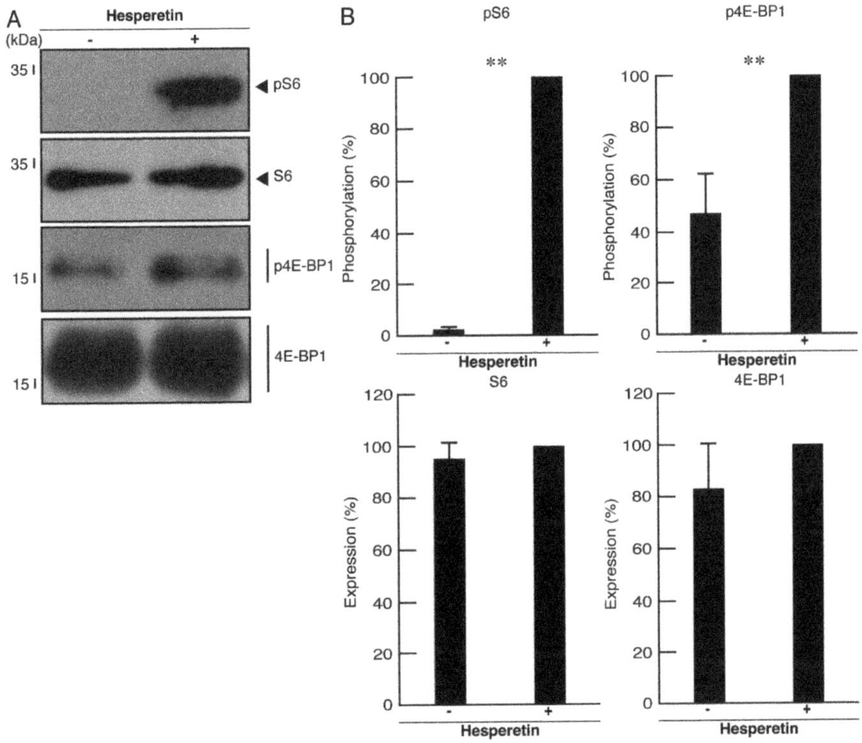

Figure 6. Hesperetin recovers decreased phosphorylation levels of ribosomal S6 and translational 4E-BP1 proteins in cells harboring mutated TMEM106B. (**A**) The lysates of cells at 5 days following the induction of differentiation in the presence or absence of hesperetin were immunoblotted with the respective antibodies against phosphorylated ribosomal S6 and translational 4E-BP1 proteins (pS6 and p4E-BP1). Total ribosomal S6 and translational 4E-BP1 protein (S6 and 4E-BP1) bands are also presented. (**B**) Quantification of immunoreactive bands, using hesperetin plus immunoreactive bands as 100%, is depicted in the respective graphs of pS6, S6, p4E-BP1, and 4E-BP1 (** $p < 0.01$; $n = 3$ blots).

In addition, following treatment with hesperetin, mutated TMEM106B was present as organelle-like punctate structures (Figure S3). As observed in the subcellular distribution of wild-type TMEM106B, treatment with hesperetin localized the mutant TMEM106B to the lysosome (Figure S4), indicating that hesperetin recovers the phenotypes observed in mutated TMEM106B.

As control experiments, we confirmed the effect of hesperetin on the phenotypes in cells harboring wild-type TMEM106B. Hesperetin did not affect the cellular phenotypes, as indicated by marker protein expression (Figure S5), nor did it influence the phosphorylation levels of the ribosomal S6 and translational 4E-BP1 proteins (Figure S6). These findings suggest that hesperetin may specifically affect cells harboring mutated TMEM106B.

4. Discussion

It is well known that lysosome dysfunction and/or dysfunctional signaling around the lysosome is broadly linked to neurodegeneration [33,34]. Mutations in lysosome gene products including the TMEM106B protein are associated with many types of glial and neurological diseases [1–6]. Recent studies on brain diseases illustrate the role of the TMEM106B protein in regulating many aspects of lysosomal function [1–6]. It is believed that this protein is indispensable for lysosomal function in glial and neuronal cells [1–6]. For example, in the *TMEM106B*-deficient Oli-neu oligodendroglial cell line, the protein expression levels of LAMP1 and cathepsins D and L are greatly decreased, revealing that the TMEM106B protein contributes to supporting the biomaterial degradation abilities in the lysosomes in oligodendroglial cells [35]. In patients with genetic dementia, the expression levels in the neuronal and oligodendroglial cells of the brain tissue are downregulated; conversely, those of dementia-associated progranulin are upregulated [35]. It is likely that the decreased expression or deficiency of *TMEM106B* is linked to some brain diseases [5,6, 36]. The TMEM106B protein is critically involved in controlling organelle function, such as the intracellular retrograde movement of lysosomes [1–6]. While the TMEM106B protein is a transmembrane protein in the lysosome [5,6], we have observed that HLD16-associated mutation causes the TMEM106B protein to affect Rab7-positive intracellular components. These components are known to correspond to late endosomes that link to the lysosomal organelle [31,32]. The HLD16-associated mutation may cause the TMEM106B protein to adopt an abnormal conformation, possibly forming small aggregates that are prone to degradation in the lysosome. This alteration could impair TMEM106B's intended role on the cytoplasmic side of the lysosome.

There exists the possibility of a toxic gain of function for the HLD16-associated TMEM106B protein. This protein is also implicated in neurodegenerative diseases such as Alzheimer's disease, Parkinson's disease, amyotrophic lateral sclerosis (ALS), and frontotemporal lobar degeneration (FTLD) [37–44]. In addition, the BioGRID website (see https://thebiogrid.org/, accessed on 1 March 2024) bioinformatically identifies more than 300 molecules of actual and putative TMEM106B-binding proteins. Among those listed are some brain disease-associated proteins. Their protein complexes appear to be present under certain conditions, such as liquid–liquid phase separation (LLPS) in cytoplasmic and/or extracellular regions [45,46]. In FTLD-related risk single-nucleotide polymorphism (SNP) carriers, as one of the examples, mutated TMEM106B protein-derived filaments are increased, precisely correlating with the dysfunction of ALS type 10 (ALS10)-associated 43 kDa nuclear RNA/DNA-binding protein (TDP-43) [44]. It is possible that the differentially localized HLD16-associated TMEM106B mutant protein could undergo denaturation and aggregation, especially in long-term cell culture. Alternatively, the differentially localized TMEM106B mutant protein might inhibit the function of TMEM106B-binding proteins or other proteins. In either scenario, future studies will help to elucidate the cellular pathological changes occurring in myelinating oligodendroglial cells, which typically have a long lifespan.

It is unclear how the HLD16-associated mutation of *TMEM106B* decreases the phosphorylation levels of the ribosomal S6 and translational 4E-BP1 proteins as the output molecules of mTOR signaling. These proteins are typically localized around the lysosome as part of a molecular complex resembling a signalosome [47–50]. The TMEM106B protein has multifunctional roles in the lysosome, contributing to the maintenance of lysosomal homeostasis [5,6]. Therefore, mutated TMEM106B, which fails to be localized in the lysosome, may affect mTOR signaling around the lysosome to decrease the activity leading to the phosphorylation of the ribosomal S6 and translational 4E-BP1 proteins. However, it remains to be established whether the function and localization of TMEM106B are indeed linked to mTOR signaling [47–50].

It is noteworthy that signaling through mTOR plays an essential role in oligodendroglial cell differentiation and myelination [15,16]. Transgenic mice overexpressing Akt kinase, a central molecule in the mTOR signaling pathway, typically experience enhanced oligodendroglial cell differentiation and myelination, causing enhanced myelination [51]. Similarly, almost all positive regulators composed of mTOR signaling around the lysosome are involved in triggering proper myelination [52–54]. These findings suggest a possible connection between TMEM106B and mTOR signaling, which is required for proper myelination [2].

The naturally prenylated flavonoid fraction from *Glycyrrhiza glabra* or astilbin, as the major flavanonol derived from *Hypericum perforatum*, has the ability to stimulate the enzymatic activity of Akt kinase as well as mitogen-activated protein kinase (MAPK) [55,56]. Although it is unlikely that hesperetin is contained in the *G. glabra* or *H. perforatum* fraction, hesperetin or its unidentified hesperetin metabolic derivatives stimulate or modulate the enzymatic activity of Akt kinase, acting upstream or downstream of mTOR in some types of cells [57,58]. These effects may also be relevant in oligodendroglial cells [13–16]. It is thought that flavonoids including hesperetin reduce neuroinflammation, rather than directly affecting cells and tissue, in neurodegenerative diseases such as Alzheimer's disease, Parkinson's disease, and ALS [59,60]. However, although the direct intracellular molecular targets related to mTOR signaling are unknown so far, hesperetin has been reported to modulate the activity of several signaling molecules. One of them is tyrosine phosphatase 1B (PTP1B), which exhibits broad substrate specificity. PTP1B is a negative regulator of tyrosine phosphorylation for insulin receptor substrate 1 (IRS1) and molecules associated with mTOR signaling and Akt kinase, acting as direct downstream molecules of IRS1 [55]. Since these molecules are important for differentiation and myelination in oligodendroglial cells [15,16], it can be assumed that hesperetin directly promotes their differentiation and myelination by regulating the activity of PTP1B. While hesperetin target molecules such as PTP1B may not be therapeutic targets for underlying diseases such as HLD16, hesperetin can promote oligodendroglial cell differentiation and possible myelination in pathological conditions and reverse disease states, at least at the molecular and cellular levels.

In the present study, we observed that the HLD16-associated TMEM106B mutant protein is localized throughout the cytoplasmic region. Cells harboring mutated TMEM106B exhibit decreased morphological differentiation along with decreased ribosomal S6 and translational 4E-BP1 phosphorylation compared to those harboring the wild type. Conversely, hesperetin recovers the mutated TMEM106B-induced phenotypes. Further detailed studies will promote our understanding of not only the mechanism by which mutated TMEM106B decreases morphological differentiation in primary cells and mice but also the ways in which hesperetin can recover defective phenotypes. Such studies will allow us to clarify the molecular picture between the HLD16-associated TMEM106B mutant protein and signaling around the lysosome. Given that TMEM106B has been identified as the receptor required for the entry of SARS-CoV-2, independently of angiotensin-converting enzyme 2 (ACE2) [61,62], and it causes oligodendroglial pathological effects [63,64], studies focused on TMEM106B may reveal a link to oligodendroglial molecular and cellular pathologies that is stronger than previously anticipated.

Supplementary Materials: The following supporting information can be downloaded at: https://www.mdpi.com/article/10.3390/cimb46080478/s1, Figure S1: Immunoprecipitation of respective antibodies against intracellular component marker proteins; Figure S2: Cells harboring mutated TMEM106B show decreased cell differentiating abilities; Figure S3: Following the treatment with hesperetin, TMEM106B mutant protein localizes to punctate structures; Figure S4: Following the treatment with hesperetin, TMEM106B mutant protein localizes to the lysosome; Figure S5: The effects of hesperetin on cells harboring wild type TMEM106B. Figure S6: The effects of hesperetin on phosphorylation levels of ribosomal S6 and translational 4E-BP1 proteins; Figure S7: Original-size images of immunoblots from figures; Figure S8: Original-size images of immunoblots from Supplemental Figure S1; Figure S9: Original-size images of immunoblots from Supplemental Figures S5 and S6.

Author Contributions: J.Y. and Y.M. organized all of the studies. S.S. and J.Y. wrote the draft. J.Y. edited the manuscript. S.S. and M.I. performed the experiments. S.S. and M.I. carried out the statistical analyses and evaluated the experimental and statistical data. All authors have read and agreed to the published version of the manuscript.

Funding: This work was supported by the Core Research for Evolutional Science and Technology (CREST) of the Japan Science and Technology Agency (JST). This work was also supported by Grants-in-Aid for Scientific Research from the Japanese Ministry of Education, Culture, Sports, Science and Technology (MEXT) and Grants-in-Aid for Medical Scientific Research from the Japanese Ministry of Health, Labour and Welfare (MHLW), as well as grants from the Daiichi Sankyo Science Foundation, Japan Foundation for Pediatric Research, Mishima Kaiun Memorial Foundation, Mitsubishi Tanabe Science Foundation, Otsuka Science Foundation, and Takeda Science Foundation.

Institutional Review Board Statement: Not applicable.

Informed Consent Statement: Not applicable.

Data Availability Statement: The datasets used and/or analyzed in the current study are available from the corresponding author upon reasonable request.

Acknowledgments: We thank Takako Morimoto and Yoichi Seki for the insightful comments that they provided throughout this study.

Conflicts of Interest: The authors declare no conflicts of interest.

References

1. Lang, C.M.; Fellerer, K.; Schwenk, B.M.; Kuhn, P.H.; Kremmer, E.; Edbauer, D.; Capell, A.; Haass, C. Membrane orientation and subcellular localization of transmembrane protein 106B (TMEM106B), a major risk factor for frontotemporal lobar degeneration. *J. Biol. Chem.* **2012**, *287*, 19355–19365. [CrossRef] [PubMed]
2. Simons, C.; Dyment, D.; Bent, S.J.; Crawford, J.; D'Hooghe, M.; Kohlschütter, A.; Venkateswaran, S.; Helman, G.; Poll-The, B.T.; Makowski, C.C.; et al. A recurrent de novo mutation in TMEM106B causes hypomyelinating leukodystrophy. *Brain* **2017**, *140*, 3105–3112. [CrossRef] [PubMed]
3. Chen-Plotkin, A.S.; Unger, T.L.; Gallagher, M.D.; Bill, E.; Kwong, L.K.; Volpicelli-Daley, L.; Busch, J.I.; Akle, S.; Grossman, M.; Van Deerlin, V.; et al. TMEM106B, the risk gene for frontotemporal dementia, is regulated by the microRNA-132/212 cluster and affects progranulin pathways. *J. Neurosci.* **2012**, *32*, 11213–11227. [CrossRef]
4. Brady, O.A.; Zheng, Y.; Murphy, K.; Huang, M.; Hu, F. The frontotemporal lobar degeneration risk factor, TMEM106B, regulates lysosomal morphology and function. *Hum. Mol. Genet.* **2013**, *22*, 685–695. [CrossRef]
5. Schwenk, B.M.; Lang, C.M.; Hogl, S.; Tahirovic, S.; Orozco, D.; Rentzsch, K.; Lichtenthaler, S.F.; Hoogenraad, C.C.; Capell, A.; Haass, C.; et al. The FTLD risk factor TMEM106B and MAP6 control dendritic trafficking of lysosomes. *EMBO J.* **2014**, *33*, 450–467. [CrossRef]
6. Feng, T.; Lacrampe, A.; Hu, F. Physiological and pathological functions of TMEM106B: A gene associated with brain aging and multiple brain disorders. *Acta Neuropathol.* **2021**, *141*, 327–339. [CrossRef]
7. Garbern, J.; Cambi, F.; Shy, M.; Kamholz, J. The molecular pathogenesis of Pelizaeus-Merzbacher disease. *Arch. Neurol.* **1999**, *56*, 1210–1214. [CrossRef]
8. Pouwels, P.J.; Vanderver, A.; Bernard, G.; Wolf, N.I.; Dreha-Kulczewksi, S.F.; Deoni, S.C.; Bertini, E.; Kohlschütter, A.; Richardson, W.; ffrench-Constant, C.; et al. Hypomyelinating leukodystrophies: Translational research progress and prospects. *Ann. Neurol.* **2014**, *76*, 5–19. [CrossRef]
9. Wolf, N.I.; Ffrench-Constant, C.; van der Knaap, M.S. Hypomyelinating leukodystrophies-unravelling myelin biology. *Nat. Rev. Neurol.* **2021**, *17*, 88–103. [CrossRef] [PubMed]
10. Torii, T.; Yamauchi, J. Molecular pathogenic mechanisms of hypomyelinating leukodystrophies (HLDs). *Neurol. Int.* **2023**, *15*, 1155–1173. [CrossRef]
11. Dhaunchak, A.S.; Colman, D.R.; Nave, K.A. Misalignment of PLP/DM20 transmembrane domains determines protein misfolding in Pelizaeus-Merzbacher disease. *J. Neurosci.* **2011**, *31*, 14961–14971. [CrossRef] [PubMed]
12. Inoue, K. Pelizaeus-Merzbacher disease: Molecular and cellular pathologies and associated phenotypes. *Adv. Exp. Med. Biol.* **2019**, *1190*, 201–216. [PubMed]
13. Baumann, N.; Pham-Dinh, D. Biology of oligodendrocyte and myelin in the mammalian central nervous system. *Physiol. Rev.* **2001**, *81*, 871–927. [CrossRef] [PubMed]
14. Simons, M.; Lyons, D.A. Axonal selection and myelin sheath generation in the central nervous system. *Curr. Opin. Cell Biol.* **2013**, *25*, 512–519. [CrossRef] [PubMed]
15. Saab, A.S.; Nave, K.A. Myelin dynamics: Protecting and shaping neuronal functions. *Curr. Opin. Neurobiol.* **2017**, *47*, 104–112. [CrossRef] [PubMed]

16. Abu-Rub, M.; Miller, R.H. Emerging cellular and molecular strategies for enhancing central nervous system (CNS) remyelination. *Brain Sci.* **2018**, *8*, E111. [CrossRef] [PubMed]
17. Yan, H.; Kubisiak, T.; Ji, H.; Xiao, J.; Wang, J.; Burmeister, M. The recurrent mutation in TMEM106B also causes hypomyelinating leukodystrophy in China and is a CpG hotspot. *Brain* **2018**, *141*, e36. [CrossRef] [PubMed]
18. Ikemoto, S.; Hamano, S.; Kikuchi, K.; Koichihara, R.; Hirata, Y.; Matsuura, R.; Hiraide, T.; Nakashima, M.; Inoue, K.; Kurosawa, K.; et al. A recurrent TMEM106B mutation in hypomyelinating leukodystrophy: A rapid diagnostic assay. *Brain Dev.* **2020**, *42*, 603–606. [CrossRef]
19. Alotaibi, L.; Alqasmi, A. Identification of a de novo mutation in TMEM106B in a Saudi child causes hypomyelination leukodystrophy. *Glob. Med. Genet.* **2023**, *10*, 38–41. [CrossRef]
20. Zhou, X.; Nicholson, A.M.; Ren, Y.; Brooks, M.; Jiang, P.; Zuberi, A.; Phuoc, H.N.; Perkerson, R.B.; Matchett, B.; Parsons, T.M.; et al. Loss of TMEM106B leads to myelination deficits: Implications for frontotemporal dementia treatment strategies. *Brain* **2020**, *143*, 1905–1919. [CrossRef]
21. Horiuchi, M.; Tomooka, Y. An oligodendroglial progenitor cell line FBD-102b possibly secretes a radial glia-inducing factor. *Neurosci. Res.* **2006**, *56*, 213–219. [CrossRef] [PubMed]
22. Okada, A.; Tomooka, Y. A role of Sema6A expressed in oligodendrocyte precursor cells. *Neurosci. Lett.* **2013**, *539*, 48–53. [CrossRef] [PubMed]
23. Chang, W.; Teng, J. Prox1 is essential for oligodendrocyte survival and regulates oligodendrocyte apoptosis via the regulation of NOXA. *Acta. Biochim. Biophys. Sin.* **2018**, *50*, 7. [CrossRef] [PubMed]
24. Fukatsu, S.; Miyamoto, Y.; Oka, Y.; Ishibashi, M.; Shirai, R.; Ishida, Y.; Endo, S.; Katoh, H.; Yamauchi, J. Investigating the protective effects of a citrus flavonoid on the retardation morphogenesis of the oligodendroglia-like cell line by Rnd2 knockdown. *Neurol. Int.* **2023**, *16*, 33–61. [CrossRef] [PubMed]
25. Famurewa, A.C.; Renu, K.; Eladl, M.A.; Chakraborty, R.; Myakala, H.; El-Sherbiny, M.; Elsherbini, D.M.A.; Vellingiri, B.; Madhyastha, H.; Wanjari, U.R.; et al. Hesperidin and hesperetin against heavy metal toxicity: Insight on the molecular mechanism of mitigation. *Biomed. Pharmacother.* **2022**, *149*, 112914. [CrossRef] [PubMed]
26. Lin, C.Y.; Chen, Y.H.; Huang, Y.C. Hesperetin induces autophagy and delayed apoptosis by modulating the AMPK/Akt/mTOR pathway in human leukemia cells in vitro. *Curr. Issues Mol. Biol.* **2023**, *45*, 1587–1600. [CrossRef] [PubMed]
27. Spagnuolo, C.; Moccia, S.; Russo, G.L. Anti-inflammatory effects of flavonoids in neurodegenerative disorders. *Eur. J. Med. Chem.* **2018**, *153*, 105–115. [CrossRef] [PubMed]
28. Wdowiak, K.; Walkowiak, J.; Pietrzak, R.; Bazan-Woźniak, A.; Cielecka-Piontek, J. Bioavailability of hesperidin and its aglycone hesperetin-compounds found in citrus fruits as a parameter conditioning the pro-health potential (neuroprotective and antidiabetic activity). *Nutrients* **2022**, *14*, 2647. [CrossRef] [PubMed]
29. Wyant, G.A.; Abu-Remaileh, M.; Wolfson, R.L.; Chen, W.W.; Freinkman, E.; Danai, L.V.; Vander Heiden, M.G.; Sabatini, D.M. mTORC1 activator SLC38A9 is required to efflux essential amino acids from lysosomes and use protein as a nutrient. *Cell* **2017**, *171*, 642–654. [CrossRef]
30. Kell, M.; Halpern, A.; Fölsch, H. Immunoprecipitation and western blot analysis of AP-1 clathrin-coated vesicles. *Methods Mol. Biol.* **2023**, *2557*, 619–633.
31. Wong, Y.C.; Kim, S.; Peng, W.; Krainc, D. Regulation and function of mitochondria-lysosome membrane contact sites in cellular homeostasis. *Trends Cell Biol.* **2019**, *29*, 500–513. [CrossRef] [PubMed]
32. Borchers, A.C.; Langemeyer, L.; Ungermann, C. Who's in control? Principles of Rab GTPase activation in endolysosomal membrane trafficking and beyond. *J. Cell Biol.* **2021**, *220*, e202105120. [CrossRef] [PubMed]
33. Ferguson, S.M. Neuronal lysosomes. *Neurosci. Lett.* **2019**, *697*, 1–9. [CrossRef] [PubMed]
34. Zhu, Y.; Liu, F.; Jian, F.; Rong, Y. Recent progresses in the late stages of autophagy. *Cell Insight* **2024**, *3*, 100152. [CrossRef] [PubMed]
35. Feng, T.; Sheng, R.R.; Solé-Domènech, S.; Ullah, M.; Zhou, X.; Mendoza, C.S.; Enriquez, L.C.M.; Katz, I.I.; Paushter, D.H.; Sullivan, P.M.; et al. A role of the frontotemporal lobar degeneration risk factor TMEM106B in myelination. *Brain* **2020**, *143*, 2255–2271. [CrossRef] [PubMed]
36. Satoh, J.; Kino, Y.; Kawana, N.; Yamamoto, Y.; Ishida, T.; Saito, Y.; Arima, K. TMEM106B expression is reduced in Alzheimer's disease brains. *Alzheimer's Res. Ther.* **2014**, *6*, 17. [CrossRef] [PubMed]
37. Rutherford, N.J.; Carrasquillo, M.M.; Li, M.; Bisceglio, G.; Menke, J.; Josephs, K.A.; Parisi, J.E.; Petersen, R.C.; Graff-Radford, N.R.; Younkin, S.G.; et al. TMEM106B risk variant is implicated in the pathologic presentation of Alzheimer disease. *Neurology* **2012**, *79*, 717–718. [CrossRef]
38. Yan, H.; Liu, M.; Gao, Y.; Yuan, Y.; Liu, X.; Wang, Y.; Li, L.; Wang, Q.; Wang, Y.; Shi, C.; et al. Assessing the impact of novel risk loci on Alzheimer's and Parkinson's diseases in a Chinese Han cohort. *Front. Neurol.* **2024**, *15*, 1326692. [CrossRef] [PubMed]
39. Vass, R.; Ashbridge, E.; Geser, F.; Hu, W.T.; Grossman, M.; Clay-Falcone, D.; Elman, L.; McCluskey, L.; Lee, V.M.Y.; Van Deerlin, V.M.; et al. Risk genotypes at TMEM106B are associated with cognitive impairment in amyotrophic lateral sclerosis. *Acta Neuropathol.* **2011**, *121*, 373–380. [CrossRef]
40. Van Deerlin, V.M.; Sleiman, P.M.; Martinez-Lage, M.; Chen-Plotkin, A.; Wang, L.S.; Graff Radford, N.R.; Dickson, D.W.; Rademakers, R.; Boeve, B.F.; Grossman, M.; et al. Common variants at 7p21 are associated with frontotemporal lobar degeneration with TDP-43 inclusions. *Nat. Genet.* **2010**, *42*, 234–239. [CrossRef]

41. Rabinovici, G.D.; Miller, B.L. Frontotemporal lobar degeneration: Epidemiology, pathophysiology, diagnosis and management. *CNS Drugs* **2010**, *24*, 375–398. [CrossRef] [PubMed]
42. Karageorgiou, E.; Miller, B.L. Frontotemporal lobar degeneration: A clinical approach. *Semin. Neurol.* **2014**, *34*, 189–201. [CrossRef] [PubMed]
43. Tropea, T.F.; Mak, J.; Guo, M.H.; Xie, S.X.; Suh, E.; Rick, J.; Siderowf, A.; Weintraub, D.; Grossman, M.; Irwin, D.; et al. TMEM106B Effect on cognition in Parkinson disease and frontotemporal dementia. *Ann. Neurol.* **2019**, *85*, 801–811. [CrossRef] [PubMed]
44. Marks, J.D.; Ayuso, V.E.; Carlomagno, Y.; Yue, M.; Todd, T.W.; Hao, Y.; Li, Z.; McEachin, Z.T.; Shantaraman, A.; Duong, D.M.; et al. TMEM106B core deposition associates with TDP-43 pathology and is increased in risk SNP carriers for frontotemporal dementia. *Sci. Transl. Med.* **2024**, *16*, eadf9735. [CrossRef] [PubMed]
45. Wang, B.; Zhang, L.; Dai, T.; Qin, Z.; Lu, H.; Zhang, L.; Zhou, F. Liquid-liquid phase separation in human health and diseases. *Signal Transduct. Target Ther.* **2021**, *6*, 290. [CrossRef] [PubMed]
46. Boyko, S.; Surewicz, W.K. Tau liquid-liquid phase separation in neurodegenerative diseases. *Trends Cell Biol.* **2022**, *32*, 611–623. [CrossRef] [PubMed]
47. Wang, S.; Tsun, Z.Y.; Wolfson, R.L.; Shen, K.; Wyant, G.A.; Plovanich, M.E.; Yuan, E.D.; Jones, T.D.; Chantranupong, L.; Comb, W.; et al. Lysosomal amino acid transporter SLC38A9 signals arginine sufficiency to mTORC1. *Science* **2015**, *347*, 188–194. [CrossRef] [PubMed]
48. Wolfson, R.L.; Chantranupong, L.; Saxton, R.A.; Shen, K.; Scaria, S.M.; Cantor, J.R.; Sabatini, D.M. Sestrin2 is a leucine sensor for the mTORC1 pathway. *Science* **2016**, *351*, 43–48. [CrossRef] [PubMed]
49. Abu-Remaileh, M.; Wyant, G.A.; Kim, C.; Laqtom, N.N.; Abbasi, M.; Chan, S.H.; Freinkman, E.; Sabatini, D.M. Lysosomal metabolomics reveals V-ATPase- and mTOR-dependent regulation of amino acid efflux from lysosomes. *Science* **2017**, *358*, 807–813. [CrossRef]
50. Condon, K.J.; Sabatini, D.M. Nutrient regulation of mTORC1 at a glance. *J. Cell Sci.* **2019**, *132*, jcs222570. [CrossRef]
51. Flores, A.I.; Narayanan, S.P.; Morse, E.N.; Shick, H.E.; Yin, X.; Kidd, G.; Avila, R.L.; Kirschner, D.A.; Macklin, W.B. Constitutively active Akt induces enhanced myelination in the CNS. *J. Neurosci.* **2008**, *28*, 7174–7183. [CrossRef] [PubMed]
52. Zou, J.; Zhou, L.; Du, X.X.; Ji, Y.; Xu, J.; Tian, J.; Jiang, W.; Zou, Y.; Yu, S.; Gan, L.; et al. Rheb1 is required for mTORC1 and myelination in postnatal brain development. *Dev. Cell* **2011**, *20*, 97–108. [CrossRef] [PubMed]
53. Dahl, K.D.; Almeida, A.R.; Hathaway, H.A.; Bourne, J.; Brown, T.L.; Finseth, L.T.; Wood, T.L.; Macklin, W.B. mTORC2 loss in oligodendrocyte progenitor cells results in regional hypomyelination in the central nervous system. *J. Neurosci.* **2023**, *43*, 540–558. [CrossRef] [PubMed]
54. Huang, H.; Jing, B.; Zhu, F.; Jiang, W.; Tang, P.; Shi, L.; Chen, H.; Ren, G.; Xia, S.; Wang, L.; et al. Disruption of neuronal RHEB signaling impairs oligodendrocyte differentiation and myelination through mTORC1-DLK1 axis. *Cell Rep.* **2023**, *42*, 112801. [CrossRef] [PubMed]
55. Li, D.; Fan, J.; Du, L.; Ren, G. Prenylated flavonoid fractions from Glycyrrhiza glabra alleviate insulin resistance in HepG2 cells by regulating the ERK/IRS-1 and PI3K/Akt signaling pathways. *Arch. Pharm. Res.* **2024**, *47*, 127–145. [CrossRef] [PubMed]
56. Lv, K.; Ren, Q.; Zhang, X.; Zhang, K.; Fei, J.; Li, T. Study of pro-angiogenic activity of astilbin on human umbilical vein endothelial cells in vitro and zebrafish in vivo. *RSC Adv.* **2019**, *9*, 22921–22930. [CrossRef] [PubMed]
57. Li, C.; Schluesener, H. Health-promoting effects of the citrus flavanone hesperidin. *Crit. Rev. Food Sci. Nutr.* **2017**, *57*, 613–631. [CrossRef]
58. Russo, M.; Moccia, S.; Spagnuolo, C.; Tedesco, I.; Russo, G.L. Roles of flavonoids against coronavirus infection. *Chem.-Biol. Interact.* **2020**, *328*, 109211. [CrossRef]
59. Khan, A.; Ikram, M.; Hahm, J.R.; Kim, M.O. Antioxidant and anti-inflammatory effects of citrus flavonoid hesperetin: Special focus on neurological disorders. *Antioxidants* **2020**, *9*, 609. [CrossRef]
60. Ali, M.Y.; Jannat, S.; Jung, H.A.; Choi, J.S. Structural bases for hesperetin derivatives: Inhibition of protein tyrosine phosphatase 1B, kinetics mechanism and molecular docking study. *Molecules* **2021**, *26*, 7433. [CrossRef]
61. Wang, R.; Simoneau, C.R.; Kulsuptrakul, J.; Bouhaddou, M.; Travisano, K.A.; Hayashi, J.M.; Carlson-Stevermer, J.; Zengel, J.R.; Richards, C.M.; Fozouni, P.; et al. Genetic screens identify host factors for SARS-CoV-2 and common cold coronaviruses. *Cell* **2021**, *184*, 106–119. [CrossRef] [PubMed]
62. Baggen, J.; Jacquemyn, M.; Persoons, L.; Vanstreels, E.; Pye, V.E.; Wrobel, A.G.; Calvaresi, V.; Martin, S.R.; Roustan, C.; Cronin, N.B.; et al. TMEM106B is a receptor mediating ACE2-independent SARS-CoV-2 cell entry. *Cell* **2023**, *186*, 3427–3442.e24. [CrossRef] [PubMed]
63. Fernández-Castañeda, A.; Lu, P.; Geraghty, A.C.; Song, E.; Lee, M.H.; Wood, J.; O'Dea, M.R.; Dutton, S.; Shamardani, K.; Nwangwu, K.; et al. Mild respiratory COVID can cause multi-lineage neural cell and myelin dysregulation. *Cell* **2022**, *185*, 2452–2468. [CrossRef] [PubMed]
64. Johnsson, M.; Asztely, F.; Hejnebo, S.; Axelsson, M.; Malmeström, C.; Olausson, T.; Lycke, J. SARS-CoV-2 a trigger of myelin oligodendrocyte glycoprotein-associated disorder. *Ann. Clin. Transl. Neurol.* **2022**, *9*, 1296–1301. [CrossRef] [PubMed]

MDPI AG
Grosspeteranlage 5
4052 Basel
Switzerland
Tel.: +41 61 683 77 34

Current Issues in Molecular Biology Editorial Office
E-mail: cimb@mdpi.com
www.mdpi.com/journal/cimb

www.ingramcontent.com/pod-product-compliance
Lightning Source LLC
Chambersburg PA
CBHW061613210926
51850CB00009B/2303
9783725850211